Childbirth
in Republican China

Childbirth
in Republican China

Delivering Modernity

Tina Phillips Johnson

LEXINGTON BOOKS
A division of

ROWMAN & LITTLEFIELD PUBLISHERS, INC.
Lanham • Boulder • New York • Toronto • Plymouth, UK

Published by Lexington Books
A wholly owned subsidiary of The Rowman & Littlefield Publishing Group,
Inc.
4501 Forbes Boulevard, Suite 200, Lanham, Maryland 20706
www.lexingtonbooks.com

Estover Road, Plymouth PL6 7PY, United Kingdom

British Library Cataloguing in Publication Information Available

Library of Congress Cataloging-in-Publication Data

Johnson, Tina Phillips, 1968–
  Childbirth in republican China : delivering modernity / Tina Phillips Johnson.
    p. cm.
  Includes bibliographical references and index.
  ISBN 978-0-7391-6440-2 (hardback : alk. paper) — ISBN 978-0-7391-6442-6
(ebook)
  1. Childbirth—China—History—20th century. 2. Maternal and infant
welfare—China—History—20th century. 3. Maternal health services—
China—History—20th century. 4. Motherhood—China—History—20th
century. I. Title.
  RG518.C6J64 2011
  362.198'400951—dc22   2011013291

To all of the midwives
whose stories remain untold

Contents

List of Figures and Tables ix

Acknowledgments xi

Introduction xv

1 Missionaries and Modernity 1

2 Reproduction Theory: Modern Childbirth and Modern Motherhood 35

3 The Midwifery Profession 73

4 National Reproduction in Republican China 125

Epilogue: Reproduction in Twentieth-Century China 167

Appendix: Translation of "Good Methods for Protecting Newborns and Infants" 183

Bibliography 185

Glossary of Chinese Terms 205

Index 211

About the Author 223

List of Figures and Tables

Figure 2.1. Advertisement for Dr. Williams' Pink Pills for
Pale People 45

Figure 2.2. Advertisement for Japanese Pharmaceutical
Chujoto 46

Figure 2.3. Advertisement for Dr. Wei's Red Pills to Improve
Health after Childbirth 47

Figure 2.4. Health Teacher Showing the Pregnant Mother
a Picture of the Foetus in Utero 51

Figure 2.5. Fetal Development 53

Figure 2.6. Guangzhou Municipal Hospital Maternity
Department 55

Figure 2.7. Visiting Bag with Equipment for Prenatal
and Postnatal Care 56

Figure 2.8. Mothers' Club, Peking Health Demonstration
Station 62

Figure 3.1. A Mother Proudly Displays How Well Her
Baby Is Growing 94

Figure 3.2. The "Kong" Makes an Excellent Table 95

Figure 3.3. First National Midwifery School Short Course
for Old-Style Midwives 96

Figure 3.4. Old-Type Midwives Teaching Demonstration 97

Figure 3.5. First National Midwifery School Class of
Trained Old-Style Midwives 99

Figure 3.6. Honor Students from the Tuqiang Advanced
Midwifery School 108

Table 2.1.   Basic Necessities for a "Small Maternity Center"   58
Table 3.1.   Curriculum for the Two-Year Midwifery Course
             of the First National Midwifery School,
             Beijing, 1932–33   89
Table 3.2.   Curriculum for Six-Month Course for Graduate
             Nurses of the First National Midwifery School,
             Beijing, 1932–33   90
Table 3.3.   Two-Month Refresher Course, First National
             Midwifery School   92
Table 4.1.   Police Department Announcement of Proposed
             Regulations for Registered Western Doctors,
             Obstetrists, Pharmacists, Prescriptions,
             Western Hospitals and the Red Cross   129
Table 4.2.   Standardized Curriculum for Two-Year
             Midwifery Training, as Set by the National
             Midwifery Board   154

Acknowledgments

This work would have not been completed without the help and support of many institutions and individuals over the previous decade. I am very grateful for the support provided by the Chiang Ching-kuo Foundation for International Scholarly Exchange, an Andrew Mellon Predoctoral Fellowship, and a Rockefeller Archive Center research grant. In addition, various entities at the University of Pittsburgh granted funds that allowed me to devote many summers and semesters to research in China, Taiwan, and the United States. These include a University of Pittsburgh Nationality Rooms scholarship, the University of Pittsburgh History Department C.Y. Hsu Summer Research Grant, and funding from the University of Pittsburgh China Council, Women's Studies Program, and Asian Studies Program. Saint Vincent College's Faculty Development Grant provided a research trip to China in 2008. I would like to thank the members of my dissertation committee at the University of Pittsburgh: Evelyn Rawski, for holding my feet to the fire; Seymour Drescher for his unbounding enthusiasm; Nicole Constable for introducing me to women's studies; and Ann Jannetta and Maurine Greenwald for trying to make me a better writer. My gratitude extends to Zhang Haihui of the University of Pittsburgh East Asian Library for facilitating research in the United States and throughout China. She opened doors that would have otherwise remained closed. Thanks to Huang Wenhong, Echo Chen, and Donna Wang for their meticulous research assistance, and to Marlo Verilla at the Saint Vincent College library for acquiring materials from far-flung places. My sincerest gratitude to the History faculty at Saint Vincent College for their mentoring and unwavering support.

Several readers have offered fruitful suggestions on parts of this manuscript and have in large and small ways helped to shape this undertaking. Suzanne Gottschang planted the seed for this project. The 2005 Women and Gender in Chinese Studies International Graduate Student Workshop at Charles University in Prague gave me indispensable encouragement and insight from scholars and fellow dissertators. Christina Gilmartin, Liu Shiyung, Hugh Shapiro, Judith Farquhar, Charlotte Furth, Janet Theiss, Allison Rottmann, and Gail Hershatter have given suggestions on related papers presented at conferences over the years. Ted Johnson, Yvonne Beninati, Sara Lindey, and Kimberley Baker read and commented on earlier drafts. An anonymous reviewer offered suggestions to make my arguments clearer. All flaws and mistakes, of course, remain my own.

This research has taken me to several archives in China and the United States. I am grateful to the staff at the Rockefeller Archive Center, especially Tom Rosenbaum and Michele Hiltzik; the Philadelphia College of Physicians; the National Archives of the Presbyterian Church in Philadelphia; the Number Two National Archives in Nanjing; the Shanghai Municipal Archives; the Tianjin Municipal Library; the Beijing Municipal Archives; the National Library of China; the Guangzhou Municipal Archives; the Guangdong Provincial Archives; and the Guangzhou Cultural Library. I would also like to thank Zhongshan University in Guangzhou and Beijing Normal University, both of which housed me for portions of my research. Thanks to Xiao Kai and Professor Shi Gexin in Beijing, and Mr. Tan Jinxiong at Zhongshan University for arranging my stays and providing the necessary introductions. Patricia Stranahan, Ed Rhodes, and Caroline Reeves offered essential advice on doing research in Guangzhou.

Friends and colleagues have helped me in so many ways throughout this journey with their scholarly and emotional support. Elizabeth Remick has been a friend and mentor since we shared jiachang doufu, large mystery fish, and the occasional pasta puttanesca in the students' kitchen at Zhongshan University; Cao Pingping and Xu Chunhua in Shanghai and Eric and Carol Lynne Barto in Beijing graciously opened their homes to me; Byungil Ahn shared excellent archival resources; Allison Rottmann in Shanghai read parts of the manuscript and hunted down the best spicy food in town; Bridie Andrews has been so encouraging and made me believe that this project had merit; and Michele Heryford was and is the most excellent traveling companion. Diana Wood, Michelle Renshaw, and Stefani Pfeiffer offered advice and shared resources. The University of Pittsburgh 'China girls' have been with me since the beginning: Rebecca Clothey, Frayda Cohen, and Vanessa

Sterling kept me company with travel escapes, great food, and American television.

This research and book has been with me for the better part of a decade, during which I had my own birth story to tell. Owen and Ella were with me in the womb as I researched gruesome obstetric events at the Philadelphia College of Physicians. As far as I can tell, they, and I, came away undaunted. Our nanny, Glenda Lickenfelt, my husband Ted, my in-laws Beth and Ted Johnson, and my mother, Karon Jeter, gave me the time and child care needed to do the research and complete the book. Thanks to Du Shimei for taking such good care of the kids in Beijing.

Introduction

BIRTH STORIES

A visitor to Peking Union Medical College Hospital's maternity ward today would have difficulty differentiating between the pregnancy and childbirth procedures practiced there and those found anywhere in the industrialized world. The expectant mother learns of her pregnancy from a take-home test kit that she purchased at the local pharmacy, and afterward she confirms her initial diagnosis at a clinic or hospital.[1] During the pregnancy, she makes regular visits to the clinic or hospital to ensure the fetus is developing properly and that any medical problems can be addressed. At each prenatal visit, a biomedically trained nurse weighs and measures the patient (for she became not only a pregnant woman but also a *patient*), and takes her blood pressure and temperature so that the hospital where she will deliver has a documented record of the patient's health and the development of the fetus. If she has money and the right connections, the expectant mother may be able to determine the sex of the fetus via ultrasound, though that practice has been illegal since 1987.[2] At home and in her spare time, she reads books and articles about how best to care for her fetus in-utero. She visualizes her child by looking at drawings and images of developing fetuses in these books. Because she has completed high school, she has a good knowledge of biology and physiology, and she is familiar with the scientific processes. She understands the terminology. She avoids alcohol and tobacco and excessive emotion, and she eats healthy foods that support her growing baby. She listens to classical music and reads to her bulging belly.

If she is financially well-off, she may choose to undergo a surgical birth via caesarean section in order to select an auspicious date for the birth based on numerological factors, to avoid the pain of labor, and to keep the slimness in her hips and the tightness in her vagina.[3] If she opts for a vaginal birth there are few options for analgesia. Acupuncture, massage, and analgesics diazepam (Valium) and pethidene (Demerol) are sometimes used to alleviate labor pains.[4] In the hospital room, the patient is attended by a biomedically trained nurse-midwife. She labors with other women or, if she has the means, she may choose to have a private room and hire a doula, a personal birth helper and advocate.[5] The nurses in starched, white uniforms come and go, checking periodically on the labor progression and writing notes in the patient's chart. The patient labors silently, for verbal expressions of pain, a yell or a scream, deplete the body's limited resources that must be preserved for successful delivery.[6] She is given an episiotomy, an incision to lengthen the vaginal opening.[7] If difficulties arise, for example a breech birth or arrested labor, a physician is called to turn the baby in-utero, perform a caesarean section, or to administer labor-inducing drugs. The newborn is weighed and measured and registered in its place of birth, and a file is opened on this new member of society.

After being released from the hospital, the new mother is confined at home for one month postpartum for the *zuo yuezi* period ("doing the month" or "sitting the month"). During this time, she does not wash her hair or touch cold water, and she eats warming foods like chickens and chicken eggs to restore her strength.[8] She rests while her family members or a hired nurse take care of the infant, either at home or in a specialized *zuo yuezi* center established for new mothers.[9] Neither infant nor mother is taken out of confinement during this time. After the month, mother and infant return to the hospital or clinic for regular postnatal checkups, and the mother may return to work. Thus begins the process of the entry of a new member into the state and society.

Childbirth in China was, of course, not always like this. As recently as one hundred years ago, women labored at home or in a stable, sometimes with help from a traditional midwife or, more often, either alone or attended by relatives or friends. A woman may have suspected she was pregnant upon the cessation of her menses, and perhaps her suspicions were aroused when she experienced "quickening," the first perceptible movements of the fetus that begin around the third month of pregnancy.[10] Her mother-in-law helped to manage the pregnancy because she was both experienced in childbirth and vested in the outcome; the birth of a grandson was a celebratory occasion that guaranteed the continuation of the family line and helped to solidify the position of the mother and the mother-in-law in the family and community. (Girls were less highly regarded, a "small happiness," since they eventually became members of their husbands' households and were unable to perform the necessary ritual sacrifices to one's ancestors.) During pregnancy, the mother-to-be was careful to follow proscriptions regarding her diet and daily activities, and she and her family members made offerings to various deities to ensure the safe birth of a male heir. The idea that the mother's actions could influence her unborn child had existed for centuries in China. *Taijiao*, translated as "fetal education" or "prenatal care," encouraged pregnant women to avoid quarreling, sudden movements, and certain food and drink. They instead should listen to soothing music, move slowly, and sit up straight in order to have healthy, intelligent, male offspring. The characteristics and temperament of the infant and child were solely the responsibility of the mother. Emotional distress and a sloppy bearing caused maternal and fetal unhappiness and difficulties during birth, such as breech or misplaced umbilical cord, or the birth of a girl. In contrast, a peaceful and well-balanced gestation ensured the delivery of a healthy child.

In the last trimester of the pregnancy, the expectant mother's family may have retained the services of a local midwife. *Jieshengpo*, or "birth grannies" (also called *wenpo, chanpo,* or *laolao,* among many other names), were older, married, or widowed women, usually multiparas (women who had given birth to more than one child) with birth experience. Like European or American midwives of the time, they received their knowledge from older, experienced women, and the most trusted midwives had successfully delivered hundreds of infants. The *jieshengpo* wore traditional padded jackets, skirts, and slippers, with their long hair parted in the middle and bound or braided at the back. Over their doorways they may have hung a placard signifying their profession: "*shousheng laolao*" (granny who attends births) or "*jixiang laolao*" (lucky granny). Some signs used more colorful language: "*kuai ma qing che, mou shi shou xi*" (fast horse and light cart [speedy birth], and housekeeping afterwards).

The *jieshengpo*'s responsibilities centered on the birth itself. During the last month of pregnancy, the *jieshengpo* may have made a prenatal visit to the expectant mother to bless the house, to try to determine the sex of the baby, and to predict the commencement of labor. When labor began, a relative or friend called the *jieshengpo* to the patient's home, where the latter may have burned incense and made offerings to various spirits. Often the *jieshengpo* was very active in the labor process, especially if it were moving slowly, by physically manipulating the mother and infant with massage or specific positioning intended to progress the labor. If the parturient (laboring) woman's labor was arrested or protracted, the *jieshengpo* may have made additional offerings and prayers to the deities, and the family may have called in other midwives to assist.

If the child was delivered alive, the midwife dressed the umbilicus with ash, mud, or animal dung. Then she buried the placenta, cleaned up the blood and detritus from the birth, and sometimes stayed to attend the mother and infant. She may have performed social functions such as helping to prepare a feast for family and neighbors, bathing and dressing the child, and offering sacrifices to gods and family ancestors. The *jieshengpo* usually oversaw the ritual bathing ceremony on the child's third day of life called *xisan*.[11] In this way, the child was officially installed as a new member of the family and the wider community. Families often used the same *jieshengpo* for several births, and the old-style midwife was an important part of local society. However, her duties within each family were brief, beginning in the last month of pregnancy and extending only to the third day after the birth. She was responsible for the period of labor and delivery, but unlike the modern midwife she performed little or no prenatal or postnatal care of mother or infant.

DELIVERING MODERNITY

It is difficult for casual observers or for young Chinese to imagine these procedures that dominated pregnancy and childbirth experiences in China just a century ago. In the twentieth century, biomedical technologies altered the process of childbirth on virtually every level. Traditional midwifery, marked by private, unregulated old-style midwives, was transformed into modern midwifery through the adoption of a highly medicalized and state-sponsored birth model that is standard in urban China today. What had been a matter of private interest, focusing on the family and lineage, became a national priority, a symbol of the new citizen who would participate in the creation of a revitalized nation. In the service of a modern nation, the state passed laws that increased its jurisdiction over reproduction. Reformers and politicians supported schools started by Western philanthropists to train new-style midwives in a highly medicalized birth model. Intellectuals and commercial presses disseminated "modern" models of childbirth and parenthood as well as "scientific" anatomical charts of wombs and fetuses. Eugenic themes infused popular literature designed to educate citizens on methods for producing healthy babies, while commodities for modern prenatal care and childbirth grew in variety and in number.

This transformation of reproduction coalesces with the broader story of China's twentieth-century revolutions, marked by an emphasis on science and modernity. This book examines the modern biomedical birth model introduced in Republican China and popularized throughout the twentieth century in relation to social, political, and cultural perturbations that helped to create it. The roles of the state and of Western medical personnel were paramount in affecting these changes, but equally important are the intense social and cultural shifts that occurred simultaneously. The dominant themes of modern reproduction in twentieth-century China are characterized by expanding state involvement, shifting gender roles, escalating consumption patterns accompanying the commercialization of private lives, and the increasing medicalization of the birth process. Although the Republican state was weak and there was no unified top-down movement for childbirth reform, the government's clear intent in its policies and legislation was to reform and control the process of reproduction. Many of the lasting changes in reproduction during this period continue or have intensified in the twenty-first century. China today is grappling with escalating caesarean section rates in urban centers, and the government still struggles to provide adequate maternal and child health care to its poorest citizens. Childbirth reform in the name of a modern nation that began in the Republican era remains a priority in twenty-first-century China.

WHY CHILDBIRTH?

Childbirth is a window into the shifting cultural and political landscape of a particular place and time. Much can be learned about a culture by examining its treatment of women and children.[12] More importantly, reproduction encompasses both a moral and a social imperative; the continuation of a society rests on childbirth. In imperial China, securing the continuation of the family line was the utmost filial act, with the family as the basic organizing unit of society and the state. Yi-Li Wu noted that "childbirth was the warp on which the fabric of society was woven" in imperial China.[13] I argue that childbirth remains so, and alterations in how childbirth is viewed and conducted merely point to larger ideological visions of social and political structures. Li Xiaojiang asserted in the preface to her anthropological study of modernization and traditional childbirth customs in rural China in the 1990s that "because of its close relationship with levels of health and disease, birth is one of the keys to understanding and constructing women's lives, but our field of vision has been blind to it."[14] Opening one's eyes to the rich material surrounding childbirth, the researcher is made aware that legislation regarding reproduction and birth, maternal and child health, and the general treatment of women and children illuminate the relative value or disregard a people carry for those women and children.

Childbirth affects everyone on some level. While the process of birth may seem mundane in that everyone has been born and thousands of births occur worldwide daily, the quality of prenatal care and the birth process may affect a person throughout his or her life. Childbirth is certainly routine on a global level, but it also affects individuals and families. Worldwide maternal and infant mortality rates are inconsequential when viewed at an individual level, when oneself or one's wife, mother, or sister is giving birth. Stillbirths and debilitating handicaps like neural tube defects may result from poor prenatal care, while a woman with osteomalacia (a deformity of the pelvis and related bones due to a Vitamin D deficiency), if given proper care and treatment, may be able to successfully bear many children.[15] Aside from this regard, childbirth in many places and times is the first encounter most people have had with modern medicine. Women in developing countries, like China in the Republican period, did not routinely seek preventive medical care, only appealing to medical authorities in case of emergency like protracted labor, and medical practitioners were often called only as a last resort. Through the normalization and routinization of reproduction, Western medical personnel thus had the opportunity to propagate their methods to a very captive audience, which, if they were successful, produced converts to modern medicine and, not incidentally, to Christianity.

One may make general assumptions about a society's treatment of and ideologies regarding women and children based on how the state proposes to take care of, or ignore, maternal and child health issues. For example, universal prenatal and postnatal care in some Scandinavian countries has proven to lower maternal and infant mortality and dramatically reduce labor and delivery complications, while lack of such care for everyone regardless of socioeconomic status exacerbates high maternal and infant mortality rates for those of lesser means, creating a perpetually underserved and more sickly segment of the population.[16] In Republican China, childbirth came to have a broader significance outside the continuation of the family. Concepts of nation and its citizenry built on earlier notions of social construction on an individual level, as personal health was stressed in the service of a healthy and vibrant national population. Childbirth is one important part of the many complicated shifts in ideas about the changing roles of women in twentieth-century China.

REPUBLICAN CHINA

By the early 1900s, the ailing Qing dynasty had lost several wars and had been subjected to a series of unequal treaties that expanded foreign presence in China, beginning with the Treaty of Nanjing that ended the first Opium War in 1842.[17] Since then, Great Britain, Japan, Russia, Germany, France, and the United States had all established concessions in treaty ports across the country, and business people and missionaries built communities inland.[18] The Qing dynasty of the conquering Manchu was reaching the end of its reign, and in 1911 the empire fell. What followed was a series of inept central governments while much of the country was controlled by warlords. In 1927, the Guomindang (Nationalist) government gained nominal control over the country, relinquished the northern Manchu capital of Beijing (literally "northern capital," renaming it Beiping, "northern peace"), setting up its new capital in Nanjing in the central part of eastern China.[19] The bulk of the midwifery reform in this period came from this Nanjing government, literally the "southern capital," though the state lacked the personnel, resources, and commitment to follow through on most of its plans. While attempting to build a new nation with a strong centralized government, the Guomindang was also trying to acquire control over fighting warlords and the Chinese communists and, after 1931, dealing with the Japanese who were slowly gaining territory in the north. Furthermore, infighting and the formation of political cliques among the Nationalists prevented a clear plan or process of reform, not only in the realm of public health but also with regard to other arenas like the military and finance.[20] Rapid and frequent turnover in the ministerial posts due to political favoritism and favors, in addition to limited and unqualified personnel, prevented consistent policy making.[21]

In the midst of all this political chaos, social upheavals were also under way. Encouraged by the promise of modernity, and equally discouraged by writers like Herbert Spencer who alluded that inferior "races" would eventually die out, reformers advocated all manner of major changes in daily Chinese life, culminating in the New Culture Movement (roughly 1915 to 1923) that targeted youth as the agents of change.[22] Modernity signified a break with traditional social, political, and economic structures, including dissolving the dynastic system and establishing a Western-style government, revamping the educational system, reforming marriage and gender customs, and eliminating superstitious beliefs.[23] The Republican era has been deemed China's "age of openness" because of the proliferation of ideas regarding nation, science, modernity, and economics, together with the publication and dissemination of an amazing array of popular journals and newspapers, including dozens on public health.[24] Many at this time considered modernity to be an inevitable force, according to Laurence Schneider "the product of a universal process of social and cultural evolution that all societies would experience unless they were blocked from following their natural proclivities."[25] China had either to move forward or else risk being swallowed up by those already modern nations, the same nations whose actions had resulted in China's century of humiliation through lost wars and unequal treaties.

Regardless of political leaning, maternal and child health reform was part of the modernizing project for many. Intellectual reformers produced an astounding array of popular materials on public health, childbirth, child rearing, and nutrition. They called upon women to have healthy pregnancies and modern births in order to improve the health of China's citizens. Warlords built maternity hospitals, local notables and politicians donated money, communists trained midwives, and the Guomindang passed laws, all to improve the health of China's citizens who would form the foundation of the new nation. Many wanted to create not only "mothers of citizens" (*guomin zhi mu*), but citizens in their own right who could help in nation-strengthening efforts outside the hearth and home.[26]

BIOMEDICINE AND TRADITIONAL CHINESE MEDICINE

"Modern medicine," "scientific medicine," and "biomedicine" are terms used interchangeably throughout this book to designate a particular set of practices and theories about the body, health, and disease that emerged in Europe beginning in the 1800s and subsequently in the United States and elsewhere. Scientific medicine is associated with the Enlightenment ideal of human progress and the scientific method of investigating, observing, measuring, and recording empirical phenomena. Especially important to scientific medicine was the pathogenic theory of medicine (germ theory) developed by Louis Pasteur and Robert Koch in the mid-1800s.[27] This theory maintains that germs are the cause of disease and illness, and that disease and illness can be prevented with proper aseptic, or sterile, methods. Specific to childbirth, in the 1840s Ignaz Semmelweis found that physicians' hands left unwashed after performing autopsies caused high rates of puerperal fever (septicemia contracted during labor or postpartum) in hospitals.[28] These theories and their related practices also greatly advanced the fields of surgery (as fewer people died of post-surgical infections), public health and hygiene, bacteriology, epidemiology, and the development of antibiotics. All of these fields are part of scientific medicine.

Because of China's recent humiliations at the hands of Western powers, many Chinese were ambivalent about what kinds of ideas and inventions to take from the West. Joseph Esherick has noted the tension between nationalism and modernity that arose as a developing nation like China searched for its own identity while aiming to make itself more like developed countries.[29] Although many in China considered science a main factor contributing to Western strength, the science and medicine that came from the United States and Europe was deemed "modern" instead of "Western." Therefore, China could, in fact *should*, modernize, without necessarily Westernizing. In its modernizing process, the Guomindang government was devoted to utilizing science, including modern medicine, to improve the lives of its people as well as to compete with Western powers. This is evident in Chiang Kai-shek's New Life Movement, and also in the establishment of science academies like Academia Sinica, research institutions, hospitals, and school curricula that included a considerable science component.[30]

The term "modern medicine," more than the phrase "scientific medicine," captures the ideal of striving for improvement that many Chinese identified with during this period. "Modern" connotes intangible characteristics of progress, enlightenment, and truth, and it just so happened that these ideas in China were associated with the West. The ambiguity between modernizing and Westernizing is evident in the Chinese terminology for medicine. The general Chinese term for medicine is *yiyao*, literally "doctor medicine." Western medicine and Chinese medicine are further distinguished by the literal terms *xiyao* and *zhongyao*, respectively. I believe that, in essence, *xiyao* denotes "modern," not necessarily "Western," medicine. "Modern medicine" is a more neutral term that accurately portrays the *scientific* nature of the field and does not allude to an inherent Westernness. Except when referring specifically to medical actions of Westerners, such as in the discussion on Western medical and philanthropic imperialism, I have therefore avoided the term "Western medicine" in this work. In keeping with the Chinese focus on modernity, the terms "modern midwife" and "modern physician" denote those who had received training in scientific medicine, whether in China or abroad. The term "traditional midwife" refers to apprenticed, usually multiparous (having had several pregnancies), married or widowed Chinese women who attended births who had not received training in scientific methods. "Retrained traditional midwives" had been retrained by Western medical personnel in basic aseptic methods like washing hands, sterilizing equipment, and tying the umbilical cord.

The use of the word "traditional" to describe these midwives as a singular group is misleading, as the ideas and methods that traditional midwives drew on during labor and childbirth varied tremendously, and these midwives did not necessarily ascribe to the theories and ideologies of their traditional Chinese medical male counterparts.[31] Likewise, the phrase "Traditional Chinese Medicine" does not comprise a uniform, codified body of medical knowledge. The Chinese terms for Chinese medicine and modern medicine do not delineate distinct or distinctly different methods or ideas, and these medical ideologies are fluid within and across time. In fact, Kim Taylor showed that the English term "Traditional Chinese Medicine" is a mid-twentieth-century construction created to legitimize Chinese medicine and make it more compatible with Western medicine.[32] In the 1920s, the distinction between modern medicine and traditional Chinese medicine was brought into sharp focus in the struggle between Chinese and Western-trained physicians for legitimacy and government patronage.[33] Modern physicians wished to eliminate Chinese physicians on the grounds that they were unscientific, superstitious, unregulated, and harmful. Modern physicians also sought medical hegemony and argued that modern medicine was the only valid form of medicine based on the idea that science equaled truth. At this time, fearful and angry at the attack on their livelihood, traditional Chinese physicians organized and lobbied, eventually successfully, for official recognition.[34] Within this struggle, Chinese medicine was rigidly defined against Western medicine as being more holistic, while Western medicine was accused of only treating the symptoms of disease rather than its root causes.

Both of these forms of medicine can be modern, however, and again this alludes to the fluidity of the terms and the lack of consistency across disciplines. Western medicine was never adopted wholesale without change from West to East; the Chinese made considerable adjustments to, for example, modern midwifery programs to better cope with China's specific needs. Bridie Andrews has illustrated that Western anatomy was adopted into the traditional Chinese medical canon early on, with resulting changes in some acupuncture meridians. Moreover, some knowledge of Western medicine among medical elites was common, even considered necessary, by the turn of the twentieth century.[35] Thus, the phrase "Traditional Chinese Medicine" is used in this book to denote native Chinese medical practices as contrasted with biomedicine, with the understanding that it is not a monolithic or unchanging system.

THE PROMISE OF SCIENCE AND MEDICINE

High rates of maternal and infant mortality around the turn of the twentieth century spurred Chinese reformers to modify and regulate pregnancy and the birth process. The so-called "sick man of Asia" (*dongya bingfu*) could become healthy again with good prenatal care and aseptic childbirth. Many famous modernizers like Kang Youwei, Chen Duxiu, Lu Xun, and Hu Shi heralded science as the savior of China and promised a linear progression towards modernity and its attendant prosperity and health for all.[36] In particular, modern childbirth was imbued with indisputable scientific discoveries and advancements that would improve lives and save thousands. Likewise, writers of fiction included tragedies of maternal and infant death. Lao She concluded his novel *Camel Xiangzi* (sometimes titled *Rickshaw Boy*) with a desperate plaintive: "At midnight, Tigress breathed her last with a dead child in her belly."[37] Two diseases caused the majority of deaths among new mothers and infants worldwide: puerperal sepsis and tetanus. Puerperal fever, known also as childbed fever, is caused by *Streptococcus* bacteria entering wounds in the vaginal canal or through the urinary tract during or following childbirth. Tetanus, caused by the bacterium *Clostridium tetani*, enters the body through vaginal lesions in the mother or via the infant's severed umbilical cord. Both ailments can cause serious illness or death, and they continue to affect women and children worldwide in areas without widespread use of tetanus vaccination or antibiotics to control sepsis.[38]

Many blamed traditional Chinese midwives' inadequate techniques for causing the deaths of China's mothers and infants. The traditional midwife's unwashed hands and frequent manipulation of the mother greatly contributed to the transmission of disease. The midwives commonly had long fingernails with which to rupture the amnion, or bag of waters, and they stretched and tore the perineum (the area between the vagina and anus) and cervix in order to "give the infant an open way" (*gei ying'er kai lu*).[39] Traditional midwives used various objects to sever the umbilical cord: a household knife, a pottery shard or pair of scissors, even her teeth. Then she dressed the cord with mud gathered from the ground, sawdust from the stable, or animal dung, all common hosts of *Clostridium tetani*.[40] The development of aseptic techniques like sterilizing instruments and washing hands minimized these risks, greatly contributing to the growing field of public health.

Ideas about public health and eugenics were at the forefront of medical science both in the United States and Europe after World War I, creating in effect the idea of *world* health based on the promises of health and hygiene rooted in scientific discoveries made in the eighteenth and nineteenth centuries.[41] Government and philanthropic organizations like the League of Nations Health Organization (LON-HO) and the Rockefeller Foundation's International Health Division devoted funds and personnel to China, focusing on disease prevention founded on improved nutrition and hygiene from the program developed at Johns Hopkins University School of Public Health in Baltimore. The Rockefeller Foundation and LON-HO efforts in China, therefore, were part of a larger campaign to improve health worldwide, and one of the main concentrations of the global health movement was the improvement of infant and maternal health.

Foreign medical missionaries had established Western hospitals and medical schools in China beginning in the early 1800s to save souls and bodies, but by the turn of the twentieth century science began to quickly replace religion as the primary ideology and motivation for modernization. This is evidenced within the ranks of the Rockefeller Foundation, one of the primary financial contributors to public health modernization in China. Frederick T. Gates, the Rockefeller Foundation's chief philanthropic officer for more than twenty years, made his goals in China very clear in 1905: "The mere commercial results of missionary efforts to our own land is [sic] worth . . . a thousand fold every year of what is spent on missions."[42] Gates' faith in Jesus Christ was replaced by a conviction that medicine was the ultimate savior.[43] He turned his attention to public health and medicine as the way to save mankind, and he devoted millions of Rockefeller dollars to that end. The Rockefeller Foundation took Peking Union Medical College (PUMC, *Beijing xiehe yixueyuan*) from under missionary control and made it into a secular, thus purportedly modern and progressive, organization. Professional organizations in China also became more secular in the twentieth century. The China Medical Journal had originally been founded as the China Medical Missionary Journal in 1887, but in 1907 "Missionary" was dropped as it transformed from a social publication into a rigorous scientific publication. Its founding organization, The China Medical Missionary Association, made the same name change.

In many cases, the Western medical schools in China like the Rockefeller Foundation-funded Peking Union Medical College trained physicians and nurses who later came to work in government ministries and create public health policy, with the result that the physicians, the schools, and policy making are oftentimes so intertwined that it is difficult to tease them apart. Dr. Yang Chongrui (Marion Yang), a graduate of PUMC's obstetrics/gynaecology and public health programs, headed the National Midwifery Board and the government-sponsored First National Midwifery School (FNMS) and was thus responsible for making and enacting maternal and child health policy.[44] Chen Zhiqian (C.C. Chen), another PUMC graduate, ran the public health program for the Mass Education Movement in Dingxian.[45] Liu Ruiheng (J. Heng Liu) was a director of PUMC hospital and held various public health-related posts in the Nationalist government. These individuals, as well as their funding institutions, were crucial to the reproductive health programs of Republican China, especially because China's political system was extremely unstable. During the best of times the central government held tenuous control over much of China, and internal and external pressures prevented the implementation of many governmental maternal and child health campaigns.

Concurrent with the rise of worldwide public health programs, the medical profession in Europe and the United States was also undergoing important changes that affected the ways that maternal and child health projects were implemented abroad. Scientific medicine was advancing so rapidly that it was impossible for one person to learn and utilize all the knowledge required to treat all conditions and illnesses, and so physicians began to specialize in particular fields. Before the twentieth century, the term "specialist" generally referred to quacks, for example, "venereal specialist" or "hernia specialist," and in the 1800s general practitioners usually delivered babies as part of their practices, most often in the woman's home.[46] The ideal of aseptic births to decrease maternal and fetal illness and death led to the specialized branch of obstetrics. Even as early as the 1870s, physicians began to establish specialized medical professional organizations, such as the American Gynecological Society (1876) and the American Association of Obstetricians and Gynecologists (1888).[47]

Germ theory taught that since birthing women and their babies are especially susceptible to septic infections and tetanus that can be present in contaminated settings, pregnancy and childbirth began to be considered illnesses, rather than natural occurrences, that required medical treatment in a hygienic environment. Abnormal fetal presentation (such as breech or transverse) or pelvic deformities caused by malnutrition may result in protracted labor. Calcium deficiencies regularly resulted in osteomalacia, a deformation of the pelvis that restricted or even prevented vaginal childbirth. If caught early through prenatal examinations, physicians could anticipate these problems and schedule necessary procedures like version (turning the infant in utero from breech or other unfavorable position), the use of forceps, or even caesarean sections. The development of antisepsis and anesthesia in the mid-1800s allowed physicians to perform caesarean sections instead of craniotomies to remove a fetus.[48] The ideal setting for such procedures was the hospital where all aspects of the birth process could be controlled.

In early nineteenth-century America, hospitals were charity institutions for the poor who could not afford physicians or nurses to treat them in their own homes. Advances in scientific medicine led more and more people to patronize hospitals, and their number in the United States grew from 170 in 1880 to over 1,500 by 1904. Independent hospitals owned by physicians, religious groups, or rich philanthropists gradually replaced poor almshouse institutions.[49] As early as 1906, physicians in the United States were calling for all women to give birth in hospitals attended by an obstetrician.[50] (Ironically, these maternity hospitals in the 1800s, before the advent of germ theory and the widespread use of aseptic methods, created near epidemic levels of puerperal fever.[51]) By 1940 over half of all births in the United States took place in hospitals, with physicians displacing midwives as the primary birth attendants.[52]

The development of modern hospitals contributed to the increased need for trained medical personnel in the United States and abroad. As the field of medicine gained more credence and began to organize and professionalize, physicians—overwhelmingly male—helped to create a subordinate "semi-profession" of nursing, and, in China, the professional subfield of midwifery.[53] It might seem that since Westerners and Western-trained personnel were the ones creating and enacting reproductive health reforms that they would follow an American or European model. However, several conditions existed that prevented a foreign model from being dropped on an unsuspecting Chinese populace. On the one hand, there was a serious lack of resources to ensure that all women delivered their babies in a hospital attended by a physician. There were few physicians and fewer hospitals. On the other, long-standing customs mandated that women should attend births, and that there was no place for men in the delivery room. Although there was a branch of traditional Chinese medicine that dealt with women's illnesses and pregnancy, delivery was left to the midwives.[54] Thus the transformation of childbirth in China took a different turn. A midwifery profession was created, and although short-lived, it was a great leap for women in many ways. Midwives had a career, one of the first for women in the Republican era; and birth was given national importance, an importance that remains.

A NEW PROFESSION

Although public health reforms were under way by the 1910s as part of China's modernization efforts, the state of medical training was still in its infancy. China had no consistent educational policy in the late Qing era, much less a standardized medical curriculum.[55] Formal education for women at this time was dismal, and women's medical education was almost nonexistent, but change was rapid and forthcoming. The idea that women could and should be educated was spreading. This major shift in gender identity, that women were worthy of an education and that they could help to build a new China, gave them more opportunities and opened the medical field to them, albeit a profession perceived as feminine because it emphasizes nurturing qualities. In addition, modern medicine and public health gradually became more widely accepted, especially in urban areas, in part because of their effectiveness in halting the North Manchurian plague epidemic in 1910-1911.[56] This success boosted people's confidence in modern medicine and proved that China could run an effective public health program.[57] The foundation laid by the medical missionaries from Great Britain and the United States, buttressed in many cases by the support of local gentry and officials, allowed the Nationalist government to rapidly adopt public health and medical education measures. By the late 1920s the Nationalist government began to release plans for a system of regulated and standardized medical schools, nursing schools, and midwifery-training programs.[58] Although many of these medical programs were never put into place or were only partially completed, they are indicative of the increasing interest in medical reforms in the name of modernization and nation-building in the early twentieth century.[59]

Gradually, Chinese women entered the medical field, often as low-level technicians, and although medicine was not a prestigious field, they gained experience that allowed them in some cases to pursue further education or to encourage others to do the same. These women opened the doors for the professional midwives who were to follow. As women became nurses and medical helpers (and later midwives), and medicine became more and more regulated under the expanding arm of the state, women too were subject to more regulation. There exists a very clear trend towards centralized government control over public health and the medical field, as well as greater cooperation between Western and Chinese institutions, during the Nationalist era. The scattered and erratic medical training in the last decades of the Qing dynasty forms the basis on which Nationalist public health policies were built.

This is not to say that the medical missionaries built medical schools and students flocked to their doors. Medical professionals in late nineteenth-century China had a difficult time recruiting suitable nursing and midwifery students. As in Europe and the United States in the 1800s and early 1900s, medicine was not a very respectable profession, and for women even less so. Caring for sick people and handling bodily fluids and flesh was looked upon as dirty work. According to one medical missionary, "Until recent years our difficulty has been in securing those whom we considered to be suitable candidates for training. Such work was considered to be beneath the dignity of most," the "most" usually referring to literate young men and women from good families.[60] Medical missions got most of their early students from affiliated orphanages and mission schools, as missionaries opened girls' schools and in some cases adopted Chinese daughters, and Chinese Christian families were more eager to send their own children to Western schools. Very few Chinese women studied medicine in the United States, Europe, or Japan. For example, in 1920, there were only 65 Chinese women studying in America in all fields, and only 11 of those studied medicine.[61] Most were educated in Western institutions in China.

STATE BUILDING AND REPRODUCTIVE HEALTH

The development of modern midwifery was inextricably tied to the modernization process under way in Republican China. The moulding of a modern city necessitated a modern public health program that began at birth and focused on women both as reproducers and as active participants—as midwives—in the birthing of a new nation.[62] As childbirth became linked with scientific medicine and defined as an essential element in the development of a strong and modern nation, local and national governments began to regulate midwives as early as 1913, demonstrating the increased importance of women in China's rebuilding process.[63] A healthy population begins at birth, and in order to create a healthy population, the Guomindang mandated particulars about reproduction—where it occurred, who could participate as mothers, and who attended these births. Under the guidance of the newly formed National Midwifery Board (established in 1929), changes in childbirth were part of a greater effort to modernize the country. Women started to enter the medical and public health fields as employed professionals, and homemakers were targeted as subjects requiring education and training in order to serve as mothers in a modern nation.[64]

Efforts to push through changes in state-run public health initiatives in China affected nearly every part of a person's life in the early twentieth century, creating a level of "hygienic modernity," to use an eloquent phrase coined by Ruth Rogaski.[65] These initiatives played a crucial role in city planning and were the cornerstone of China's modernization process in the "administration of space and populations in order to eliminate dirt and prevent disease."[66] "Hygienic modernity" is evident in the New Life Movement that included bans on public spitting and urination, while other public health advocates called for fundamental changes in Chinese living and eating habits, such as eliminating the family bed and promoting the use of individual eating utensils in place of traditional family-style dining.[67]

A strong state pursues control of people, resources, and information, and one of the Guomindang's main public health goals was improved collection processes for vital statistics. The state regulated the recording and submission of birth and death statistics to the central government in order to more effectively collect taxes, plan cities and towns, and make policies. They employed the newly trained midwives to track births and deaths and their outcomes and causes, and to actively push for childbirth reforms in local communities. Twentieth-century technology has facilitated the state's extended control over individual reproductive activities and characteristics. Medical technologies allow for prenatal intervention, in the early twentieth century by diagnosing pregnancy earlier and detecting potential problems like osteomalacia and breech position. The length of time devoted to prenatal care was therefore broadened and, in some cases, mandated by the hospital or the state.[68] Efficient record-keeping systems and expanding literacy resulting from broader educational policies allowed the state or local hospital to track patients and follow up with post-partum visits, educating new mothers on modern parenting methods and spreading knowledge about the importance of community health and nutrition. Regardless of the weaknesses of the Republican govern-ment, the policies to regulate pregnancy and birth introduced in this period set an important precedent of state control over reproduction that was taken up by later governments and remains a crucial compo-nent of policy making today.

REPRODUCTION THEORY

Central to China's reproduction revolution is the biomedical birth model created in the West and exported to developing countries be-ginning in the early twentieth century. The move to science-based births produced rapid changes in the ways people thought about births and bodies. Scientific advancements certainly lowered China's high maternal and infant mortality rates. Adherence to a scientific birth model also radically altered perceptions of motherhood, pregnancy and labor, and infant development. The biological processes of childbirth are universal. Uncomplicated labor and delivery of an infant includes amniotic fluid release, labor contractions progressing in intensity and time leading to the birth of an infant, and the delivery of the placenta. But the social characteristics and practices surrounding childbirth are particular; they markedly differ across time and between cultures. Biomedical science changes childbirth, but not, as Brigitte Jordan argues, because scientific evidence supports its methods.[69] Medical-ization does not automatically result in improved maternal and child health outcomes.[70] As an example, the United States has one of the most advanced medical systems in the world with regard to innova-tive pharmaceuticals and technology, yet the infant and maternal mortality rates are higher than in many other countries.[71] In 2004, the infant mortality rate in the United States was higher than that of 28 other countries, despite a considerable portion of the U.S. GDP being spent on health care.[72] Instead of scientific evidence, then, impelling changes in reproduction, it is the accompanying social and cultural perturbations that directly affect alterations in labor and delivery, for example barriers of race and poverty that affect maternal and infant mortality. The highly medicalized birth model introduced in the early twentieth century is driven by the creation of the pregnant woman as a *patient* to be managed by professionals. Unquestionable scientific medicine, imposed from the top down, had made birth into a medical event requiring professional assistance.[73]

Biomedicine is useful for treating abnormal pregnancies and births like malnutrition-related malformed pelves, gonorrhea, and other pre-existing diseases in the expectant mother. And in fact, in Republican China, most modern prenatal care and midwifery focused on simple hygiene and nutrition, and most births still took place at home, though midwives encouraged their patients to deliver in a hospital or clinic. However, a glance at the list of "necessary" accoutrements for a small modern maternity center in China in 1924 gives one pause: The 24 different items include pelvimeters, catheters, utensil sterilizers, needles, scissors, a craniotomy hook, and three different kinds of midwifery forceps.[74] In contrast, a century ago most Chinese women gave birth at home, either alone or surrounded by relatives, friends, and perhaps one or more midwives. The traditional midwife's tools were simple. According to one account, the midwife "never furnished anything, only borrowing the following implements from the patients: 'House hold' [sic] scissor, a piece of 'color silk' and cotton, a pair of iron coal chopsticks, and an iron hook for abnormal cases."[75] Charlotte Furth relates a Japanese account of more elaborate Chinese birth utensils, perhaps for parturition in a higher socioeconomic class: "paper toweling to catch birth blood; container for placenta; pregnancy sash for belly support; infant's swaddling wrap."[76] The scissors and hooks of the traditional and modern birth attendants were used for the same purposes, to cut the umbilical cord and to extract a deceased infant from the vaginal canal, respectively. The sterilized equipment of the modern midwife, however, modern in form and in practice, in theory eliminated infection and resulted in healthier infants and mothers.

Some of the reforms to reproductive health in Republican China were based firmly in scientific evidence, like maintaining asepsis during childbirth to prevent septic infections and tetanus in mother and infant, and the administration of silver nitrate eye drops to inhibit infection or blindness (from gonorrhea or syphilis) that the infant may contract in the birth canal.[77] Further reforms, like the starched white uniforms and caps of the nurses, were material symbols of the modern midwife. Still others, like the reclined position of the parturient during labor and birth, and the exacting, timed rigidity of the modern labor and birth model, were sometimes even harmful, causing injury or death of mother and infant.[78] Biomedicine claims superiority over other methods, and thus all resources flow to the dominant model leaving others to languish. This story is not as simple as a new model replacing an old one, however. Many traditional practices like *taijiao* and *zuo yuezi* are woven into the new biomedical forms of childbirth. Modern childbirth worked within the existing social and medical ideas about the pregnant body to form something new, a unique conception unlike what was occurring in the West. Instead of wholesale masculinization of the birth attendants (as in the United States), childbirth in China was touched by science yet remained firmly in the realm of women's activities.

Throughout this work, there are references to the sterility, cleanliness, and order of the modern birth environment, as opposed to the disorder and disarray of the "untrained" traditional *jieshengpo*. The modern midwife's aeseptic birth model did lessen infant and maternal deaths. Their starched white uniforms and bobbed hair, however, seem superfluous. Or were they? It is much easier to tell whether or not a white garment is dirty, in contrast with the drab fabrics worn by the *jieshengpo* and, indeed, most of the population. Furthermore, short hair is more easily kept out of the way—of the eyes, the hands, the patient—under a (clean, white) hat. Regardless of their effectiveness, these visual characteristics imported from the West were modern representations of the modern midwife's professionalism and educational level.

Perceptions of one's body during pregnancy and of the birth process also transformed in the early twentieth century, driven by the immutability of scientific medicine and informed by new forms of visual knowledge about fetal development.[79] The fetus in traditional Chinese medicine was "imagined as a destabilizing intruder spirit" that disrupted and weakened the mother's health, creating an opportunity for disease and other ailments.[80] However, biomedical physical depictions of the fetus eliminate the need for imagination; the fetus becomes a scientific visual image that trumps all other understandings of pregnancy and birth.[81]

SOURCES OF REPRODUCTION

When taken alone and out of context, government documents and legislation present a very optimistic story of national childbirth reform that resulted in lowered maternal and infant mortality rates. Such documents intimate that modern midwives across the country were examined, licensed, and given a uniform training curriculum. They worked in clean environments like hospitals or clinics, or in homes with sterile instruments. They followed national rules and procedural regulations. Likewise, the writings by modern midwives and physicians who were vested in defining themselves against traditional medicine paint the traditional Chinese midwives as uncontrollable, superstitious, dangerous swindlers with no formal training. Any traditional midwife could "hang up a shingle" and distribute harmful medical advice and medicines without regulation. As we shall see, there was more to this dichotomy than first glance allows.

First of all, the reality of childbirth in China does not correspond with the written documents, especially those promulgated by local and national governments. While legislation mandated that all midwives be examined and registered by the state, for example, in reality this law was unenforceable. It is certain that well into the twentieth century modern medicine reached very few people in China, and modern childbirth was even rarer. The number of Chinese who accessed, or had access to, modern medicine during this period was very small. In 1910 there were fewer than 500 modern physicians in China, most located in urban coastal areas, to serve a population of roughly 500 million.[82] The medicalization of childbirth was only beginning to take place in the early twentieth century, even in the West, and so ideas about hospital births and antenatal care were not widespread or even considered necessary. Specialized and systematic midwifery training was limited, and it did not commence in China until the late 1920s with the advent of a modern public health system and greater importance placed on maternal and child health.

Furthermore, women rarely wrote about childbirth, and certainly not about the majority of routine, uncomplicated birth stories. Childbirth was a natural occurrence that did not warrant written exposition by those who experienced or witnessed it. Few personal accounts of childbirth exist, and an egregious silence emanates from the traditional midwives, whom we only get to know through the words of modern medical personnel and legislators. Furthermore, while famous female obstetrician/gynecologists warrant biographies and memorials dedicated to their careers, the main actors in this story, the modern midwives, fell somewhere between medical elite and medical worker. Their position did not justify commemoration. Although literate and educated, they rarely left any written record of their lives, aside from the occasional entry in a local gazetteer. They did, however, write poems, plays, songs, and standard testimonies proclaiming their love of helping people and their country that were published in midwifery school yearbooks. Their images may be indistinct but are much more clear and discernable than those of their traditional sisters.

Men, however, did write about midwives. Yi-Li Wu has shown that in late imperial China (Ming and Qing dynasties, 1368–1911), "the activities of nonliterate practitioners and lower-class healers, including midwives, are heard only through the voices of male writers."[83] Traditional Chinese physicians often wrote scathingly about meddling midwives, as they interfered with the "cosmologically resonant childbirth" by hastening labor and manipulating the mother and infant.[84] Midwives in China were associated with the pollutions of birth and death, and they had access to the most intimate secrets of their female patients, access that male physicians could not hope to gain. By practice male physicians did not attend births; they remotely managed pregnancy and labor with medicines rather than manipulation. Midwives were therefore necessary, yet feared and despised.[85] By the twentieth century, not only were the writers of medical texts male, they were also often practitioners of Western medicine, and they continued the custom of lambasting the so-called superstitious and unsanitary practices of the traditional midwives. Nor did modern midwives of the twentieth century write texts on modern midwifery; those works were left to the primarily male physicians who taught them and headed their schools and hospitals. What remains is a polemic: scathing critiques of traditional births contrasted with the wonders of the modern birth model written by Chinese and foreign biomedical practitioners and reformers. In her interviews with Chinese women who were midwives in the 1950s, Gail Hershatter has begun to contrast the ideology with the reality, finding that midwives and parturient women alike distrusted the new childbirth methods forced upon them by government organizations.[86] Unfortunately, the voices of the midwives of the 1930s are silent today. Few recollections of their lives remain, and the midwives from that period have passed on.

Yet another complication to this story is that there was no unified or regulated movement to promote maternal and child health in Republican China. Several different groups of people contributed to changes in reproduction: Westerners—medical personnel, social scientists, and religious evangelists—as well as Chinese modernizers and government officials, many of whom were trained in modern medicine. Childbirth reform, therefore, disseminated from several different places, especially Beijing, the site of the First National Midwifery School; Nanjing, seat of the Guomindang government between 1927 and 1937; and Shanghai, a strong publishing center and home to a large foreign population. One finds evidence of childbirth reform in many other cities, as local notables established maternity hospitals and midwifery training programs as part of their modernizing goals; in rural locations like Dingxian where philanthropists and public health officials attempted to improve maternal and child health; and even in small towns where medical missionaries settled and established hospitals and schools.

Because of the dearth of unbiased and complete sources, and lack of a central reforming force, this book is primarily a study of printed and published official and popular materials—legislation, annual reports, medical textbooks and pamphlets, yearbooks, journals, newspapers—that must be read carefully against the polemic and taken into account alongside the shifting political and economic situations. Advertisements, scientific and popular images, short stories, plays, and self-help articles illustrate the changing nature of reproduction in relation to nation-building. Modern midwifery techniques, training curricula, and the public image of midwifery programs illustrate the appeal of science. Legislation shows the Nationalist commitment to reproductive health reform, and other accounts betray the government's limitations in achieving it.

STRUCTURE OF THE BOOK

This book is divided into five chapters, each dealing with a separate yet intertwined aspect of reproduction in Republican China, tied together with the major themes of modernization, state building, shifting gender roles in family and society, consumer culture, and the medicalization of childbirth. Chapter 1 provides the setting for the book, an overview of changes in childbirth as a result of medical missionaries' work in several treaty ports in China in the mid- to late-nineteenth century. Following the story of Lady Li and her treatment by Western missionary physicians in treaty-port Tianjin in 1879, this chapter addresses the rhetoric of modernity as applied to reproduction and maternal and child health and their importance among reformers in late Qing and Republican China. Cities became sites of modern reproduction as local politicians partnered with medical missionaries to shape modern locales. Chapter 2 continues the themes of modernity and state-building, this time in the popular imagination. It is a discussion of scientific motherhood and what I refer to as reproduction theory—the changing ideologies, assumptions, predilections, and aversions surrounding childbirth. This chapter also looks at the changing gender dynamics of parenthood and family life during this period, with particular emphases on modernity, commodification of childbirth, and the role of women in nation building as mothers. Imagery of the fetus, family, health workers, and reproductive technology are central to the understanding of the shifts in ideology about reproduction.

In chapter 3, I trace the professionalization of modern midwives that gave women a new identity and national importance as modern birth attendants. The new paramedical midwifery profession was created largely by Dr. Yang Chongrui, head of the First National Midwifery School and the National Midwifery Board. Dr. Yang and her cohorts aimed to alter the image of midwifery, transforming it from what they saw as an apprenticed vocation populated by illiterate middle-aged and older women to a high-profile profession staffed by forward-thinking, educated young women. These modern midwives formed the basis for changes in the normative birth model, for after training they were sent around the country to popularize modern midwifery. Chapter 4 examines state-regulated childbirth under the Guomindang, focusing on legislation passed, though not always implemented, during this period. Reproductive health reform would not have been possible without the resources and personnel supplied by foreign philanthropic organizations, especially the Rockefeller Foundation's China Medical Board. This chapter therefore details the connections between these organizations.

The book ends with an epilogue that extends the history of reproduction in Republican China to the rest of the twentieth century. I recount wartime reproductive health reform in the 1930s and 1940s, and in the first few decades of the People's Republic of China after its establishment in 1949. The Chinese Communist Party built on the infrastructure and reforms of the previous government, extending its reach even further into the lives of individual citizens with the population policies of the 1970s onward. The Nationalist policies to strengthen the state in the fields of medicine and public health were continued in the People's Republic of China (PRC) after 1949. Paul Cohen has examined the fallacy of the perceived "1949 divide" that was common into the 1990s.[87] This imaginary divide was created by the Chinese Communist Party in its quest to shape a new China separate from its feudal past as well as from the first half of the twentieth century and the Nationalist government. It was also supported by others. Marxists and feminists around the world heralded full social equality for all under the Chinese Communist Party, while capitalists mourned the loss of freedom and a potentially lucrative market. Recently, scholars have begun to see the continuities between the Guomindang and the CCP administrations.[88] According to the rhetoric, a revolution was supposed to have taken place in 1949 and afterwards, but the health system after 1949 was, in fact, not that revolutionary. Concurrently, a growing middle class since the 1980s has resulted in ever-increasing consumerism with regard to reproduction, while advances in science and technology have created a highly medicalized birth model in urban areas, resulting in the demise of both the traditional and the modern midwives. Nonetheless, efforts to make childbirth safer in China, as well as to bring about continued state control over births and bodies, remain.

NOTES

1. These descriptions are amalgams of stories and articles collected on childbirth in urban China in the 1990s and early 2000s, contrasted with a "traditional" birth before the widespread adoption of the biomedical model. These examples are not intended to be comprehensive in all aspects, as every birth story is different, and birth customs and practices vary widely. Instead, they are meant to give the reader an initial insight into the massive changes in reproduction that have occurred in China over the twentieth century and to set the stage for the analysis that follows.

2. Lisa Handwerker, "The Politics of Making Modern Babies in China: Reproductive Technologies and the 'New' Eugenics," in *Infertility around the Globe: New Thinking on Childlessness, Gender, and Reproductive Technologies*, ed. Marcia C. Inhorn and Frank Van Balen (Berkeley: University of California Press, 2002), 310.

3. The women who belonged to the private gym in Guangzhou, where I conducted research in 2002, wore their vertical caesarean scars like badges of honor, a visual representation of their affluence and a means to preserve their figures.

4. A 2001 study of Shanghai birthing practices in four hospitals showed that less than 27% of laboring women received any form of analgesia. Xu Qian et al., "Evidence-Based Obstetrics in Four Hospitals in China: An Observational Study to Explore Clinical Practice, Women's Preferences and Provider's Views," *BioMed Central Pregnancy and Childbirth* 1, no. 1 (2001). A 2007 study claimed that less than 1% of laboring women in China receive neuraxial (epidural) anaesthesia. Zi Tian Fan, Xue Lian Gao, and Hui Xia Yang, "Popularizing Labor Analgesia in China," *International Journal of Gynecology and Obstetrics* 98, no. 3 (September 2007): 205.

5. N.F. Cheung, "The 'Doula-Midwives' in Shanghai," *Evidence Based Midwifery* 3 (2005): 73–79.

6. Robin Kartchner and Lynn Clark Callister, "Giving Birth: Voices of Chinese Women," *Journal of Holistic Nursing* 21 (June 2003): 106; Suzanne Gottschang, "The 'Becoming' Mother: Transitions to Motherhood in Urban China" (PhD dissertation, Pittsburgh, PA: University of Pittsburgh, 1998).

7. According to a survey conducted in 2002–2003, the national episiotomy rate in China is 44.9%, though in provincial capital hospitals that rate is 68.6%. Bin Wang et al., "National Survey on Midwifery Practices in Health Facilities in China (887 *suo yiliao baojian jigou zhuchan jishu shishi*

xiankuang de fenxi)," *Chinese Journal of Obstetrics and Gynecology (zhong-hua fuchanke zazhi*) 42, no. 5 (May 2007): 306.

8. Gottschang, "The 'Becoming' Mother: Transitions to Motherhood in Urban China," chapter 6: 'Doing the Month' in Urban Beijing."

9. *Zuo yuezi* centers have become popular on Taiwan and the mainland since the 1990s. Ling-ling Wong, "Tso yüeh-tzu: The Post-natal Ritual of Han Chinese Women in Taiwan" (University of Oxford, 1998); Ngai-en Cheung et al., "'Zuoyuezi' after Caesarean in China: an interview survey," *International Journal of Nursing Studies* 43 (2006): 193–202.

10. There were many tests in imperial Chinese medicine to determine pregnancy, including taking one's pulse and ingesting drugs to induce fetal movement. See Yi-Li Wu, *Reproducing Women: Medicine, Metaphor and Childbirth in Late Imperial China* (Berkeley and Los Angeles: University of California Press, 2010), 124–135; Barbara Duden, *Disembodying Women: Perspectives on Pregnancy and the Unborn*, trans. Lee Hoinacki (Cambridge, MA: Harvard University Press, 1993), 86–96.

11. Yang Nianqun, "The Transformation of Space and Control of Birth and Death in Early Republican Beijing (*Minguo chunian beijing de shengsi kongzhi yu kongjian zhuanhuan*)," in *Space, Memory, Society: A Collection of New Historical Cultural Research* (*Kongjian, jiyi, shehui zhuanxing: 'xin shehui shi' yanjiu lunwen jingxuan*), ed. Yang Nianqun (Shanghai: Shanghai renmin chubanshe, 2001), 139.

12. Cecilia Van Hollen, *Birth on the Threshold: Childbirth and Modernity in South India* (Berkeley: University of California Press, 2003).

13. Wu, *Reproducing Women: Medicine, Metaphor and Childbirth in Late Imperial China*, 6.

14. Li Xiaojiang, "Preface: Why Do We Use Cultural Anthropology As a Starting Point in Our Research? (*Xu: Women wei shenme yi wenhua renleixue wei yanjiu qidian?*)," in *Birth: Tradition and Modernization* (*Shengyu: Chuangtong yu xiandaihua*), ed. Li Xiaojiang (Henan: Henan renmin chubanshe, 1997), 3–15.

15. Robert J. Berry et al., "Prevention of Neural-Tube Defects with Folic Acid in China," *New England Journal of Medicine* 341, no. 20 (November 11, 1999): 1485–90.

16. Brigitte Jordan, *Birth in Four Cultures: A Crosscultural Investigation of Childbirth in Yucatan, Holland, Sweden, and the United States*, ed. Robbie Davis-Floyd, 4th ed. (Prospect Heights, IL: Waveland Press, Inc., 1993).

17. Jonathan D. Spence, *The Search for Modern China* (New York and London: W.W. Norton, 1990), 158.

18. Jane Hunter, *The Gospel of Gentility: American Women Missionaries in Turn-of-the-Century China* (New Haven: Yale University Press, 1984), 6.

19. Lloyd Eastman et al., *The Nationalist Era in China 1927–1949* (Cambridge: Cambridge University Press, 1991).

20. Hung-Mao Tien, *Government and Politics in Kuomintang China 1927–1937* (Stanford: Stanford University Press, 1972), chapter 3, "Factions in Kuomintang Politics," 45–72.

21. Ibid., 22–26.

22. Vera Schwarcz, *The Chinese Enlightenment: Intellectuals and the Legacy of the May Fourth Movement of 1919* (Berkeley, Los Angeles, London: University of California Press, 1986).

23. Wen-hsin Yeh, "Shanghai Modernity: Commerce and Culture in a Republican City," *The China Quarterly* 150 (June 1997): 375–94; Frank Dikötter, ed., *The Age of Openness: China before Mao* (Berkeley and Los Angeles: University of California Press, 2008).

24. Dikötter, *The Age of Openness: China before Mao.*

25. Laurence Schneider, *Biology and Revolution in Twentieth-Century China*, Asia/Pacific/Perspectives (Lanham, MD: Rowman & Littlefield Publishers, Inc., 2003), 6.

26. Weikun Cheng, "Going Public Through Education: Female Reformers and Girls' Schools in Late Qing Beijing," *Late Imperial China* 21, no. 1 (2000): 111.

27. Irvine Loudon, *The Tragedy of Childbed Fever* (Oxford: Oxford University Press, 2000), 120–21.

28. Semmelweis's theory was initially rejected by the medical community, as germ theory had not yet been adopted at that time. Ibid., 92–99.

29. Joseph W. Esherick, "Modernity and Nation in the Chinese City," in *Remaking the Chinese City: Modernity and National Identity, 1900–1950*, ed. Joseph W. Esherick (Honolulu: University of Hawai'i Press, 1999), 1–16.

30. Schneider, *Biology and Revolution in Twentieth-Century China*; Ka-che Yip, *Health and National Reconstruction in Nationalist China: The Development of Modern Health Services, 1928–1937*, Monograph and Occasional Paper Series (Ann Arbor: Association for Asian Studies, Inc., 1995).

31. Wu, *Reproducing Women: Medicine, Metaphor and Childbirth in Late Imperial China*, 17.

32. Kim Taylor, *Chinese Medicine in Early Communist China, 1945–63: A Medicine of Revolution* (London: RoutledgeCurzon, 2005), 82–86.

33. Xiaoqun Xu, *Chinese Professionals and the Republican State: The Rise of Professional Associations in Shanghai, 1912–1937* (Cambridge: Cambridge University Press, 2001).

34. Xiaoqun Xu, "'National essence' vs. 'Science': Chinese native physicians' fight for legitimacy, 1912–1937," *Modern Asian Studies* 31, no. 4 (1997): 847–77.

35. Bridie Andrews, "Tailoring Tradition: The Impact of Modern Medicine on Traditional Chinese Medicine, 1887–1937," in *Notions et perceptions du changement en Chine*, ed. Viviane Alleton and Alexeï Volkov (Paris: Collège du France Institute des Hautes Études Chinoises, 1994), 149–66.

36. D.W.Y. Kwok, *Scientism in Chinese Thought, 1900–1950* (New Haven and London: Yale University Press, 1965); Leo Ou-fan Lee, "The Cultural Construction of Modernity in Urban Shanghai: Some Preliminary Explorations," in *Becoming Chinese: Passages to Modernity and Beyond*, ed. Wen-hsin Yeh (Berkeley, Los Angeles, London: University of California Press, 2000), 31; Ono Kazuko, *Chinese Women in a Century of Revolution, 1850–1950* (Stanford: Stanford University Press, 1989).

37. Lao She, *Camel Xiangzi*, trans. Shi Xiangzi, Bilingual edition. (Hong Kong: The Chinese University Press, 2005), 462.

38. Wu, *Reproducing Women: Medicine, Metaphor and Childbirth in Late Imperial China*, 194.

39. Chou Chun Yen, "The Female Body and Nationality: Vigorous Nation and Women's Hygiene in Modern China (1895–1949) (*Nüti yu guozu: Qiangguo qiangzhong yu jindai zhongguo de funü weisheng*)" (PhD dissertation, Taibei, Taiwan: National Chengchi University, 2008), 194.

40. Birth practices varied widely in China, even within the same city or town, depending on the midwife and local cultural practices. Here I have given a broadly typical description.

41. Alison Bashford, "Global Biopolitics and the History of World Health," *History of the Human Sciences* 19, no. 1 (2006): 67–88.

42. E. Richard Brown, "Public Health in Imperialism: Early Rockefeller Programs at Home and Abroad," *American Journal of Public Health* 66 (1976): 897–903.

43. According to Brown, Gates had been a Baptist minister but left the church when he decided that the Baptist religion was built on faulty documentation and that Jesus had no intention of ever baptizing anyone. E. Richard Brown, *Rockefeller Medicine Men: Medicine and Capitalism in America* (Berkeley: University of California Press, 1981), 124.

44. Tina Phillips Johnson, "Yang Chongrui and the First National Midwifery School: Childbirth Reform in Early Twentieth-Century China," *Asian Medicine—Tradition and Modernity* 4, no. 2 (2009): 280–302.

45. Charles W Hayford, *To the People: James Yen and Village China* (New York: Columbia University Press, 1990).

46. Charlotte G Borst, *Catching Babies: The Professionalization of Childbirth, 1870–1920* (Cambridge, MA: Harvard University Press, 1995), 139–40; Judith Walzer Leavitt, *Brought to Bed: Childbearing in America, 1750 to 1950* (New York: Oxford University Press, 1986), 61–63.

47. The first was Ophthalmology, begun in 1917. Edward Stewart Taylor, *History of the American Gynecological Society 1876–1981 and American Association of Obstetricians and Gynecologists 1888–1981* (St. Louis: C.V. Mosby Company, 1985).

48. Loudon, *The Tragedy of Childbed Fever*.

49. Ellen S. More, *Restoring the Balance: Women Physicians and the Profession of Medicine, 1850–1995* (Cambridge, MA: Harvard University Press, 1999), 105–7.

50. Borst, *Catching Babies: The Professionalization of Childbirth, 1870–1920*, 145.

51. Loudon, *The Tragedy of Childbed Fever*.

52. Leavitt, *Brought to Bed: Childbearing in America, 1750 to 1950*, 171.

53. Anne Witz, *Professions and Patriarchy* (London and New York: Routledge, 1992).

54. Wu, *Reproducing Women: Medicine, Metaphor and Childbirth in Late Imperial China*; Charlotte Furth, *A Flourishing Yin: Gender in China's Medical History, 960–1665* (Berkeley: University of California Press, 1999).

55. AnElissa Lucas, *Chinese Medical Modernization: Comparative Policy Continuities, 1930s–1980s* (New York: Praeger Publishers, 1982), 38–40; John Z. Bowers, *Western Medicine in a Chinese Palace: Peking Union Medical College, 1917–1951* (New York: Josiah Macy, Jr. Foundation, 1972), 31.

56. Carl F. Nathan, "The Acceptance of Western Medicine in Early 20th Century China: The Story of the North Manchurian Plague Prevention Service," in *Medicine and Society in China*, ed. John Z. Bowers and Elizabeth F. Purcell (New York: Josiah Macy, Jr. Foundation, 1974), 55–75.

57. Liande Wu, *Plague Fighter: The Autobiography of a Modern Chinese Physician* (Cambridge: W. Heffner, 1959).

58. Zaitong Zhang and Cheng Rijin, eds., *Selected Republican-Era Medical and Public Health Legislation (Minguo yiyao weisheng fagui xuanbian, 1912–1948)* (Shandong: Shandong Daxue Chubanshe, 1990), 79–81.

59. Ruth Rogaski, "Hygienic Modernity in Tianjin," in *Remaking the Chinese City: Modernity and National Identity, 1900–1950*, ed. Joseph W. Esherick (Honolulu: University of Hawai'i Press, 1999), 30–46; Esherick, "Modernity and Nation in the Chinese City."

60. W. Arthur Tatchell, "The Training of Male Nurses," *The China Medical Journal* 26, no. 5 (1912): 271.

61. Chindon Yiu Tang, "Woman's Education in China," *Bulletins on Chinese Education* 9, no. 2 (1923): 1–36.

62. Cheiko Nakajima, "Health and Hygiene in Mass Mobilization: Hygiene Campaigns in Shanghai, 1920–1945," *Twentieth-Century China* 34, no. 1 (November 2008): 42–72.

63. Guangdong Provincial Government Police Department, *Police Department announcement of draft regulations for registered western doctors, obstetrists, pharmacists, prescriptions, western hospitals and the Red Cross (Jingchating gongbu shixing suo ni xiyisheng chankesheng yaojishi tiaoji yaofang xiyiyuan chihongzihui ge li'an zhangcheng wen)*, vol. 23 (Guangdong Provincial Government, 1913).

64. Susan Glosser discusses the increased government control of family lives during the Nationalist era in Susan Glosser, *Chinese Visions of Family and State, 1915–1953* (Berkeley: University of California Press, 2003).

65. Rogaski asserts that the Chinese term for hygiene, *weisheng*, should in some cases be read as "hygienic modernity." Ruth Rogaski, *Hygienic Modernity: Meanings of Health and Disease in Treaty-Port China*, 1st ed. (Berkeley: University of California Press, 2004), 2.

66. Rogaski, "Hygienic Modernity in Tianjin."

67. Chinese meals are usually served "family style," in which each person uses his or her own chopsticks to serve food from communal dishes. For dining reform, see Sean Hsiang-Lin Lei, "Habituate Individuality: Framing of Tuberculosis and Its Material Solutions in Republican China" (presented at the Annual Meeting of The Association for Asian Studies, Chicago, IL, April 2, 2005).

68. First National Midwifery School (hereafter FNMS), *Fourth Annual Report, First National Midwifery School, Peiping, July 1, 1932–June 30, 1933*,

Annual Report, July 15, 1933; Neizhengbu nianjian bianzuan weiyuanhui, *Yearbook of Internal Affairs (Neizheng nianjian)*, vol. 4 (Shanghai: Shangwu yinshuguan, 1936), G234.

69. Jordan, *Birth in Four Cultures: A Crosscultural Investigation of Childbirth in Yucatan, Holland, Sweden, and the United States*, 121.

70. Brigitte Jordan's landmark study of childbirth in four cultures showed that physician-assisted births in Holland had a 12–fold higher perinatal mortality rate as compared with midwife-assisted births. Ibid.

71. World Health Organization, *World Health Statistics 2009* (Geneva, Switzerland: World Health Organization, 2009), 52, 114.

72. 15.3 percent of U.S. GDP is used on health care expenditures. World Health Organization, *World Health Statistics 2009*, 52; Nicholas Bakalar, "U.S. Still Struggling with Infant Mortality," *New York Times*, April 7, 2009.

73. Jordan, *Birth in Four Cultures: A Crosscultural Investigation of Childbirth in Yucatan, Holland, Sweden, and the United States*, 45.

74. John B. Grant, "Letter to Dr. Victor Heiser," September 20, 1926.

75. Marion Yang, "Letter [to John B. Grant?]," 1928.

76. Nakagawa Tadahide, *Observations of Qing Dynasty Customs (Shinzoku kibun)*, 1800. Edition: Tokyo: Heibonsha, 1966; as cited in Furth, *A Flourishing Yin: Gender in China's Medical History, 960–1665*, 254, Figure 16.

77. Theodor Rosebury, *Microbes and Morals; the Strange Story of Venereal Disease* (New York: Viking Press, 1971), 171.

78. Jordan, *Birth in Four Cultures: A Crosscultural Investigation of Childbirth in Yucatan, Holland, Sweden, and the United States*, 63, 125–26.

79. Duden, *Disembodying Women: Perspectives on Pregnancy and the Unborn*, 86; Frank Dikötter, *Sex, Culture and Modernity in China: Medical Science and the Construction of Sexual Identities in the Early Republican Period* (Hong Kong: Hong Kong University Press, 1995), 86.

80. Furth, *A Flourishing Yin: Gender in China's Medical History, 960–1665*, 94.

81. Duden, *Disembodying Women: Perspectives on Pregnancy and the Unborn*, 7.

82. China Medical Commission of the Rockefeller Foundation, *Medicine in China* (New York: Rockefeller Foundation, 1914).

83. Wu, *Reproducing Women: Medicine, Metaphor and Childbirth in Late Imperial China*.

84. Ibid., 182–83.

85. Furth, *A Flourishing Yin: Gender in China's Medical History, 960–1665*, 278–83.

86. Gail Hershatter, "Birthing Stories: Rural Midwives in 1950s China," in *Dilemmas of Victory: The Early Years of the People's Republic of China*, ed. Jeremy Brown and Paul Pickowicz (Cambridge, MA: Harvard University Press, 2008).

87. Paul A. Cohen, "Reflections on a Watershed Date: The 1949 Divide in Chinese History," in *Twentieth-Century China: New Approaches*, ed. Jeffrey Wasserstrom (London and New York: Routledge, 2003): 27–36.

88. Merle Goldman, "Restarting Chinese History," *The American Historical Review* 105, no. 1 (February 6, 2000): 153–64.

I

Missionaries and Modernity

Our steps were thronged with eager suppliants, who, hearing that the Viceroy's wife was undergoing medical treatment, sought for relief from the same source.[1]

In 1879, Viceroy Li Hongzhang's wife fell ill. She "had been given up by the old-style physicians," so the Viceroy sent for two Western physicians to attend her, Dr. John Kenneth Mackenzie, a Canadian of the London Missionary Society, and Dr. A. Irwin, the Customs Medical Officer.[2] Due to the nature of Lady Li's illness, "it became necessary for the patient's complete restoration to health . . . to adopt a certain line of treatment, which, according to Chinese etiquette, could only be carried out by a lady."[3] Dr. Mackenzie called for a female medical missionary working in Beijing, Dr. Leonora Howard, to hasten to Lady Li's palace. The three physicians stayed in the viceroy's palace for one month, using electrotherapy treatment (*shouyao dianji zhenzhifa*) to remedy Lady Li's affliction, diagnosed as apoplexy (*zhongfeng*), in which half of her body was paralyzed (*ban shen bu sui*).[4] This not uncommon ailment was often attributed to uncontrolled menstrual bleeding or hysteria, and was considered to be a disorder of the womb when it occurred in women. (Empress Dowager Cixi was believed to have died from apoplexy in 1908 following a terrifying "fit of rage."[5]) Electrotherapy was the most modern of Western medical treatments at the time and was used for a wide variety of illnesses and disorders, especially those, like apoplexy, thought to be neurological in nature.[6] News of Lady Li's recovery soon spread, as Mackenzie later reflected on his stay in the palace:

To reach the family apartments we had to pass through these numerous courts, and here we were beset with patients from the crowds
assembled outside the gates, and the friends of the soldiers, door-
keepers, secretaries, and attendants who had succeeded in gaining an
entrance.[7]

Viceroy Li Hongzhang was no doubt persuaded by the technological
wonders of electrotherapy, and after Lady Li's cure he devoted considerable sums to support Western medicine. The foreigners courted
Viceroy Li, who as the holder of the influential viceroyalty of Zhili,
the area surrounding Beijing, they considered to be "the most powerful mandarin in his time."[8] According to G.H. Choa, the viceroy
"firmly believed that China could only be strengthened by the full
exploitation of the benefits of Western science. With this conviction
he played a significant part in fostering medical education in China
and encouraging the acceptance of Western medicine."[9] Li Hongzhang
witnessed several surgical operations (including a tumor removal and
a harelip repair), and soon afterwards set up a room outside the gates
of the yamen (administrative headquarters) for dispensary work. The
crowds grew too large for this small space, so in a quadrangle of the
Taiwang temple to his predecessor as Viceroy of Tianjin, Qing military
general Zeng Guofan, he established a dispensary and inpatient clinic,
over which Dr. Leonora Howard later assumed control.[10] The viceroy
pledged to finance all medical work at the temple. Dr. Howard recounts that she "was called to the houses of the highest officials; their
prejudices are breaking down everywhere over the land. . . . Patients
come from the interior and take up their residence near the temple,
that they may be treated."[11]

Lady Li later built a hospital for Dr. Howard in Tianjin, and the
Viceroy's mother bequeathed a large sum to finance it, reportedly the
first inheritance from a Chinese woman to a Christian.[12]

The story of Lady Li sets the background for this book as it illustrates the entry of Western medicine into China in the 1800s, a
precursor of the changes to childbirth and reproduction that followed.
New concepts of modernity in the realm of human relationship to
disease and wellness were spreading throughout China, albeit slowly
and never comprehensively, in the nineteenth century. Gentry reformers, warlords, scholars, and officials sought to make a mark in their
communities by associating with the newly arrived Western medical
missionaries whose successes, especially in surgery, popularized them.
Not all of the missionaries' practices were accepted, nor were the missionaries trusted by all. Stories of local attacks against missionaries

and Western physicians are well known, as are the rumors surrounding the strange inclination of these foreigners to open charity hospitals and orphanages.[13]

The adoption and support of scientific medicine by reformers was a crucial part of a new and modern China. In cities around the country, local elites established public health programs and built Western-style hospitals and clinics. Inhabitants of treaty-port cities like Shanghai and Guangzhou (Canton) began to patronize Western-style or Western-trained physicians and their private and public hospitals to give birth. Training programs taught young Chinese students the new medical methods and concepts of the human body. Wives of prominent local leaders often supported these institutions, though sometimes forward-thinking men, like Li Hongzhang, actively promoted Western medicine, even medicine for women. These early experiences laid the foundation for the fundamental changes in reproduction in the twentieth-century.

GENTRY PHILANTHROPISTS

Philanthropy among Chinese officials and gentry to improve the lives of citizens has a long history in China, and so the fact that local elites supported the building of western hospitals and medical schools is not surprising. From the Tang dynasty (618–907 CE) onward, individual philanthropists (*shanren*) occasionally donated money for prescriptions and medicine to the poor and established charity infirmaries and pharmacies.[14] These "famous intellectuals" began to create organized aid institutions in the Ming and Qing dynasties, and gentry and local leaders usually contributed funds to such institutions during times of pestilence or disease.[15] It was also common in the Qing to fund the printing of medical treatises in order to bring merit on oneself and one's ancestors.[16] Furthermore, charitable halls and merchant guilds were often important philanthropic institutions that aided the poor and indigent, especially during times of famine or disease.[17] During such periods, the Qing government occasionally established dispensaries or almshouses. For example, the Yongzheng emperor in the mid-1700s ordered that charitable halls be established throughout the empire and urged the opening of foundling homes. These were private institutions that would benefit from government recognition and occasionally even financial aid. [18]

While philanthropy in China was not unique, the philanthropic activities of gentry like Li Hongzhang and others like him are very different. These local leaders gave money to fund Christian organizations and permanent Western-style hospitals established and run by foreigners. These were not indigenous solutions to temporary problems, but permanent, foreign institutions that would provide continuous services to China's citizens. Viceroy Li Hongzhang supported modern medicine in Tianjin less than a decade after the Tianjin Massacre in which Chinese attacked foreigners based on rumors and fears that foreign missionaries were kidnapping children for their orphanage.[19] Viceroy Li was supporting the very foreigners that many of his countrymen wanted dead or at least out of the country. Furthermore, modern medicine often conflicts with the traditional and more holistic Chinese paradigm of the body and its relation to the cosmos, society, the mind, health, and disease.[20] Yet many utilized modern medicine in the hopes of improvement in their lives, or out of utter desperation, and sometimes both. Western medicine was imagined to be so powerful that women went into labor—one of the most vulnerable and critical times in their lives—attended by strangers with unfamiliar dress and even more unusual ideas, methods, and tools.

Throughout China at the end of the Qing dynasty, officials and gentry had engaging experiences with Western medicine, pledging to fund hospitals and dispensaries after they or their relatives were cured. Some of these were Chinese Christians, though others were decidedly not. Thomas Cochrane, a Scottish physician with the London Missionary Society, cared for the Guangxu emperor (ruled 1875–1908) and his son, as well as the head eunuch Li Lianying and lady-in-waiting Duchess De. According to Dr. Cochrane, Duchess De wanted him to "perform a delicate and difficult operation but she feared that, when she went back to court, she would get into trouble for having allowed a man to operate on her . . . she went through a ceremony whereby I became her brother-in-law and then it was considered proper for me to operate."[21]

Cochrane reportedly then convinced the Empress Dowager Cixi of the importance of a new Western-style medical school, to which Cixi donated 10,000 taels (1,400 British pounds). Other court gentry added an additional 1,600 pounds to fund the Peking School of Medicine.[22]

In the Yangzi River valley far south of Tianjin and Beijing, the Maternity Hospital and Training Home for Midwifery opened in Hangzhou in July 1906, a joint effort between Chinese gentry and Dr. Duncan Main of the Edinburgh (Scotland) Medical Missionary Society. A Mrs. Kao, a prominent Hangzhou philanthropist, "conceived the idea of starting such an institution with [Dr. Liu Ming-ts, Dr. Main's chief assistant]."[23] Kingston DeGruche, Dr. Main's biographer, stated that Mrs. Kao, with her friends, was not only willing but anxious that some definite help for Chinese women in their confinements should be provided. These ladies were most sympathetic with the idea of training native women midwives and monthly nurses, that this appalling evil [of the sufferings of women and infants due to native childbirth practices] should be lessened as far as possible.[24]

The Training Home for Midwifery received 90 student applications its first year. Its faculty taught students to give vaccinations to children and adults and to treat cases of opium poisoning, a common method of suicide among Chinese women. The Governor of Hangzhou's wife and sister both delivered their babies at the Maternity Hospital.[25]

In nearby Suzhou, Dr. Mildred Phillips of the Methodist Episcopal Church, South, oversaw the building of the Suzhou Women's Hospital in 1888 with help from the local gentry. In 1904, Governor En Shou and various officials donated $3,000 to build a residence for one of the hospital's Western physicians.[26] The next year, two Chinese men, Mr. Zhu Baosan and Mr. Xia Zenan, raised $1,300 in Shanghai for the hospital. The donations continued. In 1906, Governor Chen gave $2,000, and a Dr. A.E. Yandell and a Mr. Si raised over $400 in the city of Wuxi. Additionally, seven families from Suzhou made monthly donations of $.50 to $5 each to the hospital, and several others gave $50 per year. In 1906, a prominent Suzhou banker, Lu Sandong, contributed $30 from his bank and raised $200 from 17 other banks.[27]

In Nanchang, Jiangxi Province, Dr. Kang Cheng (known in English as Ida Kahn) graduated from the University of Michigan and started her medical work in 1903 with much help from the locals.[28] One early patient was the wealthy wife of a reformer, a Mr. Tseo, whose wife she treated for "nervous collapse" and apparent insanity.[29] Dr. Kang and her colleague Dr. Shi Meiyu (known in English as Mary Stone) treated her physically and spiritually with daily Bible study. After her recovery, Mrs. Tseo sent her sons to the mission school in Jiujiang, and her husband donated money to the dispensary.[30] Dr. Kang went on to establish the self-supporting Nanchang Women's and Children's Hospital, with most of the donations coming from Chinese gentry and officials. In 1905, the local gentry bought Kang a piece of land worth $3,000 and built a dispensary with $2,000. Some of these funds came from a gift of grain from the public granary sold by an official to raise money for the hospital.[31]

Further west still, Changsha, Hunan, was the home of the Xiangya Medical College and Hospital, opened in 1913 under an agreement between the Yale-China Association and a group of gentry called the

Hunan Yu Chun Educational Association (HYCEA) with the support of the provincial government.[32] Along with the College and Hospital were an affiliated School of Nursing and a department to train nurses in obstetrics. The local government donated a Chinese building for the Medical College, and a new hospital building was erected across the street with Yale mission funds. During World War I, it was difficult for the hospital to secure Western physicians and other staff, and the institution was in financial trouble. However, according to a 1930 report, "it was an encouraging proof of the steadfast loyalty of the local gentry to the cause, that on several occasions, ever at their own financial loss, they raised the funds necessary to maintain the work and to put up a new medical college building on their own campus in 1919."[33] The Yale mission and the HYCEA continued joint administration of the hospital and college.

Guangzhou in southern China was a primary center of Western medicine and home to several missionary medical centers established with the support of local gentry. The Kung Yee Society (*Gongyiyuan*) was established in Guangzhou by Dr. Paul Todd of the Presbyterian Mission with substantial donations from local influential Chinese.[34] In 1909, Dr. Todd enlisted 50 Chinese men who gave $100 each to fund a men's medical school and act as a committee. In 1912, the local government gave Kung Yee 20 acres outside the city for new buildings, and the Society received $11,000 in private gifts the same year. The directors of the school and hospital were all Chinese. There were 24 faculty members, including four foreign medical men. The rest were Chinese: one educated in Edinburgh, one in Texas, two in Japan, four in Tianjin, and 12 in Guangzhou.[35] By 1914, Kung Yee had over 150 medical students, including some women, and a small hospital and dispensary on the Bund in Guangzhou. Dr. Li Shufen, a graduate of Hong Kong College of Medicine (1908) and Edinburgh University (1910), raised $100,000 during a fund-raising trip to the United States, mostly from overseas Chinese. This money was used to build a new wing of the hospital.[36] In 1923 Kung Yee became the medical department of Zhongshan University (Sun Yat-sen University Medical School, *Sun Zhongshan boshi yixueyuan*). In 1924 Mayor Sun Fo, son of Sun Yat-sen, donated nearly 20 acres of land to the hospital for its new buildings and medical school, and two years later the central government in Nanjing promised $500,000 to the new endeavor.[37]

Also in Guangzhou, the Fangbian Hospital (*Fangbian yiyuan*) was the result of local wealthy commoners' efforts at philanthropy. According to Michael Tsin, Fangbian was started as a shelter for homeless and indigent men and women (*fangbiansuo*) by local merchant guilds in

1894 in response to the plague epidemic that ravaged Guangzhou in the 1890s.[38] A local merchant with connections to Hong Kong, Chen Heyun raised money in Hong Kong to save the hospital from the verge of bankruptcy in 1899, while a merchant turned philanthropic activist in Guangzhou, Chen Huipu, coordinated efforts and funds from several local charitable halls. Donations to the hospital reached Chinese $110,000 by 1906, up from over Chinese $6,000 in 1899. It grew into one of the most well-known and modern hospitals in south China and eventually included a midwifery training school (established in 1938), and a women's ward. It too was eventually absorbed into Zhongshan University.[39]

Like Viceroy Li Hongzhang's work in Tianjin, the Hackett Medical College for Women in Guangzhou under Dr. Mary Fulton also had the support of its local leader, Zhang Renjun, the Viceroy of Liangguang (the two provinces of Guangzhou and Guangxi). He stamped the diplomas of the seven 1907 graduates, "the highest official recognition obtainable" and the only diplomas in the province to receive that distinction.[40] Viceroy Zhang also gave three gold watches to the three students with the highest cumulative grades. The following year, for the first time in the history of the Guangzhou missions, the Viceroy personally attended the commencement exercises and sent an honor guard of 500 soldiers. [41]

These few cases out of dozens more relate many things about modern medicine in China at the end of the Qing. They illustrate how local gentry leaders played a significant role in establishing and maintaining Western hospitals and training programs throughout China. What started as localized efforts to improve the health of one's family or community grew into the desire for a modern city, sometimes culminating in the goal of a modern nation. Local gentry, and later, city and national governments in China supported Western medicine in the name of science and modernity. The concurrent rise in business and consumer culture further created markets for reproductive technologies and services. These examples also form the foundation for medical and scientific developments that led to public health programs, for example germ theory that led to sanitation programs and antiseptic medical procedures. The advent of maternal and child health care, and indeed the specialization of obstetrics as a distinct field of medicine, also have their origin in the late 1800s. Women physicians like Dr. Leonora Howard and Dr. Mary Fulton opened women's hospitals and training programs for female nurses and midwives. They were training women to work in the medical field at a time when most women who had the opportunity for education would not work outside the home, and certainly not in a field associated with death and disease. By the 1930s, training programs and medical schools for women physicians, nurses, and midwives formed a fundamental part of the normative birth model.

The connection between the strength of a country and the health of its mothers and children was not lost on the medical missioners or on the Chinese leaders. Reproduction was a crucial part of the modernizing effort and the basis of new gender identities. Modernism, in turn, contributed to changing the gender dynamics of parenthood and family life in Republican China, altering the roles of women in nation building as national mothers and as professional midwives, and of men as new fathers in a reformed nuclear family structure. These efforts in China interplayed with consequent upheavals in gender dynamics that took shape in the early twentieth century. The transformations in medicine and in gender relations can be expressed in terms of a striving for modernity, or a fetish of modernity.

MEDICINE AND MODERNITY

The concept of modernity is a driving force for all participants in this narrative. More than an end product, modernity is a process, a path that rarely results in a satisfying conclusion. It is a never-ending road because to be modern means to continually strive for the next big thing, the next advancement, the newest technology. To be modern is an elusive, unattainable goal that in early twentieth-century China was entwined with foreign influence. Because of China's recent humiliations at the hands of Western powers, many Chinese were ambivalent about what kinds of ideas and inventions to take from the West, which many considered to be the font of modernity. A tension between nationalism and modernity hence arose as reformers searched for a unique Chinese identity while simultaneously aiming to make the country more modern. To reconcile this tension, the new arenas like science and medicine that came from the United States and Europe were deemed "modern" instead of "Western."[42] Therefore, China could modernize without losing its unique characteristics.

Spurred by ideas of modernism and its associate theories of social Darwinism, eugenics, and public health movements in the United States, Japan, and Europe, many Chinese intellectuals and political leaders in the early twentieth century reshaped their cities and governments in order to survive and become more competitive globally. Improvements in public health were a crucial part of the modernization process in cities worldwide, and urban China was no different.[43] Ruth Rogaski, in her study of public health in Tianjin, translates the Chinese word for hygiene, *weisheng*, as "hygienic *modernity*," which illustrates just how modern the ideas and methods of public health were at the time.[44] China's "sick man of Asia" image resulting from international humiliations would be remedied through public health initiatives like street sweeping, night soil removal, and sanitary house inspections. The spread of many parasitic and infectious diseases in China, like water-borne cholera, typhoid, and schistosomiasis; and insect-borne malaria, typhus, and bubonic plague were halted with a clean water supply and a clean environment. Reproductive health would hit at the very root of China's problem by treating diseased infants and sickly mothers. It would eliminate the sick man of Asia by creating a healthy and robust citizenry beginning at conception. This concept was the key to China's rise.

Criticisms about the health of China's population were bolstered by scientific concepts regarding sanitation that became widely accepted in the late nineteenth century. By the early 1900s the field of public health emerged to incorporate modern medical ideas and spread them to the masses.[45] A faith in cleanliness, which had first been attributed to godliness and later to health with the discovery of germ theory, was a foundation of the public health movement in the United States and abroad. This faith was buttressed by John Snow's discovery that cholera is transmitted in drinking water (1854), and by the finding that bubonic plague is carried by rats (1898).[46] Disease could be prevented by keeping one's environment clean. By the first decades of the twentieth century, fears of disease caused by dank, dark spaces mobilized Europeans and Americans to clean up their homes, use disinfectants, boil drinking water, and improve ventilation to relieve the buildup of "sewer gases."[47] The creation of modern hospitals reflected the focus on sanitation and health, as hospitals were transformed from dens of disease and illness where the indigent went to die, to sanitary houses of healing, the place of choice for the most modern treatments.[48]

Medical missionaries aimed to bring China into the modern world as part of their efforts to save Chinese souls. They would bestow on its people the new ideas of public health, medical specialization, and sanitary hospitals, and combine them in the mission fields with a quest for salvation. Such efforts professed a belief—a faith, if you will—that science would not only ensure salvation but would also solve the world's most dire health problems like infectious disease and hunger. They took to their task of saving lives with the same conviction that they had used to save souls. Medical missionaries created charity hospitals and made house calls to members of all socioeconomic classes. They sought patients and patrons from gentry and officials in order to fund their operations and garner support among the Chinese. It was the policy of these medical missionaries early on that the local Chinese would assist in building and maintaining hospitals, as well as receive medical training. The missionaries were to act as a temporary conduit of salvation and medical knowledge to be removed when the Chinese could maintain the programs and training on their own. Most hospitals and clinics operated on a sliding scale policy, with the rich Chinese paying for services which were then used to subsidize the poorer patients. Thus, "high and low, rich and poor, have been seen, both in their homes and at the hospital."[49]

Medical training was part of the modernizing process that would eventually create an independent, well-trained cadre of Chinese physicians and paramedical personnel. Missionaries attempted to remedy the perceived plight of Chinese women whom they considered bound-footed and confined to their homes, bought and sold by their families, and generally considered worthless in Chinese society. "Liberating" these women included educating them to become independent and self-sufficient members of society.[50] Missionaries complained of not being able to reach women and members of the upper classes to convert them to Christianity, as it was widely believed that women as mothers and wives had the potential to exert greater religious influence on their families and communities. Native medical personnel had the trust of their patients that the foreign missioners did not, and it followed that native *female* practitioners could attend women patients in the wards and in the patients' homes, thus bringing more people into contact with modern medicine and Christianity. Furthermore, medical missionaries simply did not have enough trained help in their hospitals and dispensaries in order to fulfill their goals of modernizing public health and fighting disease.

In the late 1800s, medical missionaries began training locals to assist them, providing unstructured lectures with hands-on apprenticeships. Lady Li's physician, Dr. Leonora Howard, was one of the first medical missionaries to train women. Between 1885 and 1890, at the Isabella Fisher Hospital in Tianjin, she trained two female students, Ms. Xu and Ms. Cai, as assistants, "one of the first institutions in China where women only were instructed in medicine."[51] Two thousand kilometers south in Guangzhou, the Canton Hospital (*Boji yiyuan*) was also training women. By 1880, its female medical students were attending female patients and making home visits to treat female diseases and disorders.[52] In 1896, 239 of the 508 home visits recorded for Canton Hospital were made by Chinese women medical practitioners trained at the hospital.[53] A few years later, Dr. Mary Fulton branched off from the Canton Hospital to organize an independent medical school for women to "train Christian women physicians to go out amongst their own countrywomen."[54] The Guangdong Medical College for Women (later renamed Hackett Medical College) and its affiliated hospital opened its doors in 1901 with nine students. Several locally trained Chinese women physicians assisted Fulton in instructing the students, including the instructor of obstetrics and gynaecology, who was a former student of the medical school at the Canton Hospital. [55] According to one contemporary, in 1915, "the operating room [at Hackett was] the best in Canton."[56]

Coupled with the increase in medical specialization, midwifery training was a logical next step to improve reproductive health in China, where the man-midwife or male physician would never succeed because of the sustaining traditions of sex segregation, especially in the women's affair of childbirth. Dr. James Boyd Neal, editor of the *China Medical Missionary Journal*, advocated short courses in midwifery for women in 1901.[57] Even illiterate women could be taught the principles of childbirth and midwifery, he claimed. Neal did not support full medical education of women because they tended to marry soon after completing training, and because family duties interfered with their work, most left the profession after marriage. Courses in the paramedical midwifery field, on the other hand, would allow women to attend classes and work despite marital and family constraints. In training midwives, Neal and his colleagues would not be restricted to teaching only young unmarried women, as was usually the case for the full medical course that lasted several years. Instead, women of all ages could participate:

> Women of considerable age might easily spare a few weeks at a time, or some months, in which to be taught the essentials of midwifery and then returning [sic] for a further course within a year or two, and after considerable practical experience, might be given certificates which would give them a certain standing at least among Christians.[58]

Some 30 years later, the Western-trained Chinese physician Yang Chongrui would adopt a short course curriculum like this to train old-style midwives in modern midwifery methods as part of a national plan to improve reproductive health, as examined later in chapter 3.

A crucial part of this modern medicine movement was the legitimization, and in many cases hegemony, of scientific medicine, which spread to encompass nearly all aspects of human life. However, the tension between Chinese and foreign philanthropists resulting from mutual distrust and disrespect led to numerous attacks on missionaries, the most well-known being the Boxer Rebellion in 1900.[59] This tension created fault lines in the last years of the waning Qing government as well because of the infighting between reformers and conservatives within its ranks.[60] The foreigners were asking, even forcing, the Chinese to give up their customs, traditions, and beliefs as superstitious, heretical, unscientific, and barbaric, even when scientific conversion superseded religious conversion. While the secularization of philanthropic work may have eased the conflicts between Western philanthropists and Chinese, as recipients of modern medical care were not always asked to renounce their religion for Christianity, the irrefutable faith in scientific medicine began to crowd out other medical and health options.

Medical hegemony notwithstanding, the methods that modern physicians used for prenatal care, parturition, and childbirth, especially around the turn of the twentieth century, were unproven and sometimes even harmful. For example, Dr. Benjamin Hobson, a missionary physician with the London Missionary Society who worked in China in the mid-1800s, recommended ice water douches to expel the placenta, although cold water in any form contradicts traditional Chinese medical beliefs of avoiding cold or cooling substances during parturition and menstruation.[61] Furthermore, some of the nutrition prescriptions prescribed by Western physicians for Chinese patients, such as consuming large amounts of red meat and dairy products, ran counter to traditional Chinese beliefs and customs about appropriate foods to consume and avoid during pregnancy.[62]

Nor were many modern childbirth techniques all that efficacious. Physicians were more apt to intervene in childbirth than were traditional midwives, both in the West and in China. After all, family members expected doctors to *do something* to aid the birth. Even well into the twentieth century, the United States Children's Bureau's Obstetric Advisory Committee's 1927–1933 study found that most of the country's 7,537 maternal deaths were caused by puerperal sepsis due to "ill-judged or botched surgical interventions by physicians."[63] Problems with cleanliness and sanitation were compounded by the use of non-sterile instruments like forceps, especially before germ theory began to gain ground in the mid-nineteenth century.[64] An ideal combination of sanitation and intervention improves normal childbirth conditions; when birth attendants moved beyond that to more invasive procedures—whether they were old or new midwives or modern physicians—maternal and infant health were jeopardized.

Additionally, the missionary literature of the nineteenth and early twentieth centuries illustrates that oftentimes the missionaries had little regard for their native patients or their practices, even though the "modern" treatments the missionaries advocated did not necessarily produce better outcomes.[65] Medical missionary writers often disregarded traditional Chinese mores and failed to accommodate the patients' customs or understanding of the world and their place in it. Only one exception from this group emerges. Dr. Browning, a medical missionary practicing in Ningbo, published an article in the *Chinese Medical Missionary Journal* supporting a traditional Chinese practice he had encountered. Browning had been called to attend a confinement case, but when he arrived the baby was already delivered and lying in a tub with its placenta still attached. The doctor, surprised at the sight, learned that in this particular area of China, midwives cut the umbilical cord only after the baby had been washed and dressed. This practice ran counter to the speedy severing and tying of the cord common in modern childbirth at the time. In the article, Dr. Browning claimed that the Chinese way was the more "natural" process, allowing for a slower transition for the baby from the womb to the outside world. He urged his fellow practitioners to consider what harm they may be doing by being too hasty.[66] Although this is a good example of the ways the Chinese and Westerners accommodated each other, this attitude was not common among medical missionaries. Most spoke of Chinese midwives—and their patients—with scorn and pity.[67]

Modern medical personnel were rarely called to attend normal births in late nineteenth-and early twentieth-century China, and usually they only saw the most gruesome examples of protracted labor and fetal dismemberment. Dr. Shi Meiyu, who had attended medical school in the United States, wrote that "from the richest to the poorest the utter lack of sanitation is so evident that the obstetrician has nothing to aid her, but on the other hand she has everything to contend with. One thing they do hold in common, and that is the ignorance of the laws of hygiene and their dread of fresh air and sunlight."[68] Dr. James Menzies, a physician in Henan, was only summoned after the wife of an official had been in labor for six or eight days, by which time "the child had evidently been dead for some time, the head having been pretty roughly used by the midwife in attendance."[69] In another case, Menzies was summoned to attend a laboring Muslim woman with an arm presentation (instead of the normal head presentation) who had been attended by no less than six midwives. Menzies "found on arrival an arm presenting with a vengeance; it was lying on the ground beneath the bed and had been torn off at midnight."[70] In both of these cases, Menzies had to perforate and dismember the infant in order to extract it from the birth canal. He administered the common abortifacient and purgative, ergot, to the mothers, who both recovered after a few days.

Yet another physician, Agnes Stewart, practicing in Hankou, complained about the commonality of uterine prolapse among Chinese women due to their methods of delivery: "On several occasions, when called to remove a retained placenta, one has found the woman sitting up, with the anterior vaginal wall and cervix outside the vulva and the midwife *still vigorously pulling on the cord*" [italics in original].[71] Another method the midwives used was tying an old shoe to the end of the umbilical cord still attached to the undelivered placenta in order to facilitate placental expulsion. The midwives also used their long fingernails to "tear anything within reach. . . . I have seen women with cervix, vagina, perinaeum all torn through—and not superficially, for the long sharp finger nails do their work thoroughly and deeply."[72] Physician James A. Greig in Jilin Province was called to aid a neighbor's wife who had been in labor for two or three days. Upon arrival by horseback, Greig found that after the midwives had been unsuccessful in delivering the child, the wife's husband had used a pair of scissors to decapitate the infant while still in the birth canal. She died several days later.[73]

The tools that modern physicians and traditional midwives had to deal with such cases of protracted labor were similar. By the time physicians were called, there was often no other option but to dismember the decaying infant to prevent the mother's death. Traditional midwives used hooks and scissors to extract infants (in one case, Menzies even borrowed one of the midwife's hooks). However, modern physicians used relatively antiseptic methods that could reduce the rate of infection from septicemia and tetanus, though these practices were not foolproof. Modern physicians rarely saw routine childbirth, and in any case such ordinary births, the vast majority of births, did not warrant inclusion in medical journals. The Western medical literature that came out of China during this time was written by nurses and physicians with an utter faith in science, and often little understanding of their patients, and is necessarily polemical.

MODERN CITIES

Regardless of outcome or real practicality, being perceived as modern was the goal of many individuals, cities, and nations. Modernity, popularized as progress, was fetishized in the early twentieth century. This force of modernity, of faith in human endeavors, drove gentry and the impoverished alike to patronize the mysterious and unknown Western medicine. Medical missionaries targeted gentry, whom they charged fees for medical service, while they also treated the poor and indigent for free.[74] Alongside the hopes of progress lay the belief in a new and modern China, one whose citizens were healthy and whose streets and homes were free of filth and debris. This desire had led medical missionaries to build hospitals in China and urged Viceroy Li Hongzhang and his countrymen to support Western science and medicine. It prompted Liangguang Viceroy Zhang Renjun to attend the Hackett Medical School graduation and sign the women graduates' diplomas.[75]

Localized modernizing efforts continued in the early twentieth century in cities around China as part of the late Qing and Republican reforms. The New Policies resulting from the Boxer Rebellion in 1900 included attempts to reform China to be more civilized (wenming) by creating a martial citizenry, a modern police force, and urban sanitation programs.[76] Cities were considered models for the rest of China's other administrative units, with provincial capitals the showpieces of the New Policies, and later for the Guomindang, who planned to establish new schools, police academies, and medical facilities in capitals throughout the country.[77] Well-planned and efficiently administered cities were the most outwardly visible components of modern nations. Previously, provincial capitals under the Qing had had no city administrations and instead were ruled through overlapping bureaucracies, thus large-scale civic programs were rare before 1895. The Republican period, according to Kristin Stapleton, is "modern China's first age of city-centered politics" as cities throughout China focused on modernizing their locales.[78] The new Republican government led by Yuan Shikai did not have widespread support, and much of the country was controlled by local warlords. This absence of central leadership allowed local leaders of Nantong, Shanghai, Chengdu, Nanjing, Beijing, and many others the relative freedom to create modern cities that included public health programs and hospitals.[79]

Many of the reforms were shaped by foreign influence. China's capital of Beijing was occupied by six nations after the Boxer Rebellion, with each nation responsible for administering a section of the city. As David Strand has related, Japan's administrative section during the occupation was controlled by Kawashima, a "self-taught China expert" with "close ties to the Japanese military."[80] Kawashima founded the Beijing Police Academy in 1901 and trained his Chinese recruits in Japanese police methods. When Japan's occupation ended in 1901, this Japanese-style police force that had been drawn from Prussian, British, and French models expanded throughout the city and controlled sanitation and regulated medical personnel.[81] This law enforcement model spread to other areas in China, including Zhili Province and its municipalities under its Viceroy, Yuan Shikai, who later became the first president of the Republic of China.[82] Thus, a Japanese-style police force, European in nature, which included oversight and regulation of public health, became the model for several cities throughout China.[83]

Similar rhetoric regarding the health of citizens and the fate of the nation accompanied reform in Japan as in China. Indeed, the very word for public health, (weisheng), was adopted in China from Japan, where it had gained shape and meaning as eisei in the late 1800s.[84] Childbirth in Japan had undergone significant change during the Meiji (1868–1912), Taisho (1912–1926), and early Showa (1926–1989) periods, with midwives receiving European-style training and state-mandated registration.[85] Traditional Japanese midwives were lambasted as abortionists and agents of death and disease (abortion was criminalized in the Meiji Criminal Code of 1870).[86] From the 1930s onward, the new midwifery methods were widely accepted in Japan as the traditional midwives (sanba) were replaced by new midwives (shin-sanba), and training and registration were brought under the control of local and national governments.[87] Japan's strong centralized government, along with willing and capable physicians, new midwives, and family members, created a medicalized childbirth paradigm much more rapidly and effectively than in China. By 1915, there were more new midwives (nearly 18,000) than old (14,000) in Japan; by 1945, only 1,864 old midwives remained, while 16,051 new midwives were registered.[88] During the occupation of Taiwan (1895–1945), the Japanese implemented similar police and public health reforms, including modern methods of midwifery training, registration, and administration.[89] Chinese midwifery reform followed a much more erratic and inconsistent path, though in the urban areas dedicated to reforming childbirth, the rhetoric and the methods were often similar to Japan's.

Following the lead of Japan, many municipal governments after 1911 incorporated public health administration into the duties of their local police forces.[90] In many cities, the police were a crucial part of the modern city who acted as "babysitters" and teachers of the new citizenry; thus local police bureaus were responsible for public health activities like licensing and regulation of medical personnel.[91] Cities like Nantong, Chengdu, and Beijing implemented modern police forces that regulated public health and sanitation projects including public toilets, ventilation systems, slaughterhouses, and the like. In Chengdu, the police initiated the examination and registration of traditional medical physicians in 1907.[92] Similarly, Beijing created a modern police force and public health unit in 1905. President Yuan Shikai reorganized the police force in 1913 and formed the city's department of public health with three administrative subsections: street cleaning, public toilets, and sewage system.[93] Poor administration and lack of a strong infrastructure in the 1910s and 1920s created serious public health problems in Beijing: public urination and littering were rampant, and nightsoil collectors were unregulated.[94] When the Guomindang relocated China's capital to Nanjing in 1927, a movement was under way to remake the old capital city as a cultural center, and the Nationalists reformed the Beijing police force and established a formal public health department in 1928.[95] This ultimately included building hundreds of public toilets, regulating nightsoil and garbage collection, and street-sweeping.

New city administrations like these targeted the "individual citizen as the basic unit" of organization and administration, thus disregarding native place associations and other traditional "unofficial mediating groups."[96] Local leaders, merchants, intellectuals, and gentry were influenced by intellectuals Tan Sitong's (1865–1898) and Liang Qichao's (1873–1929) discussions of modern society, and the necessity of China, as an emerging modern nation, to take responsibility for its citizenry.[97] Citizens supported a new form of civic duty that, according to Michael Tsin, "demonstrated the spirit of public morals by involving themselves in the affairs of the public arena *for the good of the collective*" [italics in original].[98] This was a major shift in worldview from a focus on one's family, neighborhood, or village to an awareness of China's place in the geopolitical sphere accompanied by a growing national awareness.

Many city leaders in the early Republican period established or supported hospitals as part of their modernizing projects to encourage individual responsibility for national health. Zhang Jian, the *jinshi* degree holder and primary architect of Nantong's modernization projects, along with his brother Zhang Cha, funded a hospital and medical school from their own private savings beginning in 1912.[99] They built a new hospital in 1914 containing three medical departments: internal medicine (*neike*), surgery (*waike*), and obstetrics and gynaecology (*fuchanke*).[100] The hospital buildings were spread over 16 *mu*[101] of land on the southeastern side of the medical school, with the obstetrical ward and three female patient rooms next to the morgue and infectious diseases wing, in hindsight probably not the best location for childbirth. Other cities like Guangzhou and Shanghai had no shortage of philanthropic organizations that built and/or supported local hospitals and medical schools as discussed above.

Despite the efforts of individual city planners, there were few public health departments or government-run institutions to deal with issues like sanitation, inoculation, and disease prevention, and many public health programs existed only on paper.[102] An exception is Guangzhou's very progressive Bureau of Health, established in 1912, run by Western-trained Chinese physicians who established vaccination and sanitation campaigns and set up local dispensaries and public health stations.[103] More common are thwarted plans like the proposal for a National Board of Health that was written in 1921 but still not in place by 1926.[104] When such programs were implemented, lack of funding and manpower limited their effect. Furthermore, modern medicine was available primarily in treaty ports and a few inland cities and towns where medical missionaries had settled and built hospitals and dispensaries. Well into the twentieth century modern medicine reached very few people in China, and modern childbirth was even rarer.

The Nanjing decade (1927–1937) is marked by unprecedented growth in reproductive health policies, coupled with a lack of resources and poor planning. City administration movements continued in this period, as the Guomindang issued new laws on governing cities beginning in 1927 that were "designed to centralize control over urban resources" and "promote social change."[105] Shanghai's universities began to offer urban administration courses in the 1920s so that their graduates could create and further expand modern municipal domains.[106] At the national level, the previously proposed National Board of Health (renamed the National Health Administration) was finally founded under the newly formed Ministry of the Interior to suppress communicable diseases, license physicians and pharmacists, regulate drugs, and oversee hospitals.[107] In addition, the fledgling Ministry of Education administered school hygiene programs, the Ministry of Agriculture and Commerce oversaw industrial hygiene, and local and national governments began to regulate midwives as early as 1913.[108] The rise of a new middle class directly influenced the development of cities, as shopping streets and entertainment complexes were created by and for them.[109] In Republican China, maternal and child health were low on the list of national priorities in a country ravaged by disease caused by lack of sanitation and crowded living conditions. Nonetheless, the foundations of modern medicine and public health had been laid by medical missionaries and gentry reformers decades earlier, and this partnership would continue well into the twentieth century.

CONSUMING AND REPRODUCING

The growth of cities, an increasing capitalist economy, weak governmental oversight, and a rising middle class all led to a tremendous expansion of goods and services related to reproduction and childbirth. In urban areas throughout China, the paradigm of the modern woman and new ideas about family and relationships were influenced, according to Wen-hsin Yeh, by "global forces of commerce and finance [that] resulted not only in the commodification of culture but also in the rise of new social interests and occupational classes that radically redefined what it meant to be 'Chinese.'"[110] These interests included debates on family structure and the qualities of the New Woman (*xin nuxing*), criticisms of the focus on consumerism, and an emphasis on internal qualities like patriotism and independence, or devotion to one's husband and children.[111] Emerging occupations for women, like factory work, nursing, and midwifery, defined the modern woman and allowed her to combine devotion to reproduction and the nation, topics of the following chapter. For mothers, the rising consumerism of this era meant that the New Woman, regardless of her particular characteristics, had her choice of an array of medical technologies and resources for childbirth.

Consumerism has long been linked to nationalist pursuits, with sometimes horrific results like "the conscription of consumption" in Aldous Huxley's *Brave New World* ("ending is better than mending, ending is better than mending").[112] Speaking of Deng Xiaoping's economic reforms some fifty years later, Chinese artist and intellectual Zhang Xiaogang claimed that "nationalism and commercialism can be twin brothers."[113] Republican China was also a site of the culture of consumption often linked with nationalism, as the rising middle classes, especially in urban areas, purchased modern goods and services to improve reproductive and maternal health.[114] Aside from the desire for modernity, a propelling factor in utilizing modern childbirth was the commonality that everyone wants the best for his or her children and family. Modern childbirth in urban centers like Shanghai was considered by many to be safer and to produce better outcomes for mother and child, and therefore many in the new urban middle class strived for this experience.

Intellectual reformers during this time produced an astounding array of popular materials on public health, childbirth, child rearing, and nutrition. They called upon women to have healthy pregnancies and modern births in order to improve the health of China's citizens. Some wanted to remake the Chinese family into a smaller, nuclear unit devoid of the patriarchal hierarchy of traditional extended families.[115] This conjugal family, with its educated women, eugenically chosen marriage partners, and well-bred offspring, could save the nation from further decline. As the primary consumers in the new economic unit of the nuclear family, women were urged to utilize scientific methods of prenatal care and motherhood, with all of its sometimes strange and unexpected results. Susan Glosser has illustrated the marriage of the conjugal unit and national consumerism in her study of one entrepreneur's efforts to market cow's milk as a necessary (and modern) food for healthy children.[116] Glosser's entrepreneur, You Huaigao, was not alone in his vision of a new China of happy conjugal families with healthy children. Numerous advertisements for nutritional supplements, tonics, and medicines for women's and children's health appeared in newspapers and magazines throughout this period. In some, advertisements promoting fertility clinics appear alongside those for syphilis specialists, illustrating the connection between sexually transmitted diseases and infertility (see chapter 2).[117]

Private maternity hospitals provided luxury accouchement accommodations for the rich who paid hefty sums for deluxe care, while charity organizations ran free hospitals to aid the pregnant poor. The rich and emerging middle class desired modernity for themselves, and that meant having their babies in a modern and sterile setting instead of at home attended by what they considered unlearned and unclean traditional midwives. The people who established these hospitals were part of the emerging modernizing programs, a product of the commercialization of services in treaty ports like Shanghai and Guangzhou. Modern medical pursuits at this time were largely carried out by Western medical professionals and Chinese intellectuals, politicians, and entrepreneurs, often without the support of or regulation by any particular governing body, similar to the ways that medical missionaries had worked with individual gentry and officials during the late Qing. Western and Chinese philanthropists opened free or cheap maternity clinics and hospitals in order to aid their fellow countrywomen (and men), to give the younger generations a new start with modern medicine, and to create a healthy new citizenry. Students in these schools wanted to better their own lives by practicing a new and modern profession.

By 1934, 52 private midwifery training programs in China were registered with the government, and there were countless others that never registered or were operating illegally.[118] Some of the largest and most well-known of these programs were run by foreign medical organizations. Others were established by local Chinese who had, or professed to have had, medical training abroad or in one of the Western medical schools in China. Their owners claimed sometimes dubious educational backgrounds and credentials, and they took in paying students to train them in what they asserted to be modern midwifery techniques. Shanghai's International Settlement, for example, had several such institutions under the jurisdiction of the municipal Department of Public Health. The schools ran advertisements in local newspapers to recruit students:

> Chances for Girls. The hospital provides gratis training of Students. Tuition and boarding fees and security are all exempted. Moreover, monthly allowance of about more than $10.00 is given. Candidates must be above 18 years of age, physically strong, persevering and patient. Applicants may call on Mr. Chu of the Obstetrical Hospital or CRN Honan at Haining Road daily from 4 to 6 pm.[119]

Other hospitals charged fees for their students. Hu Hsi Commoners' Obstetrical Hospital (*Huxi pingmin chanke yiyuan*, formerly Hong-kew Hospital), also in Shanghai, charged its students $100 to $400 for tuition, room, and board.[120]

By this time, municipal and national regulations controlling hospitals and medical schools were in place in China, but there was a lack of enforcement. Both free and tuition-based schools like these were the target of complaints and lawsuits filed with the local municipal authorities. The proliferation of such schools and the array of lawsuits show that the new fields of modern reproductive health were sites of extended entrepreneurial activity. Falsified medical credentials and a dearth of responsible regulating bodies created a perfect environment for ambitious businessmen (and, consequently, lawyers). The Chief Health Inspector of Shanghai wrote in 1936: "These so-called hospitals know nothing about arrangement of a hospital or clinic. They are invariably dirty, have poor equipment, insanitary kitchens and latrines." However, he found that they "probably divert poor patients from ignorant native practitioners," which, in his mind, was a good thing.[121]

Students from the Zung Wei Obstetrical Hospital (*Renhui chanke yiyuan*) on Haining Road in Shanghai brought fraud charges against the hospital, claiming that its superintendent was not a real doctor and that his hospital ran an unauthorized obstetrical school. None of the four "doctors" at Zung Wei were registered to practice medicine, nor could they produce medical diplomas, although one claimed a medical degree from "Kiao Kung" hospital in Japan and another one from Nanyang Medical College. Upon investigation, three of the "doctors," it turned out, were actually midwives trained in small, unlicensed midwifery schools in and around Shanghai. Some of the eight "nurses" on staff at Zung Wei had had some obstetrical training, again at small, unlicensed midwifery schools in the Zhejiang region. In another case, in 1936 several students went on strike against Hu Hsi Commoners' Obstetrical Hospital and demanded refunds of their tuition fees.[122]

These hospitals not only trained students but attended patients as well, some of whom also filed grievances with the Shanghai Department of Public Health. An angry husband of a maternity patient from Hu Hsi lodged a formal complaint that his parturient wife got only two young, unlicensed assistants to aid in her birth.[123] There was no midwife or physician in attendance, and the man claimed that his wife nearly died. He also asserted that the hospital was neither licensed by the municipal health authority nor adequately equipped. His family's desire for a modern birth was thwarted by inexperience and poor equipment.

Nevertheless, patients were willing to pay money for the services provided at maternity hospitals like these. Their fees varied greatly, from the cheap or free crowded charity hospitals to astronomical fees for luxury accommodations for the rich. The Hu Hsi Commoners' Obstetrical Hospital "mostly caters to the poorer classes from Zhabei who can't afford to attend the larger institutions." [124] People in the poor Zhabei district in western Shanghai, according to Hu Hsi's founder P.C. Frank Chen, suffered from a lack of hygiene, and childbirth was normally attended by "ignorant aged midwives of the old type resulting in countless unnecessary deaths."[125] He used his own money to establish the hospital and employed obstetricians to use modern obstetrical methods. There were two doctors on staff, one male and one female, along with six female and two male nursing students. A similar institution, the Ning Shao Commoners' Obstetrical Hospital (*Ningshao pingmin chanke yiyuan*, also called Kai Mai Obstetrical Hospital), established in 1922 in the French Settlement, saw 60 to 90 patients per month, half of whom received free medical care. The others paid about $1 per day.[126]

These hospitals were sometimes organized around native place or workplace ties. Ning Shao catered mostly to immigrants who had come to Shanghai from the surrounding towns of Ningbo and Shaoxing.[127] While factory workers and other laborers in Shanghai maintained their native-place ties, so did maternity patients.[128] Approximately 30 percent of the patients at San Min Obstetrical Hospital (*Sanmin chanke yiyuan*) were members of the Shanghai Laborers Union. This small hospital was established in 1935 in the Wayside district of the Shanghai International Settlement and had 10 beds, three of which were free. The poor paid 20 coppers per visit, and regular patients paid 50 cents to $1 per day. The staff included six nurses, one student nurse, and four registered physicians.[129] The Zung Wei Obstetrical Hospital used a similar sliding scale, with rich patients effectively subsidizing the poorer ones. This was a common way for medical missionaries and private hospitals alike to provide services to a wide range of the population.[130] Zung Wei charged a $4 registration fee, required in advance, and another $5 at parturition.[131] For these fees, a woman doctor would visit the patient once a month for the first seven months, and once or twice weekly thereafter until delivery. The doctor's services included providing medicines, "correct[ing] abnormalities," and notifying the family of the anticipated delivery date. After delivery, the hospital "sent doctors daily for some time free of charge" to check on the new mother and her infant.[132] Upon parturition, inpatients of the special, or highest, class at Zung Wei paid $6 per day for a private room with one female attendant (an additional attendant was another $1 per day). First class inpatients paid a daily rate of $3, second class patients $2, third class $1, and fourth class 50 cents, plus $1 per day for an additional attendant. The free ward patients had to pay 20 cents per day for meals. All fees had to be paid 10 days in advance, and a fan, stove, and medicine cost extra.[133]

An even more luxurious institution was known as the Women's Hospital (literally "parturient hospital," *chanfu yiyuan*) on Great Western Road in Shanghai. It was supported entirely by patient revenue, private gifts, and free services by physicians. The hospital had 29 paying beds and nine free beds, and a free nursery with bassinets and incubators used for premature or ill infants.[134] The hospital staffed one qualified resident physician and variable attending physicians who worked there for free, along with 12 graduate nurses. In 1937–38, the hospital received 2,608 patients. The cost of this place was $6 per day for a non-private room, up to $28 per day for a private bath and telephone. According to the Chief Health Inspector's report dated May 3, 1938, "the buildings and fittings of this hospital are positively luxurious, and it was evidently built for the accouchement of wealthy Chinese ladies."[135] An 11-bed maternity hospital run by a German woman, the Shanghai Maternity Hospital (*Shanghai furu chanke yiyuan*), was built in a "foreign style" and funded by four wealthy Chinese philanthropists. The 15 rooms were "all well equipped and nicely decorated."[136] The Shanghai Municipal Health Department rejected these hospitals' applications for charity status, which the respective hospital owners had made on the grounds that they did provide a small number of free beds for poor patients, because most of their patients paid handsomely for their services.[137]

Expectant mothers of means eagerly patronized these maternity hospitals in cities across the country. The attendance at San Ming Obstetrical Hospital, for example, had reached 11,955 in 1937.[138] The 250–bed Shanghai West Gate Women and Children's hospital (*Shanghai ximen furu yiyuan*), a facility that was jointly run by several foreign missionary outfits, accommodated 19,069 births in 1937.[139] Mary Fulton saw over 90,000 patients at her hospital and surrounding dispensaries in Guangzhou in the years 1885 to 1899.[140] Modern childbirth was linked with scientific medicine and an emerging consumer society, and it was the foundation on which to build a New Woman and a strong nation.

CONCLUSION

Modern childbirth represents a shift away from traditional ideas about health and disease and toward scientific medicine. This shift grew more pronounced by the first decades of the twentieth century. Simultaneously, while trying to reconfigure the shape of the new nation, intellectuals lamented traditional Chinese cultural ideals like the extended patriarchal family and the confinement of women. New family, New Woman, new medicine, new childbirth were all part of the modernizing reform efforts surrounding the fall of the Qing dynasty. Only massive social reform, many argued (based on modern, scientific principles), would allow China to restore its status in the world and effectively compete with the Western nations that had defeated the country in the previous century. The relationship between science and modernity is often shaky: the popularity of modern machine-rolled cigarettes, for example, and the Shanghai obsession with tight-fitting dresses, high heels, permanent waves, and dancing to jazz may be modern but not necessarily progressive or scientific or even beneficial.[141] Other reformers called for fundamental changes in Chinese living and eating habits, such as eliminating the family bed and promoting the use of individual eating utensils in place of traditional family-style dining in order to promote health and Western morality.[142] Likewise, cultural alterations like family reform, theories of racial determinism, and child rearing claimed sometimes questionable scientific backing.

Women are often defined by their reproductive capabilities, and during times of political and social turmoil these capabilities may be either called into question or strengthened.[143] In traditional China, a woman's worth was determined by her ability to produce a male heir. Her place in her family and in society was guaranteed by her relationships to men—her father, husband, and son. China's New Woman, who emerged in the early twentieth century as a separate category defined against her traditional counterpart, was burdened with additional definitions of womanhood.[144] During this period, women's importance as reproducers grew to encompass the new nation as well as the family. Major shifts in gender roles occurred with these political and social changes. The New Woman could work, select her husband, unbind her feet. However, her roles as mother and wife remained central to her definition as a woman, regardless of her modernity. The ideal New Woman was educated and may have worn makeup and cut her hair. She was liberated from the shackles of arranged marriages and bound feet. But she was still expected to marry and have children. The cultural processes of pregnancy and birth were changing, however. If her family members, especially her mother-in-law, were part of the new trend, she may have had the baby attended by a modern midwife or even in the hospital. After conceiving and utilizing the most modern methods of scientific prenatal care and childbirth, the new mother could choose to attend a "mothercraft" class to learn about the most up-to-date methods of child care. She could go to postnatal checkups. She could purchase hygienically modern products like cow's milk and nutritional supplements on which to nourish her infant.[145] These activities contrast with traditional conceptions of pregnancy that focus on women's physical weakness and emotionality, urging women to maintain a corporeal and psychological quietude to ensure a safe and healthy birth.[146] Regardless of her other roles in the new society, the New Woman was still a mother.

Men's roles changed, too. New Culture writers urged men to marry educated women with natural feet whose strong and healthy bodies were more suitable for childbirth, rather than illiterate, emotionally and physically weak and hobbled women.[147] Intellectual reformers exhorted both women and men to be active participants in their family lives, to break free of what they deemed the soul-sucking selflessness of the traditional patriarchal family.[148] Lu Xun, for example, called for modern fathers to emancipate their own children from the bonds of filial piety to create rational and independent individuals.[149] Men were redefined not as patriarch but as head of a conjugal family unit.[150] Advertisements in popular magazines like *Ladies' Journal (Funü zazhi)* featuring a happy *nuclear* family, as opposed to the traditional extended family, peddled fertility tonics and remedies for "female troubles." Men's fertility is assumed, and although science shows otherwise, women are at fault for failure to conceive. We will revisit these themes in the following chapter.[151]

Returning now to the story of Lady Li, the female physician who treated her, Dr. Leonora Howard, was typical of female medical missionaries who traveled to China to work. Treating and attending Chinese women was a goal of the missionaries from the start, but unlike Britain, where the man-midwife took over as the primary birth attendant in the 1800s, traditional ideas of gender propriety in China prevented male physicians from examining female patients like the viceroy's wife.[152] The story of Lady Li and Dr. Howard may be considered a success story. Lady Li was cured, Viceroy Li was awakened to the wonders of modern medicine, and Dr. Howard, by targeting the gentry, also gained the confidence of the "throngs of suppliants." [153] The women missioners linked spiritual salvation with corporeal salvation through modern medicine, especially cleanliness and hygiene, and believed that through women they could fundamentally improve the lives of all Chinese.[154]

Missioners worked together with local gentry and later businessmen to further their goals of a healthy, Christian China, though the focus on religion faded in the first decades of the twentieth century, replaced by science as savior. Local leaders throughout China aimed to modernize their cities nationwide, and businesspeople attempted to make a profit from the new market formed from scientific methods of childbirth. Hospitals and training programs for modern childbirth promised health and material wealth for their patients and practitioners. The Republican local and national governments began to regulate medicine and formed ministries to create and implement public health goals, while print culture spread these latest methods and ideas, instructing Chinese citizens on how to become modern in many areas of their lives.[155] The foundation for modern reproduction had been laid in the late nineteenth century, creating avenues for wider expressions of scientific childbirth throughout the twentieth century.

NOTES

1. Mary F. Bryson, *John Kenneth Mackenzie, Medical Missionary to China* (New York: Fleming H. Revell Company, 1891), 180.

2. K. Chimin Wong and Lien-Teh Wu, *History of Chinese Medicine: Being a Chronicle of Medical Happenings in China from Ancient Times to the Present Period* (Tientsin, China: The Tientsin Press, Ltd., 1932), 283.

3. Bryson, *John Kenneth Mackenzie, Medical Missionary to China*, 180.

4. Yong Ze, "English Doctor Ma Gen-Jia and Ma Doctor Hospital (*Yingyi Ma Genjia yu Tianjin Ma Daifu Yiyuan*)," *Jinwanbao: jinri tianjin huakan*, December 16, 2003.

5. "Dowager Empress Died of Apoplexy," *New York Times*, November 20, 1908.

6. David Wright, *Translating Science: The Transmission of Western Chemistry into Late Imperial China, 1840–1900* (Leiden: Brill, 2000), 90–93.

7. Bryson, *John Kenneth Mackenzie, Medical Missionary to China*, 180–81.

8. G.H. Choa, *"Heal the Sick" Was Their Motto: The Protestant Medical Missionaries in China* (Hong Kong: The Chinese University Press, 1990), 93.

9. Ibid.

10. Wong and Wu, *History of Chinese Medicine: Being a Chronicle of Medical Happenings in China from Ancient Times to the Present Period*, 283; Bryson, *John Kenneth Mackenzie, Medical Missionary to China*, 184–85.

11. Mary H. Stinson, MD, *Work of Women Physicians in Asia* (Norristown, NJ: J.H. Brandt, 1884), 20.

12. Donald MacGillivray, *A Century of Protestant Missions in China* (Shanghai: American Presbyterian Mission Press, 1907), 465.

13. Paul Cohen relates many of the rumors surrounding missionaries in Paul A. Cohen, *History in Three Keys: The Boxers as Event, Experience, and Myth* (New York: Columbia University Press, 1997), 162–67.

14. Angela Ki-che Leung, "Organized Medicine in Ming-Qing China: State and Private Medical Institutions in the Lower Yangzi Region," *Late Imperial China* 8, no. 1 (1987): 134–66.

15. Ibid.

16. Yi-Li Wu, "The Bamboo Grove Monastery and Popular Gynecology in Qing China," *Late Imperial China* 21, no. 1 (June 2000): 41–76.

17. See William Warder Cadbury and Mary Hoxie Jones, *At the Point of a Lancet: One Hundred Years of the Canton Hospital, 1835–1935* (Shanghai: Kelly and Walsh, Limited, 1935); Joseph Esherick and Mary B. Rankin, eds., *Chinese Local Elites and Patterns of Dominance* (Berkeley: University of California Press, 1990); Leung, "Organized Medicine in Ming-Qing China: State and Private Medical Institutions in the Lower Yangzi Region"; Michael Tsin, *Nation, Governance, and Modernity in China: Canton 1900–1927* (Stanford: Stanford University Press, 1999).

18. Leung, "Organized Medicine in Ming-Qing China: State and Private Medical Institutions in the Lower Yangzi Region," 148.

19. Barend J. ter Haar, *Telling Stories: Witchcraft and Scapegoating in Chinese History* (Leiden: Brill, 2006), 154–55.

20. Andrew Cunningham and Bridie Andrews, eds., *Western Medicine as Contested Knowledge* (Manchester and New York: Manchester University Press, 1997).

21. Francesca French, *Thomas Cochrane: Pioneer and Missionary States-man* (London: Hoder and Stoughton, 1956); as quoted in Bowers, *Western Medicine in a Chinese Palace: Peking Union Medical College, 1917–1951*, 8.

22. Bowers, *Western Medicine in a Chinese Palace: Peking Union Medical College, 1917–1951*, 8–9.

23. Kingston DeGruche, *Dr. D. Duncan Main of Hangchow (who is known in China as Dr. Apricot of Heaven Below)* (London: Marshall, Morgan & Scott, Ltd., 1930), 74.

24. Ibid., 73.

25. Ibid., 74.

26. MacGillivray, *A Century of Protestant Missions in China*, 419.

27. Ibid.

28. Connie Shemo, ""How better could she serve her country?" Cultural Translators, U.S. Women's History, and Kang Cheng's "An Amazon in Cathay"," *Journal of Women's History* 21, no. 4 (2009): 113.

29. Connie Shemo, ""An Army of Women": The Medical Ministries of Kang Cheng and Shi Meiyu, 1873–1937" (PhD dissertation, SUNY Binghamton, 2002), 120.

30. Ibid.

31. Ibid., 244. According to MacGillivray, the dispensary cost $1,600, and the land was valued at $6,000. MacGillivray, *A Century of Protestant Missions in China*, 466.

32. Reuben Holden, *Yale in China: The Mainland 1901–1951* (New Haven: The Yale in China Association, Inc., 1964), 124.

33. K.Y. Wang, *A Report of Hsiang-Ya Medical College & Hospital*, archival material, January 1930, series 601A, RG 1, RAC.

34. Cadbury and Jones, *At the Point of a Lancet: One Hundred Years of the Canton Hospital, 1835–1935*, 184; Robert Esper and David Bovaird, *The Problem of Medical Education in Canton*, July 1915; Wong and Wu, *History of Chinese Medicine: Being a Chronicle of Medical Happenings in China from Ancient Times to the Present Period*.

35. China Medical Commission of the Rockefeller Foundation, *Medicine in China*, 26–27.

36. Choa, *"Heal the Sick" Was Their Motto: The Protestant Medical Missionaries in China*, 166.

37. Cadbury and Jones, *At the Point of a Lancet: One Hundred Years of the Canton Hospital, 1835–1935*, 185.

38. Tsin, *Nation, Governance, and Modernity in China: Canton 1900–1927*.

39. Lu Yu, "The Fangbian Hospital of Canton (Guangzhou de fangbian yiyuan)," *Guangdong wenshi ziliao* 8 (1963): 139–50; Tsin, *Nation, Governance, and Modernity in China: Canton 1900–1927*, 27–29, 33.

40. Mary Fulton, "Hackett Medical College for Women, Canton," *Chinese Medical Journal* 23, no. 5 (1909): 324–29.

41. Ibid.

42. Esherick, "Modernity and Nation in the Chinese City," 1–16.

43. David Arnold, *Colonizing the Body: State Medicine and Epidemic Disease in 19th-Century India* (Berkeley: University of California Press, 1993); Kerrie L. MacPherson, *A Wilderness of Marshes: The Origins of Public Health in Shanghai, 1843–1943* (Hong Kong and New York: Oxford University Press, 1987); Rogaski, *Hygienic Modernity.*

44. Rogaski, *Hygienic Modernity.*

45. Cameron Campbell, "Public Health Efforts in China Before and After 1949 and their Effects on Mortality," *Social Science History* 21, no. 2 (Summer 1997): 179–218; Nancy Tomes, "The Private Side of Public Health: Sanitary Science, Domestic Hygiene, and the Germ Theory, 1870–1900," in *Sickness & Health in America: Readings in the History of Medicine and Public Health,* ed. Judith Walzer Leavitt and Ronald L. Numbers (Madison: University of Wisconsin Press, 1997), 506–528.

46. Tomes, "The Private Side of Public Health: Sanitary Science, Domestic Hygiene, and the Germ Theory, 1870–1900," 510; Carol Benedict, *Bubonic Plague in Nineteenth-Century China* (Stanford: Stanford University Press, 1996), 141.

47. Nancy Tomes, *The Gospel of Germs: Men, Women, and the Microbe in American Life* (Cambridge, MA: Harvard University Press, 1999).

48. More, *Restoring the Balance,* 105–7.

49. MacGillivray, *A Century of Protestant Missions,* 470–71.

50. Hunter, *The Gospel of Gentility: American Women Missionaries in Turn-of-the-Century China,* especially chapter 6, "Imperial Evangelism."

51. Wong and Wu, *History of Chinese Medicine: Being a Chronicle of Medical Happenings in China from Ancient Times to the Present Period,* 292.

52. Sara Waitstill Tucker, "The Canton Hospital and Medicine in Nineteenth Century China 1835–1900" (dissertation, Indiana University, 1983), 360.

53. Ibid., 364.

54. Fulton, "Hackett Medical College for Women, Canton," 326.

55. Tucker, "The Canton Hospital and Medicine in Nineteenth Century China 1835–1900."

56. Esper and Bovaird, *The Problem of Medical Education in Canton,* 2.

57. Dr. James Boyd Neal, "Training of Native Women in Midwifery," *The China Medical Missionary Journal* 15, no. 3 (1901): 221–22.

58. Ibid.

59. Cohen, *History in Three Keys: The Boxers as Event, Experience, and Myth;* Joseph Esherick, *The Origins of the Boxer Uprising* (Berkeley: University of California Press, 1987).

60. Spence, *The Search for Modern China,* 225–30.

61. Yi-Li Wu, "Introducing the Uterus to China: Benjamin Hobson's New Treatises on Women's and Children's Diseases (Fuxing xinshuo), 1858" (presented at the Association for Asian Studies Annual Conference, Chicago, IL, March 22, 2001).

62. Ibid.

63. More, *Restoring the Balance: Women Physicians and the Profession of Medicine, 1850–1995*, 154.

64. Leavitt, *Brought to Bed: Childbearing in America, 1750 to 1950*, 56, 152.

65. Jos. C. Thomson, "Native Practice and Practitioners," *The China Medical Missionary Journal* 4, no. 3 (1890): 187–88.

66. Thomson, "Native Practice and Practitioners"; Dr. Browning, "Notes of Cases," *The China Medical Missionary Journal* 6, no. 2 (1892): 82–85.

67. Mary W. Niles, "Native Midwifery in Canton," *The China Medical Missionary Journal* 4 (1890): 51–55; Neal, "Training of Native Women in Midwifery"; Marion Yang, "Control of Practising Midwives in China," *Chinese Medical Journal* 44, no. 5 (1930): 428–31.

68. Mary Stone (Shi Meiyu), "Obstetrical Outfit in China," *The China Medical Journal* 26, no. 6 (November 1912): 347–50.

69. James Menzies, "Some Interesting Obstetric Cases," *The China Medical Missionary Journal* 20, no. 1 (1906): 1–5.

70. Ibid., 3.

71. Agnes Stewart, "Gynaecological Practice in China," *The China Medical Journal* 22, no. 3 (May 1908): 145–50.

72. Mabel Poulter, "Obstetrical Experiences in a Chinese City," *The China Medical Journal* 30, no. 2 (1916): 75.

73. James Grieg, "A Case of Decapitation," *The China Medical Missionary Journal* 7, no. 1 (March 1893): 230–32.

74. Shemo, "'An Army of Women': The Medical Ministries of Kang Cheng and Shi Meiyu, 1873–1937"; MacGillivray, *A Century of Protestant Missions in China*.

75. Fulton, "Hackett Medical College for Women, Canton."

76. Tsin, *Nation, Governance, and Modernity in China: Canton 1900–1927*, 57.

77. Kristin Stapleton, *Civilizing Chengdu: Chinese Urban Reform, 1895–1937* (Cambridge, MA: Harvard University Press, 2000), 64.

78. Ibid., 2.

79. Stapleton, *Civilizing Chengdu: Chinese Urban Reform, 1895–1937*; Yang Nianqun, "The Establishment of Modern Health Demonstration Zones and the Regulation of Life and Death in Early Republican Beijing," trans. Larissa Heinrich, *East Asian Science, Technology, and Medicine*, no. 22 (2004): 69–95; Madeline Yue Dong, *Republican Beijing: The City and Its Histories* (Berkeley: Univeristy of California Press, 2003); Qin Shao, *Culturing Modernity: The Nantong Model, 1890–1930* (Stanford: Stanford University Press, 2004).

80. David Strand, *Rickshaw Beijing: City People and Politics in the 1920s* (Berkeley: University of California Press, 1989), 66.

81. Ibid., 67.

82. Ibid.

83. Que Lianyu, "The Creation and Historical Significance of the Sanitary Police in the Late Qing Dynasty (*Qingmo weisheng jingcha de chuangli ji lishi zuoyong*)," *Zhonghua yishi zazhi* (*Chinese Journal of Medical History*) 18 (1988): 97–98.

84. Rogaski, *Hygienic Modernity*.

85. Yuki Terazawa, "Gender, Knowledge, and Power: Reproductive Medicine in Japan, 1690–1930" (PhD dissertation, Los Angeles, CA: UCLA, 2001), 220–21.

86. Hidemi Kanazu, "The Criminalization of Abortion in Meiji Japan," trans. Marjan Boogert, *U.S.-Japan Women's Journal* 24 (2003): 36.

87. Yuki Terazawa, "The State, Midwives, and Reproductive Surveillance in Late Nineteenth- and Early Twentieth-Century Japan," *U.S.-Japan Women's Journal* 24 (2003): 59–81.

88. Ibid., 23.

89. Hsien-Yu Chin, "Colonial Medical Police and Postcolonial Medical Surveillance Systems in Taiwan, 1895–1950s," *Osiris* 13 (1999): 326–38; Hong Youxi and Chen Lixin, *Birth Grannies, Midwives, Obstetrician/gynecologists* (*Xianshengma, chanpo yu fuchanke yishi*) (Taibei shi: Qianwei, 2002), chapter 4, Education of Physicians (*Yisheng de jiaoyu*).

90. Frederic Wakeman, *Policing Shanghai 1927–1937* (Berkeley, Los Angeles, London: University of California Press, 1995), 346 n48.

91. Yamin Xu, "Wicked Citizens and the Social Origins of China's Modern Authoritarian States: Civil Strife and Political Control in Republican Beijing, 1928–1937" (PhD dissertation, Berkeley, 2002), 347–48.

92. Stapleton, *Civilizing Chengdu: Chinese Urban Reform, 1895–1937*, 137.

93. Xu, "Wicked Citizens and the Social Origins of China's Modern Authoritarian States: Civil Strife and Political Control in Republican Beijing, 1928–1937."

94. Ibid.

95. Dong, *Republican Beijing: The City and its Histories*; Xu, "Wicked Citizens and the Social Origins of China's Modern Authoritarian States: Civil Strife and Political Control in Republican Beijing, 1928–1937."

96. Stapleton, *Civilizing Chengdu: Chinese Urban Reform, 1895–1937*, 63.

97. Tsin, *Nation, Governance, and Modernity in China: Canton 1900–1927*; Cheng, "Going Public Through Education: Female Reformers and Girls' Schools in Late Qing Beijing," 109.

98. Tsin, *Nation, Governance, and Modernity in China: Canton 1900–1927*, 31.

99. Shao, *Culturing Modernity: The Nantong Model, 1890–1930*, 110.

100. Ibid., 59.

101. 15 mu equals 1 hectare; 6 mu equals one acre.

102. MacPherson, *A Wilderness of Marshes: The Origins of Public Health in Shanghai, 1843–1943*; Rogaski, *Hygienic Modernity*.

103. Yip, *Health and National Reconstruction in Nationalist China: The Development of Modern Health Services, 1928–1937*, 16.

104. Ibid., 15.

105. Stapleton, *Civilizing Chengdu: Chinese Urban Reform, 1895–1937*, 258.

106. Ibid., 259.

107. Yip, *Health and National Reconstruction in Nationalist China: The Development of Modern Health Services, 1928–1937*, 15.

108. Guangdong Provincial Government Police Department, *Police Department announcement*, vol. 23.

109. Sherman Cochran, ed., *Inventing Nanjing Road: Commercial Culture in Shanghai, 1900–1945* (Ithaca, NY: Cornell University Press, 2000), 57–65; Tsin, *Nation, Governance, and Modernity in China: Canton 1900–1927*, 57–65.

110. Yeh, "Shanghai Modernity: Commerce and Culture in a Republican City," 385; Louise Edwards, "Policing the Modern Woman in Republican China," *Modern China* 26, no. 2 (April 2000): 115–47.

111. Edwards, "Policing the Modern Woman in Republican China."

112. Aldous Huxley, *Brave New World* (New York: Harper Perennial Modern Classics, 2006), 33.

113. Jing Jun, ed., *Feeding China's Little Emperors: Food, Children, and Social Change* (Stanford: Stanford University Press, 2000), 17.

114. Karl Gerth, *China Made: Consumer Culture and the Creation of the Nation* (Cambridge, MA: Harvard University Asia Center, 2004).

115. Glosser, *Chinese Visions of Family and State, 1915–1953.*

116. Ibid.

117. "Liu Hanzhen, Female Physician (*Liu Hanzhen, nu yishi*)," *Guo huabao*, July 27, 1936.

118. Yip, *Health and National Reconstruction in Nationalist China: The Development of Modern Health Services, 1928–1937*, 166.

119. *Complaint re: Hu Hsi Obstetrical Hospital, 112 Markham Road, Shanghai International Settlement*, Police Report, March 20, 1936.

120. Ibid.

121. Ibid.

122. Public Health Department, "Zung Wei Obstetrical Hospital (*Renhui chanke yiyuan*)" (Shanghai Municipal Archives, 1935), 1–16–1–772, Shanghai Municipal Archives.

123. *Complaint re: Hu Hsi Obstetrical Hospital, 112 Markham Road, Shanghai International Settlement.*

124. Ibid.

125. Ibid.

126. Public Health Department, "Kai Mai Commoners' Obstetrical Hospital (*Ning Shao pingmin chanke yiyuan*)" (Shanghai Municipal Archives, 1933), 1–16–1–770, Shanghai Municipal Archives.

127. Ibid.

128. Emily Honig, *Sisters and Strangers: Women in the Shanghai Cotton Mills, 1919–1949* (Stanford: Stanford University Press, 1986).

129. Public Health Department, "San Ming Obstetrical Hospital (*Sanmin chanke yiyuan*)" (Shanghai Municipal Archives, 1935), 1–16–1–771, Shanghai Municipal Archives.

130. Shemo, "'An Army of Women': The Medical Ministries of Kang Cheng and Shi Meiyu, 1873–1937"; MacGillivray, *A Century of Protestant Missions in China.*

131. Dr. Hou-ki Hu, "Letter from Dr. Hou-ki Hu to County Hospital, Shanghai," n.d., 1–16–1–772, Shanghai Municipal Archives.

132. Ibid.

133. Ibid.

134. Public Health Department, "Women's Hospital (*Chanfu yiyuan*)" (Shanghai Municipal Archives, 1935), 1–16–1–773, Shanghai Municipal Archives.

135. Ibid.

136. Public Health Department, "Shanghai Hospital for Women and Children (*Shanghai furu chanke yiyuan*)" (Shanghai Municipal Archives, 1935), 1–16–1–856, Shanghai Municipal Archives.

137. Public Health Department, "Shanghai Hospital for Women and Children (*Shanghai furu chanke yiyuan*)"; Public Health Department, "Women's Hospital (*Chanfu yiyuan*)."

138. Public Health Department, "San Ming Obstetrical Hospital (*Sanmin chanke yiyuan*)."

139. Public Health Department, "Shanghai West Gate Hospital for Women and Children (*Shanghai ximen furu yiyuan*)" (Shanghai Municipal Archives, 1937), 1–16–1–866, Shanghai Municipal Archives.

140. Cadbury and Jones, *At the Point of a Lancet: One Hundred Years of the Canton Hospital, 1835–1935*, Appendix A, 276–79.

141. Tani Barlow, "Wanting Some: Commodity Desire and the Eugenic Modern Girl," in *Women in China: The Republican Period in Historical Perspective* (Germany: LIT Verlag Munster, 2005), 312–50; Edwards, "Policing the Modern Woman in Republican China."

142. Lei, "Habituate Individuality: Framing of Tuberculosis and Its Material Solutions in Republican China."

143. Philip C.C. Huang, "Women's Choices under the Law: Marriage, Divorce, and Illicit Sex in the Qing and the Republic," *Modern China* 27, no. 1 (January 2001): 3–58; Susan Mann, "The Cult of Domesticity in Republican Shanghai's Middle Class," *Historical Research on Modern Chinese Women* (*Jindai zhongguo funü shi yanjiu*) 2 (1994): 179–201.

144. Edwards, "Policing the Modern Woman in Republican China."

145. Rogaski, *Hygienic Modernity*.

146. Yi-Li Wu, "Ghost Fetuses, False Pregnancies, and the Parameters of Medical Uncertainty in Classical Chinese Gynecology," *Nan NÜ* 4, no. 2 (2002): 170–206; Charlotte Furth, "Concepts of Pregnancy, Childbirth, and Infancy in Ch'ing Dynasty China," *Journal of Asian Studies* 46, no. 1 (February 1987): 7–35.

147. Sally Borthwick, "Changing Concepts of the Role of Women from the Late Qing to the May Fourth Period," in *Ideal and Reality: Social and Political Change in Modern China, 1860–1949*, ed. David Pong and Edmund S.K. Fung (Lanham, New York, London: University Press of America, 1985), 63–91.

148. Schwarcz, *The Chinese Enlightenment: Intellectuals and the Legacy of the May Fourth Movement of 1919*, 111.

149. Lu Xun, "What is Required to be a Father Today (*Women xianzai zenyang zuo fuqin*)," *Xin Qingnian* 6, no. 6 (1919): 558–59.

150. Glosser, *Chinese Visions of Family and State, 1915–1953*, 12.

151. Lisa Handwerker, "The Hen That Can't Lay an Egg (*Bu Xia Dan de Mu Ji*): Conceptions of Infertility in Modern China," in *Deviant Bodies: Critical*

Perspectives on Difference in Science and Popular Culture, ed. Jennifer Terry and Jacqueline Urla (Bloomington: Indiana University Press, 1995), 358–86.

152. Lisa Forman Cody, *Birthing the Nation: Sex, Science, and the Conception of Eighteenth-Century Britons* (Oxford: Oxford University Press, 2005), 11.

153. Bryson, *John Kenneth Mackenzie, Medical Missionary to China*, 180–81.

154. Shemo, ""An Army of Women": The Medical Ministries of Kang Cheng and Shi Meiyu, 1873–1937."

155. Lee, "The Cultural Construction of Modernity in Urban Shanghai: Some Preliminary Explorations."

2

Reproduction Theory: Modern Childbirth and Modern Motherhood

Because childbirth is a public act in which a mother, as heaven's surrogate, gives birth to a human being, the surroundings naturally have to be prepared in full by society.[1]

Social and economic forces in Shanghai and other urban areas in Republican China converged to allow a broad discourse on how women would fit into the larger framework of a new China. Industrialization, separation of work and home, and a growing urban bourgeoisie fed the rhetoric of a 'cult of domesticity' that infused the writings in new magazines and print materials.[2] The burgeoning popular press included conversations about the importance of maternal and child health that appeared in women's and family magazines and public health publications as part of a larger emphasis on urban sanitation and hygiene.[3] These discussions drew upon varied Western sources like the republican motherhood campaigns in colonial America that had exhorted women to raise diligent sons for the new nation, as well as Japanese 'good wife and wise mother' (*liangqi xianmu*) vocabulary.[4] Especially during the Nanjing decade under the Guomindang, this literature was imbued with fascist German and Italian pro-motherhood arguments that called for women's reproduction for nationalistic purposes.[5] It is important to note that there was no unified call for national motherhood, as some eschewed reproductive duties in favor of joining a productive female workforce, and indeed many women who entered the modern medical profession remained single or stopped working once they married, as chapter 3 addresses. Nonetheless, the appeal of contemporary eugenics and scientific themes idealized modern reproduction for mothers of a new post-dynastic China, while visual and descriptive images of motherhood permeated New Culture literature and popular magazines.[6]

Although print media as public propaganda dates back to at least the Han dynasty (202 BCE–220 CE) in China, a new type of popular press emerged in the early twentieth century and proliferated in treaty ports by the 1930s and 1940s.[7] Shanghai was the nexus of these publications that had a national distribution and readership, and home to new entrepreneurial publishers who aimed to make a profit, expand circulation, and further their readership.[8] The Commercial Press (shangwu yinshuguan), for example, was headquartered in Shanghai and published journals and textbooks for the purpose of enlightening its reading public on how to become a modern nation.[9] Many of its professional and lay titles concerned modern reproduction, including the textbooks Shengchan yu yuying (Childbirth and Nursing), Taichan xuzhi (Essentials of Obstetrics), and Taijiao (Fetal Education).[10] Their popular journals like Dongfang zazhi (Eastern Miscellany) and Liangyou huabao (Young Companion) were riddled with advertisements and articles highlighting the health and well-being of families and children, as "an entire imaginary of urban modernity was constructed in [their] pages."[11]

Issues of science and modernization were at the forefront of political and social conversations about China's future, and much of the discussion was carried out in print. According to Leo Ou-fan Lee, "the public imagination of the nation depended on print . . . these commercial ventures in publishing were all in the name of introducing the textual sources of modernity."[12] The new print media imbued reproduction—pre- and postnatal care, childbirth, and the postpartum period—with new ideas of modernization, which in turn were meant to modernize China at large. Modernization discourse in the Chinese popular press called upon women to utilize scientific prenatal care, eugenics, and taijiao (literally "fetal education," but also translated as prenatal care), in order to have healthy babies. Images of reproduction exposed the visual realities occurring inside women's pregnant bodies. Midwifery schools and maternity hospitals distributed pamphlets and other advertising material to promote their institutions' modern reproduction services and child-rearing classes. These essays, pamphlets, handbooks, and advertisements for scientific reproduction shed light on changing ideologies about maternal and child health and women's roles as social reproducers as endorsed by the Chinese government and intellectual modernizers. The selections utilized in this chapter are not meant to be comprehensive of all the modernizing literature on public health and reproduction in print at this time, yet the advertisements and images here are typical and indicative of a growing awareness of and importance attached to the reproductive process.[13]

This literature that sprung from many different sources was perhaps more widespread than if it had come from a single unified establishment. Newspapers and journals exploded in number around the turn of the twentieth century. By 1898 there were 60 periodicals published in China; in 1912, that number had grown to 487.[14] Information about science, modernity, and nation building—including treatises on modern prenatal care and child-rearing methods—was readily available, especially in the cities. Of 345 magazines published by the Shanghai Magazines Company (*Shanghai zazhi gongsi*) in 1935, 27 had titles related to "Medicine and Hygiene," while in 1936 the Life Publications Company (*Shenghuo shudian*) had 24 titles on "Medicine and Hygiene" (13) and "Woman and the Home" (11) out of a total of 255.[15] K. Huang has found that between 1912 and 1926, approximately one-third of advertisements in the newspaper *Shenbao* (*Shanghai News*) dealt with medical topics.[16] The urban reading public devoured popular literature, newspapers, bulletins, and fiction, and then passed along worn copies for use in less developed areas.[17] Storytellers related the information to the illiterate.

Women formed a new audience for the contemporary print culture that emerged around the end of the Qing dynasty. Although gentry women had been reading for centuries, new print materials like newspapers and magazines targeted lower- and middle-class women, along with merchants and peasants.[18] They sometimes used a pictorial format and either vernacular or a simplified form of *wenyan*, classical Chinese, in order to make the literature more accessible to a broader, less educated audience. Some specifically catered to a female readership, often featuring images of reading women, thus helping to define and describe these new readers.[19] The very existence of magazines for women was "revolutionary," as previous literature for women such as the *Lienü zhuan* (*Biographies of Exemplary Women*) did not bring news from the outside world.[20] Popular print material for women in Republican China was based on Western newspapers and was thus new and modern.[21] In her extensive study of print culture in China, Barbara Mittler notes the parallels between the content of Western women's magazines and those for Chinese women, namely what she calls the "three C's of the traditional female role: cooking, cleaning, caring."[22] A reading public was modern, and so were women's issues.

That said, however, the number of women who read (or were read) articles and advertisements about childbirth and child rearing was a small but significant minority, though the rate was probably higher in urban areas. Late nineteenth-century female literacy is estimated at 1 to 10 percent, but that figure probably rose somewhat by the 1920s or 1930s with the increase in female education.[23] In addition, literacy rates for women varied greatly by region, and women's access to print materials on maternal and child health often depended upon their proximity to a city or a clinic or midwifery school that published and/ or distributed them. Most of these institutions were in or near urban areas, like the Chinese-run Nantao Christian Institute in Shanghai. Their weekly bulletin, published in Chinese and English and posted and distributed in their area, contained notices of Mothers' Club meetings, baby clinics, and child-rearing classes, as well as information on healthy modern living.[24] In literature such as this, women were called upon to help strengthen the race and build the nation, often as "mothers of citizens" (*guomin zhi mu*).[25] Reformers stressed the importance of education for women so they would in turn create and educate new citizens of China.

BIOLOGICAL DETERMINISM, EUGENICS, AND FETAL EDUCATION

Representations of health and disease in advertisements and articles reflect a society rapidly shifting and adjusting to external and internal pressures, in this case foreign influence and economic and political upheaval. Fear of disease was related to social decay resulting from the introduction of Western values and a perceived decline in Chinese morality. Visual and verbal imagery in these works define who is diseased and who is well. Prostitutes and their johns, for example, were characterized by their sickly state in advertisements for curing sexually transmitted diseases, while robust nuclear families embodied the ideal of physical and emotional health in articles and advertisements concerning childbirth, motherhood, and child rearing.[26]

Scientific models of evolution and eugenics disrupted the Chinese public's views of society, replacing Confucian philosophy with human biology, according to Frank Dikötter, "as the epistemological foundation for social order."[27] Evolutionary theories proposed infinite progress instead of the cyclical rise and fall of dynasties or the changing of the seasons. Widespread belief in the early twentieth century of the low physical and mental quality of the Chinese population led to explorations of eugenics policies. These policies were never widely enacted, though there is a considerable amount of popular literature on the subject. Chinese modernizers who believed there was an urgent need to improve China's racial makeup were most influenced by Herbert Spencer's theories of group evolution.[28] Many Chinese saw the Chinese race and nation as running the risk of further degeneration or even extinction unless extreme measures were taken to improve the racial makeup. As in Nazi Germany, eugenics ideas were combined in China with a call of duty to the nation-state.[29] Republican modernizers called upon women to fulfill their biological reproductive duties in order to strengthen the race and ultimately improve the nation. It was not only science that replaced Confucianism: another layer of responsibility to the nation—the nation-family duty—was added to women's reproductive obligations.

In this literature, women were redefined and restricted through reproduction and motherhood. Radical visionary Kang Youwei (1858–1927) imagined a healthy utopia of gender equality, with a considerable focus on motherhood, in his treatise *Datong shu* (Great Harmony), of which he dedicated a large part to relieving the burdens of women. Kang called for limited contract marriages agreed upon by both parties, as well as a "human roots institution" to care for expectant and parturient women and their infants.[30] Pregnant women would enter a motherhood institution and receive prenatal care and education. After the birth, they would remain with the child there until successful weaning at three to six months, at which time the mothers would be honored for their great deed. The children would be placed in a "child-rearing institution" until the age of six when they entered primary school, while the teachers were honored for assuming the care and educational responsibilities of these children. This vision was progressive, indeed, but not feasible for a country ravaged by war and unstable governments.[31]

In other literature, women's responsibility for *taijiao*, fetal education, became the means to a scientifically eugenic, superior end. It was incorporated with new concepts of telegony and biological determinism that maintained the necessity of strict morality and the natural inferiority of women. These ideas of *taijiao* and women's submissiveness may have had roots in China's past, but in the early years of the Republic they came to be imbued with modern science. Traditional ideas were infused with scientific rationale to re-legitimatize them, while the traditional definitions of these concepts were deemed superstitious as biomedicine gained credence as the normative paradigm and eliminated or restricted those less powerful, such as traditional lay healers and midwives.

The theory of *taijiao*, that the fetus was highly impressionable by outside forces, developed scientific legitimacy in early twentieth-century China. Traditional knowledge paradigms of pregnancy had advised pregnant women since the Zhou dynasty (1045–256 BCE) to avoid strong emotions and horrific sights for fear of causing the fetus to be born with epilepsy or another malady. The *Liji* (Collection of Treatises on the Rules of Propriety and Ceremonial Usages) written during this period elaborates on *taijiao* in the chapter *Neize* (The Pattern of the Family): "A pregnant woman when sleeping shall not sleep on her side, shall not sit askew, shall not slouch or stand askew, shall not eat unhealthy foods, nor eat food that is cut irregularly, nor sit in a crooked chair or at a crooked table."[32] The Han dynasty (202 BCE–9 CE) *Lienü Zhuan* (Biographies of Exemplary Women) explained the principles of *taijiao*: "A pregnant woman's eyes shall not see revolting colors, her ears shall not hear obscene sounds, her mouth shall not speak perverse words; this is *taijiao*."[33] Later exhortations to avoid frog and rabbit meat were to prevent a colicky baby or one born with a harelip, respectively.[34] Poetry and music, on the other hand, could engender peaceful and intelligent offspring.

By the Qing dynasty, as Yi-Li Wu explores in her study of reproduction in late imperial China, "pregnancy loss was always rooted in identifiable human error or negligence. The pregnant woman was thus simultaneously liable and powerful, held responsible for miscarriage yet ultimately endowed with full power to ensure the healthy development of her unborn child."[35] By following rules of *taijiao*, which were by no means universal or codified but instead varied regionally and over time, a woman would have a smart, handsome (and ideally male) child. If she bore a female child, or one with a disability, it was because she did not follow *taijiao* proscriptions; she had performed a bad deed, was being punished for errors from a previous incarnation, or had had licentious or evil thoughts. The pregnant mother was held ultimately responsible for the health of the fetus.

During the Republican era, a new and modern *taijiao* emerged distinct from the *taijiao* of the past. Modern *taijiao* maintained that the fetus was still impressionable, but the traditional Chinese beliefs were justified in medical and scientific terms. *Taijiao* developed from traditional beliefs—those very beliefs denounced by modernizers as superstitious—into a modern ideology based on scientific principles, in much the same way that the new *zhuchanshi* (modern midwives) displaced the old-style midwives. Chinese modernizers justified schooling women in methods of *taijiao* to improve the race-nation, using paternalistic and subordinating language that utilized women as "public wombs."[36]

In a 1923 article on women's physical culture, Xie Siyan proffered that women "bear a great responsibility for childbirth and must understand proper reproductive health" and that they must improve their "hygienic habits [in order to] ensure that their future children have a proper role model."[37] Similarly, along with her discussion on avoiding sex, spicy food, and hard work during pregnancy, Yun Qin discusses the importance of environment on the fetus. It is "very important for pregnant women to be careful to maintain an emotional balance, no matter the time or place, in order to give the fetus favorable emotional effects."[38] Yun goes on to explain the scientific basis for *taijiao*: "Sociological research has shown that when a person is happy his muscles become tensed, the heart beats rhythmically and excitedly, the blood circulates vigorously, and the appetite is stimulated."[39] Sadness or worry causes the opposite, adverse effects. Blood vessels shrink, muscles wither, and appetites wane, all factors contributing to unhealthy fetuses. According to Yun, the evidence is quite clear: the offspring of loving and harmonious couples who pay attention to *taijiao* are simply smarter than the children of couples who do not have loving relationships and who do not practice it.[40] A loving and harmonious family life will keep the woman's extreme emotions in check; she will maintain emotional balance throughout pregnancy and thus will engender the same in her offspring.

Not everyone claimed to subscribe to modern scientific notions of *taijiao*, however, although their criticisms ring similarly to the praises of *taijiao*'s advocates. Huang Shi, writing in the *Ladies' Journal* (*Funü zazhi*) in 1930, asserted that there is "absolutely no 'medical' base" to *taijiao*.[41] Furthermore, biologist Chen Jianshan dismissed *taijiao* as superstition in his 1930's writings on Mendelian theories of inheritance, and asserted that children inherit their mother's nature (characteristics) "as the grass and trees receive the effects of the soil."[42] According to Chen, therefore, although the sounds and sights an expectant woman is exposed to do not affect the fetus, it is still important for mothers to care for themselves with a good diet and regular moderate exercise. Genetics and heredity are of utmost importance too. With good genes from both father and mother, combined with a healthy lifestyle, mothers are able to bear vigorous and intelligent children. Choosing a suitable marriage partner was essential, not only because a nuclear family reduced traditional reliance on the patriarchal extended family, but also for selection of favorable eugenic traits. Men were encouraged to marry healthy women with natural feet and to create an independent and modern conjugal unit.

Biology was also the basis for social proscriptions. There was a widely held belief in telegony in China, brought from Europe and the United States, that a woman's previous sexual partners could affect her offspring with later partners.[43] The semen was believed to remain in the woman's bloodstream and reappear again during pregnancy. Therefore, in order to improve the race or prevent racial degeneration, women should most certainly be virgins upon marriage because, after all, one could never know the true characteristics of a woman's previous lovers, or whether a potential wife was being honest about her prior sexual experiences.

As Song dynasty texts focused on women's reproductive capabilities, so did Republican reformers. Biology additionally offered a scientific explanation for the general inferiority of women and supported her primary role as reproducer. A woman was defined biologically as a reproducer of national citizens. As many Western scholars have noted, the female body in scientific literature of the nineteenth and twentieth centuries is often presented as a deviant form of the male body.[44] In fact, men were at the top of the evolutionary scale, while women and "savages" fell below the male ideal. Women's skulls were smaller; thus, they had less brain capacity than men. Women's relatively diminutive bodies contained less life- and strength-giving blood, making them naturally weaker. This literature influenced Chinese scientific and popular writing in the Republican era. According to Gu Shi,

> The body of man has been shaped for movement, whereas that of woman is made for reproduction. Man is dominated by action, woman by patience. Man has a tendency to go to extremes: he can become a genius, a psychotic or a moron. Women are generally more constant and are not subject to extreme changes. These are due to the structural differences which exist between male and female.[45]

The message is the same in traditional and Republican *taijiao* texts: the mother is responsible for the well-being of the fetus and infant. Although other women in her family, especially her mother-in-law, may have had considerable input, if something went wrong with the pregnancy or birth, the blame almost certainly rested upon the mother herself. Even among detractors like Huang Shi and Chen Jianshan, mothers alone remained responsible for the health of their offspring.

COMMODITIES OF REPRODUCTION

Once women internalized their reproductive duties toward the family and the nation, they could select from a wide array of commodities related to reproduction, from medicines and tonics to regulate their hormonal cycle, to hospitals in which to give birth, to classes and books to teach the latest methods of child rearing. Modernity is a commodity to be produced and consumed; its presentation and consumption is in itself an aspect of modernity. According to Qin Shao, "Modernity is a fashion that requires validation—to be modern is to be seen, judged, consumed, and thus legitimized as modern by the public."[46] In Republican China, most notably in treaty-port cities like Guangzhou and Shanghai, advertisements tempted the public with images of the modern woman, some with bobbed hair, in furs and silks and high-heeled shoes, strolling along avenues lined with high-rise buildings.[47] Several scholars have begun to examine the ways that globalization and international trade intersect with the rapidly modernizing urban culture of Shanghai, for example Susan Glosser in her study of the modern small, milk-fed family.[48] The new *xiao jiating* (nuclear family) consumed milk, the Western product made local through the advertising genius of You Huaigao, a Cornell graduate, dairy farmer, and self-styled family reformer. In order to promote the consumption of his foreign product, You wrote and published a weekly pamphlet, *Jiating xingqi* (Family Weekly) that featured a prosperous and happy ideal family nourished by cow's milk. This magazine that illustrated the modernity of consuming dairy products addressed other modern issues like home economics and "scientific" child care within a nuclear family, an example of Shanghai's emerging "commodified popular culture." [49]

The culture of consumption is applicable both to modern obstetrics wards and obstetrical methods, as well as to the modern mothers and midwives with their fashionable hairdos and hygienic child-rearing methods. There were widespread visual advertisements for improving reproductive health in China in the 1920s and 1930s, though images featuring Western medical techniques like surgeries appeared even in the late 1800s. Many medicines, both foreign and Chinese, were aimed at regulating women's hormonal fluctuations and reproductive functions, like the ubiquitous Dr. Williams' Pink Pills for Pale People (marketed in 82 countries between 1890 and the 1930s), and medicines for infertility.[50] Many of these early advertisements were in fact addressed to husbands, as Barbara Mittler has noted.[51] For example, in an advertisement for a fertility medicine the husband addresses the reader: "After more than 10 years of trying, [my wife] has not become pregnant," but after treatment with Dr. Shen's medicine, she gave birth to a son.[52] In another case, this time a treatment for yeast infection, the advertisement states that women suffering from such an affliction are infertile and informs the husband "how to recognize certain symptoms of an incapacitating disease in his wife and what to do in case such symptoms appear."[53] After the turn of the twentieth century, Mittler found that such ads dealing with reproductive issues began to speak directly to women, illustrating the increasing numbers of reading women.[54]

Many of these ads, including those for Dr. Williams' Pink Pills for Pale People (see figure 2.1), and the similar product Hormotone, utilized Western medical technology or terminology. Both of these American patent medicines were used to treat "women's illnesses" (funü jibing).[55] Dr. Williams' Pink Pills drugs were meant to cure nervous headache and tremors, and Hormotone was used to regulate the menstrual cycle, specifically addressing problems of amenorrhea and dysmenorrhea. Other advertisements were for Japanese products, like Chujoto, "the best medicine for female complaints in the world," which pictured a happy family as well as English transliterations of Japanese words, as seen in figure 2.2.[56] In the Chujoto image, a man is shown holding a happy baby while the woman looks on. This Japanese herbal supplement, used to help restore women's hormonal balance and promote relaxation, is still sold today. Chinese versions of these foreign medicines also garnered advertising space in women's magazines. Advertisements for Dr. Wei's Red Pills, a native version of Dr. Williams' Pink Pills, for example, featured a seated woman in traditional Chinese dress holding a robust male infant in her lap. Figure 2.3 shows that Dr. Wei's pills were marketed to pregnant and postpartum women to improve their health after childbirth by replenishing the blood.[57] This medicine draws both on Western and traditional Chinese medical beliefs. It is an obvious play on the Western Dr. Williams' Pink Pills, yet the focus on the color red conjures the traditional medical theory that menstruating and postpartum women should replenish their lost blood by consuming red or dark-colored foods like red Chinese dates (jujubes) and liver.

These products, some of which were widely marketed in the United States and abroad, are not so different from the advertisements in women's magazines in the twenty-first century that peddle pharmaceuticals to combat depression, obesity, allergies, and headaches. Women's hysteria and moodiness could be brought under control with hormonal regulators to ensure health and happiness for all members of the nuclear family. In other words, a happy, sedate mother engenders a calm, intelligent child, and a loving husband directly involved with his family, perhaps even participating in the realm of child care. The family problem is fixable, as it must all be in the wife's head, and if properly remedied perchance the husband will not be inclined to visit his mistress or prostitute, thereby risking the health of other family members by returning with a nasty ailment resulting in infertility or

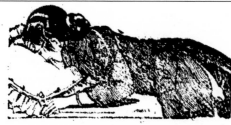
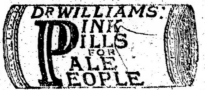

Figure 2.1. Advertisement for Dr. Williams' Pink Pills for Pale People. *Ladies' Journal* (*Funü zazhi*) 1.1 1915. Courtesy of the Library of Congress.

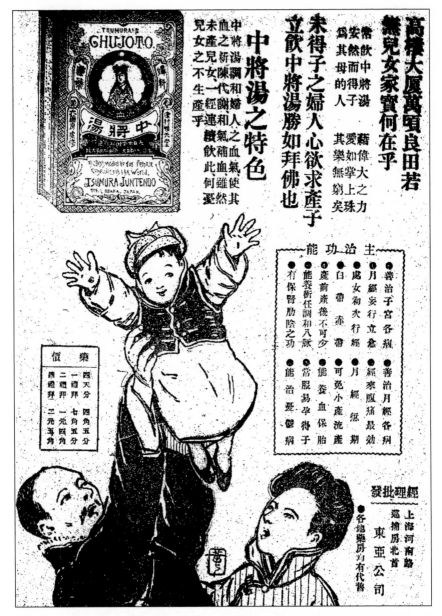

Figure 2.2. Advertisement for Japanese Pharmaceutical Chujoto. *Ladies' Journal (Funü zazhi)* 1.1 1915. Courtesy of the Library of Congress.

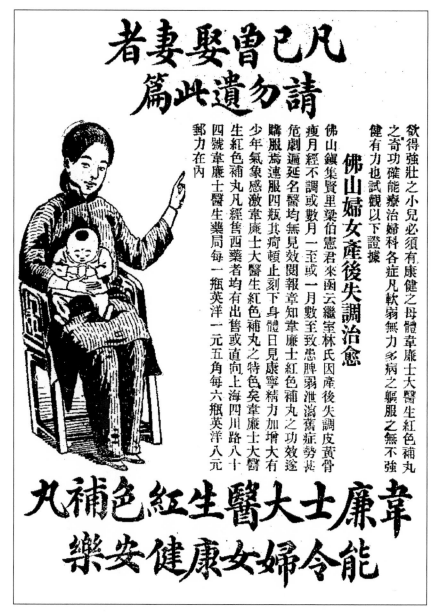

Figure 2.3. Advertisement for Dr. Wei's Red Pills to Improve Health after Childbirth. *Ladies' Journal (Funü zazhi)* 1.9.1915. Courtesy of the Library of Congress.

disease. These images must certainly be targeted towards the expanding readership of women.

The appeal of foreign medical products is clear in these advertisements, as Western medicine was deemed by many to be the most modern and scientific means to remedy common and complicated ailments.[58] According to Sze Szeming, General Secretary of the Chinese Medical Association in the 1940s, education through radio broadcasts, theatrical performances, publications, storytellers, and advertisements about the benefits of Western medicine would automatically decrease the popularity of native remedies: "As the health education of the masses is improved, the demand for native medicine will undoubtedly decrease," one of his goals for the modernization and regulation of medicine in China.[59]

VISUALIZING REPRODUCTION

Closely tied with the consumption of reproductive health is the visualization not only of healthy babies and the modern family, but also of physiology and technology. Chinese notions about reproductive health institutionalized in imperial China during the Song dynasty (960–1279 CE) shifted in the twentieth century with the advent of scientific medicine. Song-era reproductive health was based on an androgynous view of the body that corresponded to the cosmos and stressed the balance of yin and yang. In the field of *fuke*, literally "women's medicine," that meant a focus on Blood, the yin (predominantly female) aspect of one's vital force, or *qi*.[60] Much of *fuke* dealt with regulating the menses and ensuring fertility. Charlotte Furth and Francesca Bray have each found that during this period and afterwards, women alone were responsible for gestation and the reproduction of male heirs.[61] Song and later *fuke* texts focus on menstrual cycles and fertility, indicating women's important social roles as reproducers of the family. The rise of Neo-Confucianism during the Song period further reinforced women's social role as reproducers of the family and propagated cultural constructions of gender propriety.

Late imperial Chinese medical thought regarding reproduction emphasized a "cosmologically resonant" childbirth that made manual intervention unnecessary.[62] This ideology, according to Yi-Li Wu, included "two possible ways of envisioning gestation: cosmological frameworks that explained women's bodies in terms of a bodily economy of yin and yang forces, and a set of agricultural metaphors that portrayed the child as a ripening fruit whose development could be terminated or impeded at any moment by perturbations in the maternal environment."[63]

Knowledge of anatomy and bodily functions in scientific terms presented an entirely different worldview in the twentieth century. Anatomical depictions of the developing fetus in utero, x-rays of internal cancerous growths, and photographs of dissections of tumors removed from patients all present a visual knowledge that had not previously existed. Traditional Chinese medical practitioners had shied from surgery and dissection, and the new optic images of the twentieth century provided a concreteness of anatomy and physiology that were astoundingly different from earlier conceptions.[64]

Gender relations in traditional China were such that male physicians rarely touched or even saw their female patients and had to rely on a third person to relay information about the patient's illness. Childbirth was the domain of women and midwives, and Chinese physicians generally did not attend laboring women. However, if problems arose during the pregnancy or birth, the physician may provide specific pharmaceutical preparations that would restore the balance of yin and yang in the body. If these measures failed, then the fault lay with the patient and her insufficient *taijiao* or poor moral constitution.[65]

In contrast, modern medical constructions of female disease focused on the physical womb, complete with detailed imagery, and on childbirth as a disease or disruption to be physically managed and manipulated, the parturient as patient. The modern medicine used and taught by Westerners advocated manual intervention like monitoring cervical dilation and the use of forceps or caesarean sections for problematic births. This physically invasive approach is radically different from the traditional, intellectual methods of the traditional physicians. Nonetheless, in both modern and traditional childbirth, the knowledge is held by the male physicians, and the parturient and her attendants are only secondary. In traditional medicine, men were equated with cosmological birth on a philosophical and intellectual level; intervention and problems arising in childbirth took place in the women's quarters with the parturient and her attendants. In the Western birth model, the women are pushed out altogether, and it is up to the biomedically trained (male) physician to usher new life into the world. In both cases, women are unable to handle their own births without the knowledge of the men. Furthermore, the two approaches to childbirth bring up interesting questions about gender and masculinity. The intellectual model favored by the Chinese was disparaged by the Westerners who advocated the physical paradigm. Westerners considered Chinese men to be weak and effeminate in their intellectualism, while Western doctors manipulated and controlled childbirth, an outward sign of their physical masculinity. Chinese physicians, on the other hand, denigrated the physicality of midwives during birth and, ostensibly the actions of the brutish Westerners too.

The depictions of fetuses and the focus on autopsy and dissection in the Western birth model stress the visual, physical knowledge of modern medicine as contrasted with traditional Chinese medicine. Fetal growth charts, pregnancy handbooks, and articles on modern childbirth and child rearing proliferated in the 1920s and 1930s so that mothers could be modern and understand themselves and their pregnancies scientifically, thus joining the "scientific thought collective."[66] As early as the 1880s, illustrated periodicals like *Shenbao* and *Dianshizhai Huabao*, both founded by English entrepreneur Ernest Major, carried illustrations of modern medical marvels, for example a Western physician performing a caesarean section on a Chinese woman in a reclined birthing chair.[67] The accompanying text relates the story of a pregnant woman in arrested labor who was taken to Canton Hospital and safely delivered of a baby girl by a "miraculous" caesarean section performed by a Western male physician. Other images of surgeries from the *Dianshizhai Huabao* include a mastectomy, an ovariotomy, and the removal of a testicular cyst. Still others relate deliveries of "monstrous births" like conjoined twins and a "turtle baby." These images were consumed by middle-class urbanites interested in contemporary Western material culture and sensational stories.[68]

By the 1900s, one of the primary producers of such images was the *China Medical Journal* (formerly *China Medical Missionary Journal*), a joint Chinese-Western publication of the China Medical Society affiliated with Peking Union Medical College. The journal was established in 1887 by medical missionaries in Guangzhou and was initially run solely by Western medical personnel. In its early years it focused largely on social issues among medical missionaries: marriage, death, and birth notices; arrivals and departures of medical men and women; problems of doing medical work in (invariably backward, dirty, uncivilized, heathen) China. However, as it grew and became multicultural with Chinese contributors and editors, its focus shifted by the 1900s to become a scientific-minded publication, and "missionary" was removed from its name. As the *Chinese Medical Journal*, it published scientific articles on sanitation and public health, obstetrics and gynaecology, cancer, nutrition, and all other manner of health-related topics. The journal also came to include columns for hospital reports from various missionary institutions as well as a forum for the Nurses' Association of China.

During the tenure of editor Dr. S.K. Lim, also president of the Chinese Medical Association, the journal devoted entire issues to improving maternal and child health.[69] A related journal, *The National*

Medical Journal of China that in 1932 merged with the *Chinese Medical Journal*, devoted an entire issue to obstetrics and gynecology in December 1930. Images of gargantuan ovarian cysts, shaven vaginas with protruding pelvic fibromas, x-rays of pubic structures and peritoneal cysts accompany descriptions of new methods of surgery and anesthesia.[70] In the process, the journal helped to modernize these fields, imbuing them with scientific legitimacy. The *Chinese Medical Journal's* readers included obstetric, nursing, and midwifery students and faculty, and in many cases it is possible to trace the flow of information from the journal to the women on the street (see figure 2.4).

The image in figure 2.4 is a photograph, dated 1931, of a modern health worker from Peking Union Medical College's First National Midwifery School (*zhonghua di yi zhuchan xuexiao*) visiting a pregnant woman in her home. On a clipboard between the two women is a drawing of a developing fetus.[71] This image is similar to those found in the *Chinese Medical Journal*, and also to those in nursing and midwifery classrooms at the First National Midwifery School in Beijing. The mechanistic view of the female reproductive process is jarring when taken out of the classroom or the professional medical text. These images may even be considered frightening, perhaps even more

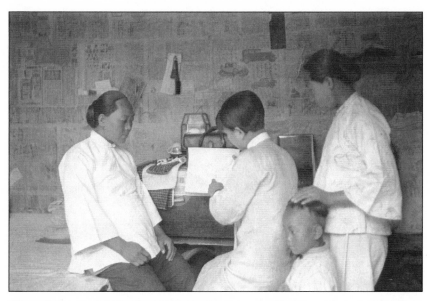

Figure 2.4.   Health Teacher Showing the Pregnant Mother a Picture of the Foetus in Utero. "MCH-PH Visiting Report," Health Station Annual Report, 1931, 100. Courtesy of the Rockefeller Archive Center.

so to the majority of Chinese women who had not been desensitized, as the Western public has today, through physiology and dissection classes in school and in the graphic depictions of bodies in entertainment mass media. By the Nationalist era, education for women was still not widespread, and for those women who did attend school, biology and physiology were not standard subjects of study. In fact, most students—male or female—would not have received education in these subjects unless they were of the small minority attending preparatory courses to enter medical school.[72]

In the photograph, the expectant mother is seeing what she is not meant to see—the inside of a body and an unborn fetus. This "skinning" of the woman, to use Barbara Duden's term, marks a shift in the ways that pregnancy and childbirth are regarded in the popular imagination. The "foundry-cast body" displayed in anatomical charts eliminates individual characteristics and processes, creating a standard incontrovertible body (and fetus) across race and class and time, deviations from which are deemed abnormal or aberrant.[73] When their bodies or their babies did not measure up, women could choose to take steps to bring them back in line with the new normative body. The photograph also represents the transformation of the parturient from an ordinary pregnant woman into a medical patient—a passive, objective, usually weakened body, disembodied from other concepts of self.[74] The modern midwifery student looks professional and scientific enough in her white coat and hat. She has the images and documents to back up her stories about fetal development, childbirth, and child care. On the other hand, the modern midwives were, for the most part, young, unmarried, and childless. Many women questioned what these midwives could possibly know about birth.

Most graphic images of fetal development, however, were reserved for midwifery, nursing, and obstetrics students and are absent from the pamphlets, journals, and handbooks geared to the layperson. Diagrams like those in figure 2.5 are found primarily in medical and paramedical school textbooks like *Essentials of Obstetrics* and *Childbirth and Nursing*.[75] *Essentials of Obstetrics* was a common small textbook for midwifery and nursing students, published by The Commercial Press, which went through several editions from the 1910s to the 1940s. The images here are arrayed in a controlled fashion—because all know that childbirth is anything but controllable—illustrating that science has won over the human body.[76] Science has taken over the baby-making machinery, and here is its proof: the images are captured for all to see, imbuing the modern medical professionals with enigmatic knowledge and power over birth and the human body.

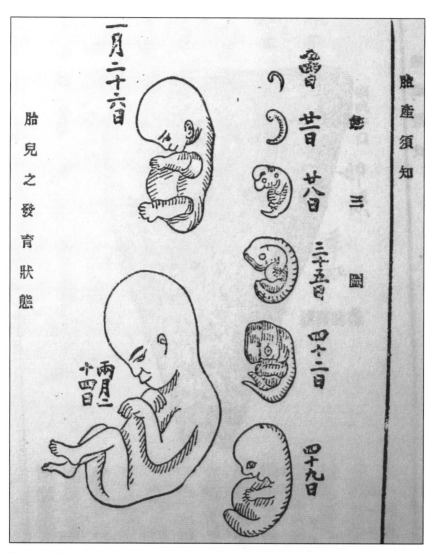

Figure 2.5. Fetal Development. Reproduced from Su Yaochang, *Taichan Xuzhi* (*Essentials of Obstetrics*), 6th ed., Medical Series. Shanghai: Commercial Press, Ltd., 1929, 8.

After learning about the inner workings of her body and the proper development of her fetus, the expectant mother, if she had the money and means, could decide to give birth in an accouchement hospital like those illustrated in chapter 1, or to be attended in her home by a modern midwife or physician. If she chose the medicalized route, either at home or hospital, she was likely subjected to a series of tests and measurements. Republican-era scientists and pseudo-scientists took measurements of every possible bodily characteristic that represented the physical and mental ideal of the strong, healthy, intelligent human. Male and female infants, children, and adults were not exempt from this scrutiny of cranium size, breast size, amount of body hair, pelvic dimensions, body odors, height, weight, length of menstrual cycle, and so on.[77] Babies in health clinics were weighed and measured, schoolchildren were subjected to extensive physical exams, and adults who patronized modern hospitals underwent sometimes embarrassing and uncomfortable tests, all in the name of nation building and modern scientific progress. The body and the birth are controlled by measuring, photographing, illustrating, describing, and drawing, as biological processes are modernized and recorded.[78]

For in addition to the written word, by the 1930s China also had a growing cadre of newly trained midwives to instruct and inform Chinese women about the science of reproduction and child rearing, while measuring and recording data for modern science. By the 1930s, the number of women enrolled in midwifery schools was very small. Most programs had fewer than 30 students in each class, and while the number of such schools was growing, modern midwifery still affected only a small minority of women. However, these women were a significant force in spreading ideas about modern childbirth, maternal and child health, and child rearing.

The midwifery schools advertised their very modern equipment and facilities through journals, annual reports, and yearbooks. For example, figure 2.6 is a collage of the Guangzhou Municipal Hospital's Maternity Department from its 1935 Annual Report. The collage features photographs (clockwise from top left) of a modern birthing room, department head Dr. Huang Gongkun, the obstetrics ward, a physical examination of a pregnant woman, and a newborn check-up. What young woman considering the medical profession or modern childbirth would not want to be associated with this prestigious facility and its modern equipment? Institutions like this adopted the most modern and scientific Western medical practices and equipment as they became available.

Similarly arrayed, the midwifery equipment in figure 2.7, from the First National Midwifery School in Beijing, is arranged neatly on the sterile, white cloth-covered table. The kit includes a razor for episiotomy or other small incisions, a pair of scissors for cutting the umbilical cord, artery clamps in case of heavy bleeding, hypodermic needle and medicine dropper to administer medication to the mother and baby, sterile pads to clean or to halt bleeding, a scale to weigh the

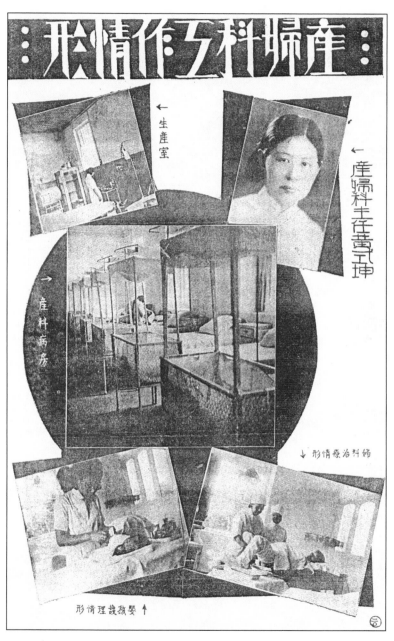

Figure 2.6. Guangzhou Municipal Hospital Maternity Department. Reproduced from the *Written Report of the Guangzhou Municipal Hospital*, 1935 (*Guangzhou shi shili yiyuan baogao shu*). Courtesy of the Guangzhou Provincial Archives.

infant and possibly the placenta, and silver nitrate eye drops to prevent infants' eye infections. As in the fetus illustrations, there is a flattening of the images—two-dimensional representations of three dimensions, laid out for all to see—for modern medicine to co-opt and control. There are no known extant photographs of the old-style midwife's equipment and its arrangement; from written descriptions she most likely carried with her some special medicines, herbs, and charms, perhaps some rope or cloths. Her tools were probably fashioned from whatever household utensils the family had: a pan of boiling water, a sharp knife. She certainly had no sterile table on which to work. The tools, if any, would have been placed on a table, the floor, or the *kang*, a multipurpose platform that served as a bed and seating area and was heated from below with fire from the cooking stove.

MODERN EQUIPMENT

Considered to be a patient in need of medical expertise, the Republican-era parturient had all manner of modern equipment at her disposal if she delivered at a hospital. The modern midwives generally carried the kit described above. However, in their classes they were taught to

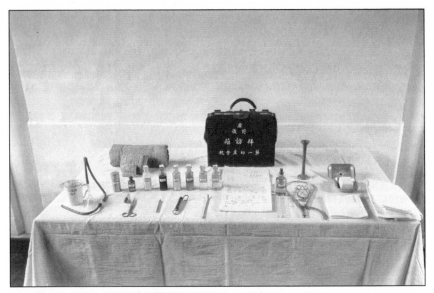

Figure 2.7. Visiting Bag with Equipment for Prenatal and Postnatal Care, First National Midwifery Training School, Peking. Courtesy of the Rockefeller Archive Center.

use most of the technical equipment listed below as the basic necessities of a "small maternity center" listed in table 2.1. The first part of this list reads like the scene of a tragedy: craniotomy forceps, perforator, decapitating hooks, curved scissors. These tools were most often used in cases in which the infant had died in labor, for example when the mother's pelvis was too narrow to allow the infant passage, or in the case of "monsters," grossly abnormal or underdeveloped fetuses. Many early medical missionaries recounted horrible tales of prolonged labor during which the infant had died and had to be decapitated and removed in pieces.[79] Narrow or deformed pelvis from osteomalacia (also known popularly as rickets) was a common cause of maternal and infant mortality due to the lack of calcium and Vitamin D in Chinese diets.[80] This situation could be more easily managed if caught early during prenatal visits so that a caesarean section could be scheduled. Sometimes the *jieshengpo* would attempt such a removal, or in trying to speed things along pull too hard on the infant and end up retrieving a disembodied arm, or leg, or a head.[81] This naturally caused great distress—not only psychologically—to the mother, as a decomposing infant in the vaginal canal is a sure incubator for septic infection. With such an extensive list of required implements for even a small maternity center, one wonders how a *jieshengpo* could have affected any type of labor and delivery given her "'house hold' scissor, piece of 'color silk' and cotton, pair of iron coal chopsticks, and iron hook."[82]

The newly minted modern midwives from the First National Midwifery School in the 1930s had to follow a delivery room and labor routine, a common curriculum issued from the National Midwifery Board and part of the more general regulations controlling midwifery education.[83] As soon as labor commenced, the patient was to be assigned to a labor room and watched continuously by the assigned student. When labor pains were strong with a four-centimeter cervical dilation, the patient was transferred to the delivery room. Depending on whether or not this was the mother's first birth (primipara), she may have been able to walk around if certain conditions were met: "slight pain, membranes intact, head engaged," and a less than four-centimeter cervical dilation.[84] If the primipara or multipara experienced bleeding or membrane rupture, then she was to lie in bed. In addition, the parturient was not allowed any food after the first stage of labor, for if a caesarean section or other surgical procedure had to be performed it increased the risk of pulmonary aspiration. After the membranes ruptured, the midwife was to monitor the fetal heart every hour. She was also instructed to perform an internal (rectal) and external exam upon admission to the labor room and then every two hours

Table 2.1. Basic Necessities for a "Small Maternity Center." John B. Grant, letter to Victor Heiser, September 20, 1926.

Sterilization

- Bramhall Deane, United States A, Sterilizing outfit with petroleum heating and No. 1 B Dressing Sterilizer
- Utensil sterilizers, No. 3, to be heated by petroleum

Instruments

(a) Two sets of instruments for in and out use, consisting of:

- Barnes' midwifery forceps with Simpson's handles and Neville Axis Traction
- Simpson's straight perforator
- Sharp decapitating hook
- Barnes' craniotomy forceps
- Churchill's craniotomy forceps
- Braxton Hicks' cephalotribe
- Blunt hook and crochet
- Long curved scissors, 10 inch.
- Chapetier de Ribes' bag and introducer, 2 bags

(b) Diagnostic instruments consisting of:

- Martin's Pelvimeter, three
- Williams' Pelvimeter, three

(c) Minor instruments for labors in and out, as follows:

- 4 rubber catheters
- 4 metal female catheters, long
- 12 pairs Rochester Carmault clams
- 6 pairs blunt pointed scissors
- needles
- 3 needle holders
- 12 sponge holding forceps
- 4 pinch forceps with teeth

(d) Other instruments, as follows:

- Apparatus for infusion of saline
- Uterine packers, two

Maternity outfits

Cases, etc. for outside work. Two.

Teaching apparatus

- Phantome (Maison Matheiu, Paris)
- Foetus, with compressible head
- Female pelvis
- Foetal head at term

Delivery bed

Operating table and instruments

until delivery. The midwife or other deliverer was to soak her hands in a Lysol solution before the internal examinations and also every half-hour regardless of her activities. The first stage of labor was allowed to "go on indefinitely" provided the following conditions were met: "membranes intact, general condition satisfactory, foetal heart well heard, temperature under 37.4 C."[85] If no progress had been made after two hours at the second stage of labor, or if the placenta had not been delivered a half-hour after delivery, then the attendant was to report the case to her supervisor or physician. After the baby was born, the midwife was to clean its mouth with gauze and add one drop of silver nitrate 1% in each eye as soon as the cord was tied, then give baby a routine bath. The baby's name was to be attached to the right wrist, and the baby was transferred to the nursery where she would then be weighed, measured, and recorded.

The ward routine was similar. All patients had to provide a urine specimen, have their temperatures and blood pressure readings taken, and their diets adjusted. Patients with skin lesions, a respiratory illness, or sexually transmitted disease were isolated from the other patients. All patients who had been examined outside the hospital (presumably by an old-style midwife) had to be isolated to prevent the spread of infection. Clothing was furnished by the maternity department, and the patients' own clothing was sent back home. Although patients could walk around in the courtyard, they were not allowed to leave the hospital grounds. The regulations also stipulated very detailed methods of postpartum patient and infant examination in the clinic and hospital.[86]

The questions of which Chinese women chose to give birth on the dusty *kang* or in the sterile delivery room at the First National Midwifery School or the Guangzhou Municipal Hospital with the accoutrements of a modern midwife, and why, are difficult to answer. The written record consists primarily of two types: personal accounts of difficult (and often solitary) childbirth gleaned from local and oral histories; and essays, short stories, and plays that lament the desperation, filth, and pain of traditional labor and childbirth in China. Chinese women's lives in their own words, collected by Li Xiaojiang, portray childbirth as frequent and lonely.[87] Daniang described one of her 13 pregnancies, of which only three survived to adulthood: each time, she gave birth alone at home on the *kang*, tied the umbilical cord, buried the placenta, and afterwards cooked dinner for her bad-tempered husband.[88] Similarly, descriptions of traditional births from a special selection of articles in *Funü zazhi*, titled "Childbirth Customs in My Hometown" (*Wu xiang de shengchan fengsu*), mock traditional birth practices. From Beijing to Henan, Jiangsu to Anhui, Fujian, Zhejiang,

Guangdong, Yunnan, and Guizhou—nationwide, it seems, from every location in China emerged the persistent threat of painful and lonely childbirth, malicious midwives, deformed infants, protracted labors, superstitious family members, and meddling neighbors.[89] Detailed records of labor and birth with favorable outcomes either do not exist or have not been found, evidence of the "eating bitterness" genre so often iterated in oral histories.[90]

As discussed in chapter 1, the women who delivered in Western hospitals or were otherwise attended by a Western-trained physician were from both the poorest and the richest classes. The former usually had been in labor for days and sent for a Western doctor only as a last resort; the latter, if they were urban, forward-thinking, and "modern," could afford to patronize one of the new elite lying-in hospitals or secure a modern physician to attend them in their homes. The successful deliveries by modern or traditional midwives, however, are only succinctly recorded in hospital records, if at all. The personal voices remain silent.

THE MODERN MOTHER

Modern methods of child rearing and family life were spread through the popular press in Republican China. Like milk entrepreneur You Huaigao, other Chinese emulated and spread Western ideas about home economics and family life. In 1930, Zhang Xiaohuai translated into Chinese a popular parenting book by Dr. Frank Howard Richardson, a prolific author and a specialist in child and family health.[91] In his preface, Zhang wrote that sex, childbirth, and love for one's spouse and children are all natural and instinctual processes, yet the Chinese sages never wrote about these issues and so the people's knowledge in this arena is lacking. Youth in schools are taught minimal sex education but instruction in proper child-rearing is absent. Child rearing, according to Zhang, is the culmination of marital sex and a crucial part of a harmonious society. He asserted that "the capitalism and imperialism of Europe and the United States is already a curse on the weak nations of the East, but we can still more or less trust the results from their patient scientific research."[92] Western science was the key to national survival. The literature on science and eugenics included exhortations, lessons, and instructions for women to assume the burden of improving the Chinese nation through healthy births and modern child rearing. Theories of acquired inheritance, the belief that improvements to oneself could be passed on to one's offspring, were common as well. Educated and active women who were free from the tethers of bound feet would engender strong, healthy, educable offspring.

After the mother successfully delivered her infant, she could choose to attend Well-Baby Clinics or Mothers' Club meetings to learn the most modern methods of infant and child care. Such meetings were held in both urban centers and in rural areas that had Western clinics or hospitals, mostly established by Western missionaries. Mothers-in-law meetings were also popular, for these matriarchs often had control over their daughters-in-law and were seen as more resistant to change. Figure 2.8 shows such a meeting with grandfather in attendance in the far back right of the photograph, perhaps to make sure nothing suspicious was underfoot in this gathering of women. These clubs, which were usually run by hospitals or midwifery or nursing schools, were intended to reduce the high infant mortality rate and to introduce septic and modern methods of childcare. In addition to baby weight checks, cursory physical examinations, and inoculations, the mother could learn how to care for her child. For example, figure 2.8 exhibits a clothesline with clean clothes, a baby bathtub, crib, bassinet, and diapering paraphernalia. Some of these organizations, like one at the Shanxi Hua County Public Health Station, distributed clean gauze with which to wrap the umbilical cord instead of the typical mud or dung, a common method of tetanus transmission.[93] The Mothers' Club attached to the Qilu (Cheeloo) Medical School in Jinan, Shandong Province, intended to "[lay] the foundation stone for the child's habits."[94] They gave demonstrations and lectures on suitable food and clothing; daily routine at birth, six months, and 12 months; clean water and its appropriate vessels; infant skin care; infant formula preparation; fresh air and sunshine; dental hygiene; and child development.

The Mother's Association in Nanjing, financed and staffed by the Nanjing Public Health Bureau, taught weekly classes in mothercraft, including "marriage problems, child welfare, family budget and house-keeping, general hygiene, disease prevention, first aid, and other kindred subjects."[95] The First National Midwifery School, under the Beiping Child Health Institute, began similar classes in 1930 because "it is the mothers who can actually practice child health and it is the mothers who build toward 'school' and 'adult' health. Before the mothers can be expected to undertake this responsibility they must be 'health conscious.'"[96] The mothers were expected not only to learn modern methods of health and child care, but also to spread this knowledge in their communities. The First National Midwifery

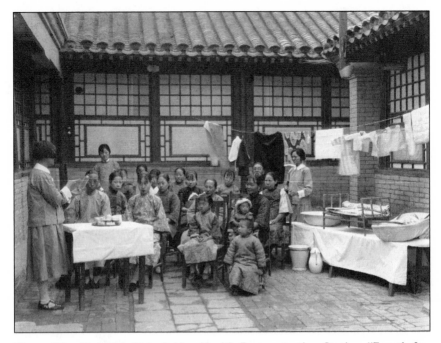

Figure 2.8. Mothers' Club, Peking Health Demonstration Station. "Fourth Annual Report of the Peking Health Demonstration Station, 1929." Courtesy of the Rockefeller Archive Center.

School distributed informational leaflets on maternal and child health with such titles as "Important Hints for Expected Mothers, Parturient Mothers and On the Care of Infants," "How to Maintain Health and Prevent Abnormalities for Antepartum, Partum, and Postpartum Mothers," and "Hints on Proper Food During Pregnancy [with] Special Emphasis on Osteomalacia."[97] The institute encouraged its graduates to form additional mothercraft classes in their own neighborhoods.

A similar organization in Changsha, Hunan, distributed fliers titled "Good Methods for Protecting Newborns and Infants" (aee appendix for a complete translation). It instructed mothers on caring for their infants' eyes and umbilical cord, gave advice on proper bathing, nursing, feeding, sleeping, environment (including fly elimination), and treating illness. It is hard to say which of these exhortations were excessive and which were necessary based on the environmental conditions at the time. For example, the flier describes how to clean the infants' eyes with a boric acid solution. Eye infections were rampant in 1920s China among children and adults, as evidenced by the large number of ophthalmic ailments treated at hospitals like Peking Union Medical College. The routine use of silver nitrate eye drops at birth to prevent the transmission of eye diseases was just becoming common in China among trained midwives during this time. It also instructs caregivers to bathe the infant daily, which may be unnecessary, not to mention impossible due to lack of water or time. Lesson number six tells parents to provide fresh air for their infant at all times regardless of season or time of day. This is contrary to traditional Chinese beliefs about illness being caused by drafts, and the lack of air circulation was one of the main complaints that Western medical personnel had about Chinese households: they were too stuffy and claustrophobic and thus ripe for breeding disease. In contemporary medical discourse, whether or not fresh air prevents disease, or causes it, is still up for debate.

Articles promoting these clubs in Western publications like *The Chinese Medical Journal* were extremely patronizing: "Women are even in greater need of enlightenment on the duties and responsibilities of motherhood."[98] These classes sought to teach Chinese women Western methods of childcare, while further burdening them with being solely responsible for the health of the fledgling Chinese nation. Both the Chinese modernizers and the Western medical personnel targeted Chinese mothers with their messages of national responsibility.

CONCLUSION

Modern images and descriptions of childbirth, midwives, and midwifery schools as put forth in the Republican-era press served to both create new methods of childbirth and maternal and child health, and they reflect rapidly occurring changes in these fields. Scientific medicine attempts to mechanize and control the human body and its functions, which may be considered a form of cultural imperialism. The assumed intrinsic goodness of Western medicine has been challenged by the degrees of contestation and syncretism between colonizers and colonized.[99] For instance, the ineffectiveness of some nineteenth- and early twentieth-century medicine, such as the English physician Benjamin Hobson's prescribed ice water douches to bring down the placenta, may have hindered its acceptance in China.[100] Furthermore, much Western obstetrics was counterintuitive to Chinese traditional cultural norms and ideas about the body and health, like the Chinese emphasis on avoiding cold water during pregnancy.[101]

New technologies were (and still are) used to explain racial and cultural differences in biological instead of social terms, "endow[ing] medical authorities and government with greater powers of intervention in the regulation of reproduction."[102] Social problems in China are often attributed to scientific causes even today, namely the "poor quality" of lower class and minority groups.[103] The focus on biological explanations for social problems moves the responsibility of China's development and modernization from the state onto the people. The irrefutability of science beginning in the Republican era and persisting today reinforces racial, cultural, and gender stereotypes.

In holding biology as the embodiment of physical and mental worth or deviance, and the physical body as the site of technological change, differing perceptions of the body, sexuality, and reproduction emerge. These new technologies and perceptions have led many scholars to explore the social framework on which scientific language and culture is based. Whereas in the past, "nature" was the moral and ethical norm, in Republican China science and technology began to take on that role and were often considered unassailable and irrefutable. However, scholars have begun to deconstruct the ways that biological processes are portrayed, not in Republican China per se, but in the West, uncovering cultural biases that often reveal gender and class prejudices. Emily Martin paved the way in this field with her analysis of the "romance" of the egg and the sperm.[104] She shows how biological processes are endowed with gendered characteristics, with slower or passive elements endowed with feminine qualities (the egg), and masculine qualities ascribed to faster or stronger components (the sperm). In addition, active characteristics of the feminine elements were downplayed, while the passive parts of the masculine segments were highlighted. In early twentieth-century China, bodily functions and elements also had gendered anthropomorphic characteristics, taken in part from the patriarchal scientific medicine in the West, and also from China's traditional patriarchal views of passive women and active men.[105] As biology became more important in discourses of health and the body, the paradigms of reproduction and fertility shifted, while women's social roles as reproducers for the family were overlaid with responsibilities to the nation-state.

The Western Enlightenment ideal that man could understand and control reproduction displaced earlier notions that childbirth was woman's work and that it was strictly a family affair. As reproduction became central to the public and fundamental to social identity, it had to be controlled by the strongest, smartest, and best-equipped. Like eighteenth-century Britons, the "scientific authority over reproduction vitally affected the well-being of the nation-state," as ideas of sex and conception and reproduction and birth intertwined with concepts of nation, gender, and identity.[106] That trend continued in the United States, so that by the 1920s and 1930s, physicians were already beginning to displace midwives in the birthing room, which largely came to mean the hospital.[107] Unlike Britain and the United States, however, women in China, as mothers and as midwives, remained central to the redefinition and reconstruction of childbirth.

NOTES

1. Kang Youwei, *Great Harmony (Datong shu)*, 1898, as quoted in Kazuko, *Chinese Women in a Century of Revolution, 1850–1950*, 43.

2. Jiang Na, "The 'New Virtuous Wife and Good Mother': Women Intellectuals' Group Identity and the Funü Zhoukan *(Women's Weekly)*, 1935–1937," *Women's History Review* 16, no. 3 (July 2007): 447–61; Mann, "The Cult of Domesticity in Republican Shanghai's Middle Class," 186.

3. Nakajima, "Health and Hygiene in Mass Mobilization: Hygiene Campaigns in Shanghai, 1920–1945."

4. Linda Kerber, "Foreword," in *Chinese Visions of Family and State, 1915–1953*, by Susan Glosser (Berkeley: University of California Press, 2003), ix–xiv; Sally Taylor Lieberman, *The Mother and Narrative Politics in Modern China* (Charlottesville: University of Virginia Press, 1998), 26–27.

5. Robert Culp, *Articulating Citizenship: Civic Education and Student Politics in Southeastern China, 1912–1940* (Cambridge MA, and London: Harvard University Asia Center, 2007), 202–4.

6. Lieberman, *The Mother and Narrative Politics in Modern China.*

7. Stephen R. MacKinnon, "Toward a History of the Chinese Press in the Republican Period," *Modern China* 23, no. 1 (January 1997): 3–32.

8. Ibid., 7.

9. Lee, "The Cultural Construction of Modernity in Urban Shanghai: Some Preliminary Explorations."

10. Yao Changxu, *Essentials of Obstetrics (Taichan xuzhi)*, 6th ed., Medical Series (Shanghai: Shangwu yinshuguan, 1929); Hong Shilu and Wu Mai, *Childbirth and Nursing (Shengchan yu yuying)*, 1st ed., Medical Science Series (Shanghai: Shangwu yinshuguan, 1930); Chen Jianshan, *Fetal Education (Taijiao)*, vol. 75, 1st ed., Universal Library (Shanghai: Shangwu yinshuguan, 1925).

11. Lee, "The Cultural Construction of Modernity in Urban Shanghai: Some Preliminary Explorations," 52.

12. Ibid., 33.

13. The images and texts used here were gleaned from extensive perusal of several popular journals, mostly from the first half of the twentieth century. The handbooks and textbooks are merely those found in archives and libraries in Tianjin, Beijing, Shanghai, Nanjing, and Guangzhou.

14. R.S. Britton, *The Chinese Periodical Press, 1800–1912* (Taipei: Chengwen, 1966), 127.

15. Lin Yutang, *A History of the Press and Public Opinion in China* (Chicago: University of Chicago Press, 1936).

16. K. Huang, "The Medical, Cultural, and Social Life of Shanghai: A Study Based on Advertisements for Medicines in Shenbao, 1912–1926 (*Cong Shenbao yiyao guanggao kan min chu Shanghai de yiliao wenhua yu shehui shenghuo*)," *Bulletin of the Institute of Modern History, Academia Sinica* (*Zhongyan yanjiuyuan jindaishi yanjiusuo jikan*) 17, no. 2 (1988): 141–94.

17. Britton, *The Chinese Periodical Press, 1800–1912*.

18. Dikötter, *Sex, Culture and Modernity in China: Medical Science and the Construction of Sexual Identities in the Early Republican Period*; Susan Mann, *Precious Records: Women in China's Long Eighteenth Century* (Stanford: Stanford University Press, 1997).

19. Barbara Mittler, *A Newspaper for China? Power, Identity, and Change in Shanghai's News Media, 1872–1912* (Cambridge, MA: Harvard University Asia Center, 2004).

20. Charlotte Beahan, "Feminism and Nationalism in the Chinese Women's Press, 1902–1911," *Modern China* 1, no. 4 (1975): 379–416.

21. *Shenbao*, for example, one of the most well-known Chinese newspapers, was founded in 1872 by Ernest Major, a British merchant. Mittler, *A Newspaper for China? Power, Identity, and Change in Shanghai's News Media, 1872–1912*, 255; MacKinnon, "Toward a History of the Chinese Press in the Republican Period."

22. Mittler, *A Newspaper for China? Power, Identity, and Change in Shanghai's News Media, 1872–1912*, 255.

23. Evelyn S. Rawski, *Education and Popular Literacy in Ch'ing China* (Ann Arbor: University of Michigan Press, 1979), 6–8.

24. For example, Jin Wuzhou, "How to be a good republican citizen? (*Zen yang zuo yi ge zhonghua minguo de lianghao gongmin?*)," *Nantao Christian Institute Bulletin* (*Puyi zhoukan*), March 20, 1925; Jie Ping, "A discussion of improving marriage (*Hunli gailiang de shangque*)," *Nantao Christian Institute Bulletin* (*Puyi zhoukan*), December 4, 1924.

25. Joan Judge, "Citizens or Mothers of Citizens? Gender and the Meaning of Modern Chinese Citizenship," in *Changing Meanings of Citizenship in Modern China*, ed. Merle Goldman and Elizabeth J. Perry (Cambridge, MA: Harvard University Press, 2002), 23–43.

26. Cui Yang and Brian G. Southwell, "Dangerous Disease, Dangerous Women: Health, Anxiety and Advertising in Shanghai from 1928 to 1937," *Critical Public Health* 14, no. 2 (June 2004): 149–56.

27. Dikötter, *Sex, Culture and Modernity in China: Medical Science and the Construction of Sexual Identities in the Early Republican Period*, 9.

28. Dikötter, *Sex, Culture and Modernity in China: Medical Science and the Construction of Sexual Identities in the Early Republican Period*.

29. Frank Dikötter, "Race Culture: Recent Perspectives on the History of Eugenics," *American Historical Review* 103, no. 2 (1998): 467–78.

30. Kazuko, *Chinese Women in a Century of Revolution, 1850–1950*.

31. The closest thing to Kang Youwei's vision in China were the kindergartens established in 1930s Guangzhou as part of the city's progressive Three-

Year Plan. Edward Bing-Shuey Lee, *Modern Canton* (Shanghai: The Mercury Press, 1936), Appendix III, 153–68.

32. *"Furen renzi, qin bu ze, zuo bu bian, li bu bi, bu shi xie wei, bu zheng bu shi, bu zheng bu zuo,"* as quoted in Yun Qin, "Hygiene and Fetal Education during Pregnancy *(Renshen de weisheng yu taijiao),"* *Far Eastern Miscellany (Dongfang Zazhi)* 34, no. 7 (1937): 258.

33. *"Jiqi you shen, mu bu jian shi e se, er bu ting yin sheng, kou bu chu ao yan, neng yi taijiao,"* from Liu Xiang, "Scroll 1, Mothers of Zhou *(Juan yi, Zhou shi san mu),"* in *Biographies of Exemplary Women (Lienu zhuan),* 18 BCE, http://etext.lib.virginia.edu/chinese/lienu/browse/ scroll1.html.

34. The word for frog, *wa,* has the same pronunciation in Mandarin as the word for a baby's cry, *wa.*

35. Wu, *Reproducing Women: Medicine, Metaphor and Childbirth in Late Imperial China,* 13.

36. Sarah E. Stevens, "Making Female Sexuality in Republican China: Women's Bodies in the Discourses of Hygiene, Education, and Literature" (PhD dissertation, Indiana University, 2001), especially chapter two, "Fetal Education and the Public Womb," 70–75.

37. Xie Siyan, "The Question of Women's Physical Culture *(Nüzi tiyu wenti),"* *Ladies' Journal (Funü zazhi)* 9, no. 7 (1923): 2–5; as cited in Stevens, "Making Female Sexuality in Republican China: Women's Bodies in the Discourses of Hygiene, Education, and Literature," 89.

38. Yun Qin, "Hygiene and Fetal Education during Pregnancy *(Renshen de weisheng yu taijiao),"* 257–58.

39. Ibid., 259.

40. Ibid.

41. Huang Shi, "What Is Fetal Education? *(Shenme shi taijiao?),"* *Ladies' Journal (Funü Zazhi),* 1931.

42. Chen Jianshan, *Fetal Education (Taijiao),* 75: 4.

43. Dikötter, *Sex, Culture and Modernity in China: Medical Science and the Construction of Sexual Identities in the Early Republican Period,* 72.

44. Elisabeth Fee, "Nineteenth-Century Craniology: The Study of the Female Skull," *Bulletin of the History of Medicine* 53, no. 3 (1979): 415–33; Emily Martin, *The Woman in the Body: A Cultural Analysis of Reproduction* (Boston: Beacon Press, 1992); Stephanie A. Shields, "The Variability Hypothesis: The History of a Biological Model of Sex Differences in Intelligence," *Signs: Journal of Women and Culture in Society* 7 (1982).

45. Shi Gu, *Man May Live Two Hundred Years (Rensheng erbainian),* 1st ed. (Shanghai: Shangwu yinshuguan, 1929), 38–39; as cited in Dikötter, *Sex, Culture and Modernity in China: Medical Science and the Construction of Sexual Identities in the Early Republican Period,* 38–39.

46. Shao, *Culturing Modernity: The Nantong Model, 1890–1930.*

47. Yeh, "Shanghai Modernity: Commerce and Culture in a Republican City," 388.

48. Glosser, *Chinese Visions of Family and State, 1915–1953.*

49. Yeh, "Shanghai Modernity: Commerce and Culture in a Republican City," 387; Susan Glosser, "The Business of Family: You Huaigao and the commercialization of a May Fourth Ideal," *Republican China* 20, no. 2 (1995): 80–116.

50. Kansas State Historical Society, "Dr. Williams' Pink Pills for Pale People," *Cool Things*, n.d., http://www.kshs.org/cool3/pinkpills.htm.

51. Mittler, *A Newspaper for China? Power, Identity, and Change in Shanghai's News Media, 1872–1912*, especially chapter four, "Fair-Sexing It," 246–311.

52. Shenbao 30.4.1877, as cited in Ibid., 260.

53. Ibid., 261.

54. Shenbao 23.5.1902, as cited in Ibid., 262.

55. *Ladies' Journal (Funü zazhi)* 1.1.1915. Also see Stevens, "Making Female Sexuality in Republican China: Women's Bodies in the Discourses of Hygiene, Education, and Literature," 140–41.

56. *Ladies' Journal (Funü zazhi)* 1.1.1915.

57. *Ladies' Journal (Funü zazhi)* 1.9.1915.

58. Szeming Sze, *China's Health Problems* (Washington, DC: Chinese Medical Association, 1944), 22–24.

59. Ibid., 22.

60. Blood in Chinese medicine, as contrasted with the red physical matter flowing through the veins, comprises not only menstrual blood, but also other vaginal discharges as well as breast milk. Furth, *A Flourishing Yin: Gender in China's Medical History, 960–1665*, 47, 73.

61. Furth, *A Flourishing Yin: Gender in China's Medical History, 960–1665*; Francesca Bray, "A Deathly Disorder: Understanding Women's Health in Late Imperial China," in *Knowledge and the Scholarly Medical Traditions*, ed. Don Bates (Cambridge: Cambridge University Press, 1995), 235–50.

62. Wu, *Reproducing Women: Medicine, Metaphor and Childbirth in Late Imperial China*, 266.

63. Ibid., 13.

64. Dissection was considered a desecration of the human body, a gift from one's parents. It was legalized only in 1913. Harold Balme, *China and Modern Medicine: A Study in Medical Missionary Development* (London: United Council for Missionary Education, 1921), 156.

65. Wu, *Reproducing Women: Medicine, Metaphor and Childbirth in Late Imperial China*.

66. Duden, *Disembodying Women: Perspectives on Pregnancy and the Unborn*, 68.

67. "Caesarean Section (Pou fu chu er)," *Dianshizhai Pictorial (Dianshizhai huabao)*, 1892.

68. Xiaoqing Ye, *The Dianshizhai Pictorial: Shanghai Urban Life, 1884–1898* (Ann Arbor: University of Michigan Press, 2003).

69. C.C. Chen and Frederica M. Bunge, *Medicine in Rural China: A Personal Account* (Berkeley: University of California Press, 1989), 63.

70. *The National Medical Journal of China* 16, no. 6, December 1930.

71. *MCH-PH Visiting Report* (Health Station Annual Report, 1931), 100, folder 472, box 67, RG IV2B9, RAC.

72. For a discussion of women's education in early Republican China, see Shou Shang Hsu, Hsiao Lan Ou Yang, and Yoehngoo Tsohsan Wu Lew, "Education of Women in China," in *Education in China: Papers Contributed by the Members of Committees of the Society for the Study of International Education*, ed. T.Y. Teng and T.T. Lew (Peking: Society for the Study of International Education, 1923), 1–35; Schneider, *Biology and Revolution in Twentieth-Century China*.

73. Barbara Duden, *The Woman Beneath the Skin*, trans. Thomas Dunlap (Cambridge, MA: Harvard University Press, 1991), 46.

74. Michel Foucault, *The Birth of the Clinic: An Archaeology of Medical Perception* (New York: Vintage, 1973).

75. Yao Changxu, *Essentials of Obstetrics (Taichan xuzhi)*; Hong Shilu and Wu Mai, *Childbirth and Nursing (Shengchan yu yuying)*.

76. Judith Farquhar, "For Your Reading Pleasure: Self-Health *(Ziwo baojian)* Information in 1990s Beijing," *Positions* 9, no. 1 (2001): 105–30.

77. Gordon Huang, "The Development of Health Centres," *Chinese Medical Journal* 55 (June 1939): 546–60; Eula Eno, "Chinese Female Pelvis: A Study in the Pelvic Measurements of 2,260 Chinese Women, with Suggestions as to the Probable Normals," *Chinese Medical Journal* 47 (1933): 179–86; Y.T. Ho, Marian Manly, and Gladys Cunningham, "Measurements of Chinese Female Pelvis and Fetal Heads in Relation to Labor," *Chinese Medical Journal* 48 (1934): 47–55; Gordon King and Yu Teh T'ang, "Obstetrical Criteria in North China: The Weights and Measurements of the Mature New-Born Child," *Chinese Medical Journal* 52 (October 1937): 501–6; K.H. Uttley, "The Birth Weight of Full Term Cantonese Babies," *Chinese Medical Journal* 58 (November 1940): 582–91; Su Tsu-fei and Chueh-ju Liang, "Growth and Development of Chinese Infants of Hunan Province," *Chinese Medical Journal* 58 (July 1940): 104–12.

78. Farquhar, "For Your Reading Pleasure: Self-Health *(Ziwo baojian)* Information in 1990s Beijing"; Sarah Franklin, "Postmodern Procreation: A Cultural Account of Assisted Reproduction," in *Conceiving the New World Order: The Global Politics of Reproduction*, ed. Faye D. Ginsburg and Rayna Rapp (Berkeley: University of California Press, 1995), 323–45; Martin, *The Woman in the Body: A Cultural Analysis of Reproduction*.

79. Josephine Bixby, "Obstetric Cases," *The China Medical Missionary Journal* 14, no. 3 (July 1900): 160–62; E. Gough, "Difficulties and Discouragements of Obstetric Work in China," *The China Medical Missionary Journal* 15, no. 4 (1901): 249–54; Marian Manly, "Outpatient Obstetrics in China: A Review of 1000 Cases," *Chinese Medical Journal* 51 (1937): 237–44; Poulter, "Obstetrical Experiences in a Chinese City"; W.E. Macklin, "Notes on Cases," *The China Medical Missionary Journal* 7, no. 1 (1893): 101–3.

80. Dr. J.P. Maxwell and Dr. Lee M. Miles, "Osteomalacia in China," *The Journal of Obstetrics and Gynaecology of the British Empire* 32, no. 3 (1925): 433–441.

81. Macklin, "Notes on Cases."

82. Yang, "Letter [to John B. Grant?]."

83. *Regulations of the First National Midwifery School* (Beiping: First National Midwifery School, 1930), folder 372, box 45, series 601, RAC.

84. Ibid.

85. Ibid.

86. Ibid.

87. Li Xiaojiang, *Women Speak for Themselves (Rang nuren ziji shuohua)* (Beijing: Shenghuo, dushu, xinzhi san lian shudian, 2003).

88. Ibid., 317–18.

89. Zi Yun (pseud.), "Childbirth Customs in My Hometown: Beijing (*Wu xiang de shengchan fengsu: Beijing*)," *Ladies' Journal (Funü zazhi)* 11, no. 7 (1925): 1173–1200.

90. Gail Hershatter, "Birthing Stories: Rural Midwives in 1950s China."

91. Zhang Xiaohuai, "Translator's Preface (*Yi zhe xu*)," in *Fumu zhi dao* (Shenzhou guo guang she chuban, 1930), 1–2.

92. Ibid.

93. Neizhengbu nianjian bianzuan weiyuanhui, *Yearbook of Internal Affairs (Neizheng nianjian)*, vol. 4.

94. Annie V. Scott, MD, "Well Baby Clinic: Its Organization and Aim," *Chinese Medical Journal* 50 (1936): 620–22.

95. "Mother's Association in Nanking," *Chinese Medical Journal* 47 (1933): 418.

96. League of Nations Health Organization, *Collaboration with the Government of China: First Report of the Central Field Health Station*, May 10, 1934.

97. FNMS, *Fifth Annual Report, First National Midwifery School, Peiping, July 1, 1933–June 30, 1934*, Annual Report, September 15, 1934.

98. "Mother's Association in Nanking."

99. Arnold, *Colonizing the Body: State Medicine and Epidemic Disease in 19th-Century India*; Cunningham and Andrews, *Western Medicine as Contested Knowledge*; Philip D. Curtin, *Disease and Empire: The Health of European Troops in the Conquest of Africa* (New York: Cambridge University Press, 1998); Lewis Pyenson, *Cultural Imperialism and Exact Sciences: German Expansion Overseas 1900–1930* (New York, Berne, Frankfurt am Main: Peter Lang, 1985); Bridie Andrews, "Judging Western Medicine by Chinese Values: Zhang Xichun and His Work," in *Association for Asian Studies Annual Conference* (Chicago, IL, 2001); Wu, "Introducing the Uterus to China: Benjamin Hobson's New Treatises on Women's and Children's Diseases (*Fuxing xinshuo*), 1858."

100. Wu, "Introducing the Uterus to China: Benjamin Hobson's New Treatises on Women's and Children's Diseases (*Fuxing xinshuo*), 1858."

101. Ibid.

102. Frank Dikötter, "Reading the Body: Genetic Knowledge and Social Marginalization in the People's Republic of China," *China Information* 13, no. 2 (1998): 1–99.

103. Dikötter, *Sex, Culture and Modernity in China: Medical Science and the Construction of Sexual Identities in the Early Republican Period*; Frank Dikötter, *Imperfect Conceptions: Medical Knowledge, Birth Defects, and Eugenics in China* (London: Hurst & Co., 1998); Ann Anagnost, "A Surfeit of Bodies: Population and the Rationality of the State in Post-Mao China," in *Conceiving the New World Order: The Global Politics of Reproduction*, ed. Faye D. Ginsburg and Rayna Rapp (Berkeley: University of California Press, 1995), 22–41.

104. Martin, *The Woman in the Body: A Cultural Analysis of Reproduction*.

105. See Dikötter, *Sex, Culture and Modernity in China: Medical Science and the Construction of Sexual Identities in the Early Republican Period*.

106. Cody, *Birthing the Nation: Sex, Science, and the Conception of Eighteenth-Century Britons*, 11.

107. More, *Restoring the Balance: Women Physicians and the Profession of Medicine, 1850–1995*, 49; Leavitt, *Brought to Bed: Childbearing in America, 1750 to 1950*, 171.

The Midwifery Profession

Midwifery is one of the professions. It can only be controlled by government through registration and enforcement of regulations. The situation requires governmental schools of good standards. Cooperation should be effected with missionary hospitals and other private institutions who however should have their training schools comply with government standards and regulations.[1]

In a matter of decades, midwifery in China transformed from an apprenticed vocation into a scientifically trained profession. Accordingly, normative childbirth in twentieth-century urban China underwent dramatic change from a home-based experience attended by a granny midwife to a controlled event in a hospital or clinic setting supervised by a modern childbirth professional. While the United States and Great Britain developed a biomedical reproductive method that focused on male physicians that they later attempted to export to other countries, many adapted the new methods to better accommodate specific cultural norms and values. Childbirth is one of these arenas in which cultural norms won out over the dominant biomedical form. Regardless of the changes in the structure, setting, and practices of childbirth, midwives in China remained at the center of this event.

In the midst of dramatic social and political change during the Republican era, the First National Midwifery School (*Zhonghua di yi zhuchan xuexiao*) was the nucleus for these unprecedented modifications in childbirth and for the development of the midwifery profession, supported by the Nationalist government, local modernizers, and foreign philanthropists. The school and its goals were created during a time of great optimism for many of China's intellectuals, yet were hindered by the Guomindang's lack of a central vision and a shortage of resources for improving public health. The school was affiliated with Peking Union Medical College (PUMC, *Beijing xiehe yixueyuan*), which served as China's modern medical model in the 1920s.[2]

The Rockefeller Foundation-supported PUMC actively shaped the nature of modern medicine in China and brought important changes in the medical field. In fact, before PUMC, there was no medical *profession* in China. Medicine was not legalized, institutionalized, or standardized. PUMC granted the first government-sanctioned medical diplomas in China. Its physicians and administrators promoted medical professionalism and opened careers for women.[3] PUMC trained physicians as well as paramedical staff like nurses and midwives. Its administrators discouraged the hiring of male nurses, who had been common in China before the 1920s, over female nurses. This decidedly American characteristic enforced a gender hierarchy at PUMC, like its role model Johns Hopkins University in Baltimore, Maryland, whereby female nurses were subordinate to primarily male physicians as the nursing profession was feminized.[4] In the American model, traditional midwives were also displaced by more highly trained and primarily male physicians. One of the chief consultants of the First National Midwifery School was Dr. J. Whitridge Williams, Dean of the Johns Hopkins School of Medicine from 1911 to 1923. Williams had widely lectured and published on the abhorrent state of maternal and child health in the United States (his *Williams Obstetrics* is still in print in its 23rd edition), and he started the first academic department of obstetrics in the United States at Johns Hopkins University, with an emphasis on hospital births attended by male doctors.[5] However, the medical model adapted in China in the 1920s comprised a deliberate attempt to create a new and respected female midwifery profession that grew out of the shortage of Western-trained physicians.

The PUMC-affiliated First National Midwifery School thus developed programs to create a modern professional midwife with the new moniker, *zhuchanshi*. The women trained as *zhuchanshi*, although highly educated, were largely young, unmarried, and childless, lacking the extensive personal experience of the traditional midwives, traditionally called *jieshengpo, chanpo,* or other similar terms that denote a granny birth helper. The *zhuchanshi*'s legitimacy was conveyed in their scientific training and educational curricula, in their appearance and the equipment they were taught to use and carry to all deliveries, and in the photographs and glossy brochures extolling the benefits of modern childbirth that advertised their education and their services.

These modern midwives were part of the Chinese state-building process as the purveyors of a national modernity.

The development of the medical profession, like the fields of law and architecture, began in the nineteenth century in Europe and the United States when members of various medical fields began to organize and create cohesive educational systems, ethics codes, and licensing and registration requirements. A rich field of literature, especially in the discipline of sociology, exists on the development of professions in the West and their ability to influence and control various segments of society, often using science and rationality as the basis for their expertise.[6] In his book on professionals in Republican Shanghai, Xu Xiaoqun presents "an analysis of professionalization as a historical process mediated by class structure, the role of the state, and the acquisition and use of power by professions."[7] He argues that while the professions of law, medicine, and journalism did not simultaneously meet all attributes of belonging to a profession, these professions developed as part of a continuum. By following Xu's lead, one may examine the process of professionalization among modern midwives in China. It is certain that at various times midwives had at least some of the necessary attributes of a profession. They organized to form professional organizations, sought government regulation of curricula and licensing, and created and upheld a code of ethics. This was a complex process that ultimately led to the demise of traditional midwives.

The midwifery profession in China is unique. Unlike the factory workers of Shanghai or the silk weavers of Guangzhou, China's modern midwives had more education, yet they were not of the educational elite like the women physicians trained in missionary schools and sent abroad for advanced schooling.[8] Comparable to the nursing profession in the United States, paramedical professions in China provided for young women a way out of their current social situations.[9] Midwives on one hand could improve their social standing and their earning power by associating with modern medicine, yet at the same time were faced with the hurdles of traditional taboos about the pollution of childbirth and of women working outside the home.[10] However, many similarities between the urban factory worker and the modern midwife do exist. Both groups of women were independent, and some had nationalistic ideals to join the workforce and help further China's social and economic growth. They were consumers with independent and disposable income who by and large were single and lived at home with their natal families. Akin to Emily Honig's more affluent female factory workers in Shanghai, the midwives too bobbed and curled their hair, wore cosmetics, and dressed in fashionable clothing and high heels.[11] Like the silk weavers in Guangdong and the factory and white-collar workers in Shanghai, modern midwives in these cities and elsewhere created sisterhoods in the form of professional associations.[12]

The study of women's work in Republican China has primarily focused on vocations like home- or factory-based textile labor, or the 'illicit' work of women in opium houses and brothels.[13] There is a dearth of information regarding white-collar work for women during this period, though some institutional histories of medical missions, professional organizations, and hospitals which women ran or worked in do exist.[14] Biographies in English and Chinese of famous Chinese women physicians like Shi Meiyu, Kang Cheng, Yang Chongrui, and Lin Qiaozhi delineate the trials and successes of women in the medical profession in the nineteenth and twentieth centuries.[15] The study of modern midwifery in China is the history of the development and growth of a new profession, positively distinct from nursing, public health, and medicine, though with strong ties and similarities to these occupations. The First National Midwifery School administration made a concerted push to keep nursing and midwifery separate, to create a specialization in midwifery.

This profession was short-lived yet fundamental in many ways. By the end of the twentieth century, professional midwives had been replaced by obstetric nurses and obstetricians. But the professional midwives of Republican China successfully introduced and promulgated a new birth model that has changed little in the several decades since its inception. The profession also forged a path for women's work in the medical and paramedical fields, and it maintained women as the primary national caregivers, for the obstetric nurses and obstetricians who attend childbirth are almost invariably still women.

MEDICAL EDUCATION FOR GIRLS

Several changes took place around the beginning of the twentieth century that allowed women to enter the medical profession, especially as nurses. Secular education for girls became more widespread, and they were encouraged to assume traditionally "feminine" roles as caregivers and teachers. Modern medicine became more efficacious, especially with the spread of germ theory, and hospitals started to become places for healing and treatment instead of homes for the indigent and terminally ill. Finally, as the field of medicine gained more credence and began to organize and professionalize, physicians—overwhelmingly male—helped to create a subordinate "semi-profession" of nursing, and eventually other professional subfields like midwifery.[16] With this process the nursing profession in the West gradually became feminized beginning around the turn of the twentieth century. In the 1800s, nursing was a predominantly male field, as strong men were needed to lift and move patients, and women were not supposed to physically touch or handle male patients. However, nursing eventually became feminized by the twentieth century, with role models like Florence Nightingale as the archetypal caring nurse.[17]

Although public health reforms were under way by the 1910s as part of China's modernization efforts, the state of medical training was still in its infancy. China had no consistent educational policy in the late Qing era, much less a standardized medical curriculum. In 1872, warlord administrators Zeng Guofan, Li Hongzhang, and Yong Hong had convinced the Qing court to send 30 students per year to study abroad. Between 1872 and 1881, only 120 had gone to the United States, a total of 30 to England and France, and none to Germany.[18] The program ended in 1881 because some court advisers thought the students were neglecting Chinese learning and losing their Chinese identity. In contrast, in 1870 the Meiji emperor of Japan sent the first government-sponsored students to study in Germany, and by 1900 Japan had three imperial government medical colleges with a national standardized curriculum: Tokyo (established in 1877), Kyoto (1897), and Kyushu (1903).[19] Japan had graduated over 15,000 practicing state-registered doctors from its medical education system by 1913, whereas China had only 500 medical students in training in all the missionary apprenticeship programs, hospital-schools, and union medical schools throughout China.[20] After the Boxer Rebellion and China's defeat in the Sino-Japanese War, the Qing government made belated reforms. The New Policies in 1909 "ordered every Chinese provincial capital to establish 'government medical schools' with hospitals, similar to the special medical schools in Japan," though this would not happen for decades.[21]

Public education of any kind for girls was a new phenomenon in China in the early 1900s, one that many reformers encouraged at the end of the Qing dynasty and especially around the time of the New Culture Movement.[22] This movement's participants aimed to bring China into the modern world with social reforms that sought, in part, to redefine the family and society. Included were goals of public education, free marriage, equality for women, and the end of footbinding.[23] In 1907, the Chinese government issued regulations for girls' normal and elementary schools. They deemed the highest level of education for girls the normal school, which, depending on the school, was roughly equivalent to the American junior high or high school. There were no colleges for women aside from those run by foreign missions. The curriculum for girls' elementary education was one year shorter than that for boys, and elementary co-education was allowed if there were not enough girls to form their own class.[24] This was a significant step forward for educating women and girls, as previously there was little education for them, although the classes were still mostly sex segregated until the early 1920s.

In 1912, after the Republic was founded, the newly created central Ministry of Education revamped the educational system to include at least theoretical equality of male and female education. The term for school, *xuetang*, was changed to *xuexiao*, which "signifies a democratic turn in the conception of education" and stressed the importance the new government placed on basic public primary education.[25] Throughout this period, the various governments stressed the move from traditional Confucian education based on traditional, individual morality to a public, civic morality, especially during the Nanjing decade.[26] The new ministry divided the educational system into 18 years containing four years of lower primary, three years of higher primary, four years of middle school, and six years of college. Students began school at age six or seven, and those graduating from college were 26 or 27 years of age. According to national education statistics for China, between 1907 and 1918–19 the number of girls in elementary schools rose from 11,936 to 215,626. Still, in 1918–19 girls comprised only 5.4 percent of all students in elementary schools.[27] By 1923, the percentage of all female students in non-mission schools was 6.3 percent, an increase from .07 percent in 1906.[28]

The Ministry of Education passed the University Act in 1912, which standardized a four-year medical curriculum and established provincial medical schools in Beijing and Hangzhou the same year, with two more the following year in Suzhou and Wuchang. These Medical Special Colleges (for men only) were staffed mainly by Chinese graduates of Japanese four-year second-grade medical colleges.[29] The Ministry of Education standardized their curriculum in 1912 and included obstetrics and gynecology, with practical obstetrical training using manikins.[30] The Medical Special Colleges came under attack in the 1920s by League of Nations Health Organization advisers, Chinese medical leaders, and Nationalist government administrators critical of the quality of the Chinese medical personnel who ran them. They began to close in the late 1920s.[31] Regulations for special medical schools (*yixue zhuanmen xuexiao*) were also enacted. The course of study was for four years preceded by one year of premedical and more than one year of postgraduate studies.[32] In 1912, medicine was divided into the fields of medicine and pharmacy, and premedical courses were required for admission to either. In 1917, the medical course of study was raised from four to five years.[33]

The 1921 and 1922 conferences of Provincial Educational Associations, held in Guangzhou and Jinan, respectively, restructured the educational system and included provisions for four-year national technical colleges. Co-education was allowed and was common in the lower primary grades. Several national colleges adopted co-education, though in practice upper primary and middle schools were still sex segregated.[34] Even in national co-educational colleges and universities, the number of female students was very small; for example, there were 11 female and 2,246 male students at the National University of Beijing in 1923.[35] The conference members also encouraged the creation of more elementary and secondary vocational schools for girls, which were on the same standing as girls' normal schools.[36] Vocational colleges included specialty curricula in midwifery, nursing, and medicine, as well as in business and handiwork like embroidery and dressmaking. The number of girls' vocational schools, mostly private institutions, grew from 21 in 1916 to 158 in 1922. In 1923, the Joint Conference of Education and Industry in Jiangsu passed a resolution to establish a provincial girls' vocational school.[37]

The majority of colleges were in urban areas. In 1923, Beijing had 37 colleges, and Jiangsu had 15. Eleven provinces had either only one or no colleges. Beijing had the largest number of female college students, with 653. Nationwide, there were 847 female college students of a total of 34,880 college students in China. Women comprised 7.13 percent of all students in secondary vocational schools, with 1,452 of 20,360 total students. Again, Beijing had the largest number of these students, 617. The number of females in elementary vocational schools was greatest in Jiangsu, perhaps because of the large missionary influence and silk industry there. There were none in Beijing. Female students of this kind comprised 1,757 of a total of 20,467 vocational students nationwide.[38]

By this time, China had eight union medical schools for men, at Mukden, Beijing, Jinan, Hankou, Chengdu, Nanjing/Hangzhou, Fuzhou, and Guangzhou. In addition, there were three medical schools for women: Hackett in Guangzhou, Suzhou under Margaret Polk, and the Union Medical College for Women in Beijing.[39] Out of the 815 students enrolled in medical schools in 1923, 17 were girls. They were all in urban areas, leaving the vast majority of China's population untouched by Western medical influence. Furthermore, there were no enforced national standardized curricula or registration, thus no uniformity among admissions requirements or training. In addition to these legitimate schools, there was still unofficial training of medical personnel in various hospitals throughout China.[40] None of these schools had many students. Some Chinese women studied medicine in the United States, Europe, or Japan, though these were few. In 1919, there were 63 Chinese women studying in America in all fields, and 65 in 1920, and most overseas Chinese students did not choose to study medicine.[41]

Boxer Indemnity money that the United States remitted to China between 1908 and 1917 was used to found Qinghua (Tsinghua) University and to send Chinese men and women to study in the United States. Qinghua was established in 1911 as a junior college to prepare students for study in the United States on Boxer scholarships. In the first 18 years of the program 1,300 men and women were sent abroad.[42] The program was initially designed to send 10 female students for a five-year course of study in America every other year, but those numbers were not met.[43] No students were sent in 1920 or 1922, and as of 1923, Qinghua dedicated only three percent of its total scholarship money to sending women students abroad and proposed to stop sending women altogether. Several educational and women's organizations challenged this proposal, so Qinghua planned to send five female students in 1923.[44]

Formal education for women, even by the 1920s, was dismal, and women's medical education was almost nonexistent, but change was rapid and forthcoming. The idea that women could and should be educated was spreading. This major shift in gender identity, that women were worthy of an education and that they could help to build a new China, gave them more opportunities and opened the medical field to them. The cooperation between European and American medical missionaries and local gentry and officials allowed the Nationalist government to rapidly adopt public health and medical education measures in the 1930s.

Gradually, Chinese women entered the medical field, often as low-level technicians trained by the medical missionaries discussed in chapter 1, and although medicine was not a prestigious field, they gained experience that allowed them in some cases to pursue further education or to encourage others to do the same.[45] These women opened the doors for the professional midwives who were to follow. As women became nurses and medical helpers (and later midwives), and medicine became more and more regulated under the expanding arm of the state, women too were subject to more regulation. There exists a gradual but definite move towards centralized government control over public health and the medical field, as well as greater cooperation between Western and Chinese institutions, during the Nationalist era. The scattered and erratic medical training in early twentieth-century China formed the basis on which Nationalist public health policies were built, and the foundation for childbirth reform in the twentieth century.

THE FIRST NATIONAL MIDWIFERY SCHOOL

The seed of modern maternal and child health in China was developed by Dr. John B. Grant, a member of the Rockefeller Foundation's International Health Division and chairman of Peking University Medical College's Department of Public Health; and Dr. Yang Chongrui, a Western-trained obstetrician. Grant was born in Ningbo, China, to medical missionary parents, and then educated at the medical schools of the University of Michigan and Johns Hopkins University.[46] A staunch public health advocate, Dr. Grant was the primary supporter of public health activity in and around Beijing. Grant focused on improving school hygiene and establishing community health centers like Beijing's First Health Demonstration Station.[47] He was also instrumental in getting funding and approval from the Rockefeller Foundation for midwifery training, writing that the high infant mortality rate caused by tetanus neonatorum was "one of the outstanding public health problems" facing China, one easily controllable by creating midwifery training programs.[48] Grant noted that several governmental and private midwifery schools had been established in China in the previous 15 years, but that the best government-run one (in Taiyuanfu, Shanxi Province) "would not qualify for the lowest standards of midwifery schools in northern Europe."[49] Likewise, the private schools run by Hackett Medical School in Guangzhou and St. Elizabeth's in Shanghai produced "moderately well-trained graduates."[50]

In the 1920s, Grant urged the establishment of a midwifery division within the municipal health department in Beijing to help control infant and maternal mortality. Until that time, there had been no agency to train or supervise old-style midwives, widely considered the leading cause of maternal and infant death. In one 1200-person village outside of Beijing that he had visited, Grant found an 80 percent infant mortality rate over a 10-year period "due solely to the peculiarly dirty habits of the single midwife of the village."[51] In a letter to his colleague Dr. Victor Heiser, Grant recounted the story of a merchant from that same village who had come to his office "with tears in his eyes—an unusual thing for Chinese men—and stated he had lost all of his six consecutive sons within the first week of life from 'wind' disease."[52] According to Grant, the three previous governors of Beijing had been interested in solving the midwife problem by controlling traditional midwives, but because of political instability the China Medical Board had been hesitant to collaborate on any significant municipal public health efforts.[53] By 1926, Grant believed that the local government was stable enough to move forward with a plan to develop a midwifery division within the health department. He repeatedly prodded the Rockefeller Foundation's International Health Division to support and fund the fledgling midwifery program. The following year, Beijing cooperated with the Guomindang government to open a municipal midwifery training school. [54]

With Grant's support, Dr. Yang Chongrui pioneered midwifery training in early twentieth-century China and helped to transform childbirth in China from a family-centred, unregulated event into a state-controlled institutional practice. Born in 1891 at the American Board Mission in present-day Tong County of Beijing to a wealthy Christian family, Yang's educational opportunities were remarkable. Her father taught her to read at an early age and sent her to American mission schools in Beijing, and she went on to graduate in 1917 from the Women's Union Medical College, a precursor to Peking Union Medical College, where she eventually specialized in obstetrics and gynecology.[55]

In an autobiographical essay reflecting on her career, Yang recounted two experiences that solidified her commitment to community maternal and child health work.[56] The first incident occurred when a pregnant woman came to her Qihuamenwai clinic in Beijing after being in labor for several days. She was carried to the hospital, but by then it was too late. Nothing could be done to save her because her uterus had ruptured. According to Yang, this tragedy could have been prevented if the woman had had access to modern prenatal care, even at a small rural clinic. The second experience was the receipt of a letter written in 1924 by a man in the Beijing countryside to PUMC's surgical department that read, "Your surgical skills are good. But we don't know how to safely deliver babies, to keep children from dying, or what medicine to take."[57] Long discussions with Grant about this letter led Yang to make a connection between general public health and infant and maternal health. These two events—the woman's dying in labor and Yang's receipt of the letter—spurred Yang to undertake the "virgin territory" of public health work, and she began by conducting two rural tetanus neonatorum studies to determine how best to go about preventing this primary cause of infant death.[58]

Yang continued to work and study at Peking Union Medical College, combining obstetrics and gynecology with an interest in public health. In 1926, she received a one-year fellowship to the United States to study obstetrics and gynecology at the Johns Hopkins University School of Hygiene and Public Health in Baltimore, Maryland, and followed that with a six-month tour of Canada, England, Scotland, Germany, France, Denmark, and other European countries to observe their obstetrics/gynecology and public health education programs. After returning to Peking Union Medical College with greater knowledge of public health problems and programs worldwide, Yang assumed a joint post as assistant professor of public health and head of the First Health Demonstration Station in Beijing, an urban experimental health center that included maternal and infant health work.

Among her patients, Yang repeatedly encountered cases of tetanus neonatorum and puerperal sepsis, two preventable diseases that greatly contributed to China's high infant and maternal mortality rates. Asserting that the six million annual preventable deaths in China occurred primarily among infants and childbearing women, and that "the main responsibility for the excessive deaths among the mothers and babies may be laid on the untrained group [of old-style Chinese midwives, or *jieshengpo*]"—which she estimated to number 400,000—Yang knew that maternal and infant health were crucial factors in improving the general health of any population.[59] Thus with the help of the Nationalist government and colleague John B. Grant, Yang began to formulate a national program of midwifery reform for China, beginning with midwifery education and culminating in the creation of a government agency to regulate midwifery, the National Midwifery Board, which is discussed in more detail in chapter 4.

Yang's approach to midwifery education was a unique adaptation from medical training in the United States and was meant to address China's immediate needs. China had neither the money nor the physicians necessary to deliver all its babies in the manner that Yang and others were advocating, that is, in a clinic or hospital setting attended by a highly trained physician. She also recognized that the continued use of current birthing practices and traditional midwives would not easily be displaced. She and Grant originally thought to recruit women with elementary school educations and give them abbreviated basic midwifery training, perhaps for two to six months. However, they worried that these women would soon be lost to social and scientific advances, and that these semi-trained midwives would quickly become antiquated. Therefore, Yang established a plan for a national midwifery school, which she presented at the Seventh Annual Meeting of the Chinese Medical Association in 1928, along with a proposed dual-level midwife training structure. The lower level training consisted of short midwifery courses of two and six months' duration that stressed quantity and basic modern maternal and child health knowledge. Some of these courses aimed at retraining the *jieshengpo* in aseptic birth procedures. Upon completion of this course, the *jieshengpo* were required to register with the government and apply for a license to practice. Yang promoted the training courses as an efficient way to quickly reduce the high death rates associated with childbirth.

However, the Chinese had an enduring distrust and superstition surrounding childbirth, and of midwives as unscrupulous old hucksters; as we have seen, distrust of midwives in China is evident in writings from the seventh century onwards.[60] If Yang and her cohorts did not improve the image of midwives, these commonly accepted biases would continue, both preventing talented women from entering the profession and sustaining midwives' poor public image. To address this social and cultural problem, Yang proposed the creation of a higher level training program with entrance requirements that included a high school-level education. The higher level midwifery course, which stressed quality education, comprised a two-year course for a smaller number of higher level students that provided more detailed training in midwifery and required an internship. The proposed midwifery school would thus have to have its own, or an affiliated, maternity hospital in order to meet the practicum requirements. Graduates of this program would be well-educated and well-trained, could keep up with advances in medicine, and would "stand on their own two feet" (*keyi liwen liang jiao*).[61] Yang hoped to create a midwifery profession with increased legitimacy, effectively eliminating the need for lower-level training in three years' time.[62] This professional training would first begin at the school Yang helped to establish, the First National Midwifery School, affiliated with Peking Union Medical College and funded largely by the Rockefeller Foundation's China Medical Board.

The purpose of the First National Midwifery School, as Yang Chongrui had outlined, was to serve as a "higher normal" school for other midwifery schools nationwide, a training center for midwives who would in turn train others around the country. According to Yang, "the development of midwifery practice in China should be an integral part of maternity and child health, rather than merely an obstetrical procedure as [is] the common practice in other countries."[63] In other words, proper midwifery techniques were crucial to improving general maternal and child health. While Yang's new midwifery utilized all the technological advances and scientific medicine, it was not to be detached from the larger national public health goals. Nor was it to be removed to the hospital whereby only those with money, connections, or in close proximity would be able to take advantage of scientific midwifery. Yang would bring her midwifery to the people, through clinics, community centers, home visits, and especially the Beiping Child Health Institute and the local Health Demonstration Stations.

The school saw rapid growth and expansion. In 1929, the First National Midwifery School had facilities to house 40 midwifery students. By 1934, the number of students and patients in the maternity hospital increased so much that the school had to be enlarged. The school purchased and remodeled new grounds and buildings for a new 120-student dormitory. Some maternity patients then moved into the previous dormitory site for a total of 70 to 80 beds.[64] During the 1934–35 school year, the school purchased an additional seven *mu* of land with several buildings on it used to house a 20-student library, and to add two classrooms, a school health room, an infirmary, two offices, a 350-seat auditorium, and dormitory space for an additional 100 students. The cost of the land, buildings, remodeling, and new furniture was $53,867.49, all of which came from local gifts to the school.[65] This addition brought the total number of hospital beds to 76, of which 58 were public beds, 14 special beds for septic cases in isolation wards, and four semi-private beds. The clinic space grew from two to five examination rooms, and the clinic records room and laboratory were enlarged, while the waiting room was reduced in size since it was not necessary for patients to wait as long because of the increased number of examination rooms.[66]

TRAINING MODERN MIDWIVES

The new midwife and her profession required a new name to distinguish her from the midwives of the past—*zhuchanshi*. The terminology that the First National Midwifery School created to describe and delineate the activities of the new midwives is significant. *Jieshengpo* literally means "old woman who receives the birth." This term refers to a likely illiterate peasant woman with no institutionalized training, her knowledge gained from personal experience and as an apprentice. On the other hand, *zhuchanshi*, which was the name applied to graduates of the First National Midwifery School's higher-level course, literally means "birth helper," with the suffix *shi* denoting a scholar or an educated person, similar to the new terminology for nurse, *hushi*, literally meaning "caring scholar" or "professional caregiver."[67] This dramatic change in naming is an important characteristic representative of the process to create the new, modern, scientifically trained *zhuchanshi*, separating them from the activities of the old, illiterate, and superstitious *jieshengpo*.

The curricula that modern midwifery schools created and instituted were based on Western scientific principles of childbirth in which the mother's body was treated as a reproductive machine and the pregnant body as ill or diseased. The six-month advanced maternity course offered by the First National Midwifery School illustrates the focus on the scientific nature of childbirth. The 136 hours of coursework included anatomy and physiology of female reproductive organs, embryology, abnormal labors, hemorrhage, puerperal sepsis, pregnancy toxemia and eclampsia, heart disease, tuberculosis, the use of instruments, labor induction, caesarean section, reconstructive operations, use of drugs during pregnancy and labor, extrauterine pregnancy, twins and "monsters" (fetal neural tube defects), antenatal care, urinalysis, and diseases of the newborn.[68]

This contemporary view of pregnancy set the modern midwives apart from their traditional counterparts, who largely viewed pregnancy and birth as normal social events. It is clear that modern beliefs were adopted in midwifery school curricula in China, though it is unclear whether or how much the modern midwives altered their daily practices when treating their pregnant and parturient patients. Judging from some of the midwifery school yearbooks that contain writings by their students, the new midwives seem to have wholeheartedly adopted modern medical beliefs. These publications are necessarily polemical, as they are, after all, the official products of modern midwifery schools. There were no courses in psychology, bedside manner, grief counseling, pain management, or other means to make the birth more comfortable for the mother or her family members. The graduated midwives were not allowed to use instruments or attempt version unless the mother's life was in jeopardy and no other medical help was available.[69]

The First National Midwifery School took a multifaceted approach to delivering modern childbirth to China, which is reflected in the different courses aimed at students and midwives with varying levels of education. The curricula of some programs were adjusted over the years "to meet practical conditions," while some programs like a six-month fast-track course were discontinued with no reason given in the annual reports.[70] The higher-level courses of six months and two years formed a cadre of professional modern midwives, and various shorter programs were aimed at lower-level midwifery students and *jieshengpo*. In addition, courses were offered not only at the school itself, but also at community public health centers throughout Beijing, which served to rapidly disseminate modern methods of midwifery. The curricula for the higher level courses varied, but all courses were taught in Chinese and included "party principles," sociology, and Chinese language, in addition to the science courses and practicum. The students performed physical exercises for 15 minutes every morning and attended a monthly two-hour hygiene lecture with the intention to mold the physical body as well as the mind.[71]

The higher-level courses aimed to create a modern midwifery profession, as reflected in the entrance requirements. Students entering the six-month and two-year programs were required to be unmarried middle school graduates of "good character and in good health" who had successfully passed the First National Midwifery School entrance examinations.[72] There were few differences between the six-month candidates and the two-year candidates. The two-year program required previous primary school courses in Chinese and basic science, while the six-month program only specified graduation from higher primary or junior middle school. In addition, the age requirements for each program varied. Six-month course candidates had to be between 25 and 35 years of age, while the two-year program accepted 20 to 30 year olds. The six-month course candidates would have accrued work experience and study of nursing or midwifery before matriculating at the First National Midwifery School, which may explain the higher age range. No tuition was charged for First National Midwifery School students, but each student had to pay $10 for her own board and lodging for a one-month probationary period. Those who passed probation had to pay $100 for board and lodging, $50 for miscellaneous expenses, and $6 for physical exercise and medical expenses, for a total of $156 per year. Students also had to provide their own textbooks and uniforms. Furthermore, they were required to supply a letter of guarantee with a deposit of $20 to be refunded upon graduation. The letter of guarantee stated that if a student was dismissed for violating the regulations or left the school before her studies were completed, the student or her guarantor would be responsible for paying the school for expenses incurred by the student, equivalent to $30 per semester.[73] The two-year course was the most expensive of the programs, costing the school $3,036.30 per student.[74] The total cost for the school per student for the six-month course was $759.08.[75]

The Two-Year Midwifery Course was the backbone of the First National Midwifery School, intended to "safeguard the qualification and the standard of the midwifery profession."[76] This course, along with the six-month course, represented "permanent national instruction for qualification considered satisfactory" and was under the auspices of the national Department of Education.[77] Its graduates "would be-come leaders—teachers, organizers, and supervisors of 'quantity' short course schools" throughout China.[78] By 1932, 30 students had enrolled in this course.[79] The curriculum was rigorous, consisting of 148.5 hours of anatomy and physiology, 142 hours of normal midwifery, and more than 3,500 hours of practical experience in the antenatal clinic, delivery room, and postnatal ward (see table 3.1). Upon completion, these midwives would be able to attend even abnormal emergency cases. Each student was required to examine 50 antenatal, postpartum, and well-baby cases each, and to attend 25 deliveries. There were eight students in the Two-Year Course in 1931 and 14 in 1932.[80] By 1932, there were more applications than spaces available for students, so the school increased the rigor of the entrance examination. Seventy was the passing grade for all subjects, and failure in one course prevented graduation. Upon graduating, the students were eligible for registra-tion with the National Midwifery Board. In 1935, the Ministry of Education increased the mandatory training period for midwives from two to three years at the suggestion of the National Midwifery Board.[81]

In addition to training modern midwives, the First National Midwifery School extended its reach throughout China by providing supplemental training to graduates of other nursing and midwifery schools. Through Yang Chongrui, the First National Midwifery School worked closely with the Nationalist government to create a national maternal and child health program. As a founding member of the Na-tional Midwifery Board, Yang helped to construct the education and licensing requirements for both *jieshengpo* and modern midwives. Thus, although numerous private and provincial nursing, medical, and midwifery schools existed throughout China, the First National Mid-wifery School was the center of midwifery training, effectively setting national curriculum standards and providing specialized midwifery courses for those who had received training elsewhere in order to meet the new national requirements.

The Graduate Courses for Nurses and Midwives helped to spread the ideas of the First National Midwifery School and standardize maternal and child health training and practice nationwide. By 1929, there were more than 142 nurse training schools in China, 18 of which operated a "nurse-midwifery" course consisting of one year's training in a maternity ward after completing the regular nursing classes. The Nurses' Association of China "granted a special certificate to gradu-ates of this course."[82] When the First National Midwifery School was founded, the Nurses' Association of China turned midwifery train-ing over to the National Midwifery Board. To meet the government

Table 3.1. Curriculum for the Two-Year Midwifery Course of the First National Midwifery School, Beijing, 1932–33. Reproduced from FNMS, *Second Annual Report*, Peiping, July 1, 1930–June 30, 1931.

	First Academic Year		Second Academic Year		Total	Total hours for each subject
	First Semester	Second Semester	First Semester	Second Semester		
	Hours per week		Hours per week			
Anatomy & Physiology	5	4			9	148.5
Nursing	2				2	41
First Aid	1				1	20
Bacteriology	2				2	50
Materia Medica	4				4	82
Party Principles	1	1			2	40
Chinese	1	1	1	1	4	80
Sociology		2			2	30
Urinalysis		1			1	21
Midwifery (normal)		4	3		7	142
Care & feeding of children		2	2		4	82
Hygiene		2			2	41
Gynecology			2		2	41
Midwifery (abnormal)				2	2	41
Dietetics				1	1	20
Dermatology				1	1	20
Bedside instruction			2		2	40
Model demonstration			2		2	40
Clinic practice (antenatal)		6	6	6	18	369
Delivery room practice (midwifery)			4	4	8	190
Ward practice (postnatal)	30	30	42	42	144	2,952
	46	53	64	57	220	4,526.5*

Hours: theory   = 1,015.5
Hours: practice = 3,511.0
Total hours   = 4,526.5

*These numbers are not accurately calculated in the original table.

requirements for midwife registration, the First National Midwifery School began a special course for nurses and nurse-midwives who were members of the Nurses' Association of China. The Six-Month Course for Graduate Nurses admitted students who had already completed nursing school and desired specialized instruction in obstetrics (see table 3.2). The curriculum was an accelerated form of the Two-Year Course. The first class opened in July 1931 and focused on delivery room practice and community health work, for a total of 132 hours of coursework and practicum combined.[83] Even these nurses were taught to refer abnormal cases to physicians.

A special Six-Month Graduate Course for Midwives was started in 1932 to give additional training to graduates of provincial or other registered private midwifery schools, as the First National Midwifery School was the first place in the country to provide complete midwifery training with required practical field work. Upon graduation, the students were to return to their home institutions to continue their work. The First National Midwifery School was thus able to extend its reach beyond Beijing. As Yang stated, "It was felt that this would be helpful in raising midwifery standards throughout the country and

Table 3.2. Curriculum for Six-Month Course for Graduate Nurses of the First National Midwifery School, Beijing, 1932–33. Reproduced from FNMS, *Second Annual Report.*

	1st and 2nd month Hours/week	3rd and 4th month Hours/week	5th and 6th month Hours/week
Abnormal midwifery			3
Midwifery	6	6	
Urinalysis	3		
Care and feeding of children	2	2	
Dietetics	2		
Party Principles	1	1	
Chinese	1	1	
Sociology	2	2	
Hygiene	1	2	2
Gynecology		2	
Antenatal clinic	6	8	18
Delivery room practice	20	10	10
District work		10	11
Total	44	44	44

would also help the Central Government to enforce registration regulations of midwifery schools."[84] The National Health Administration offered fellowships to selected students. The course was limited to 10 students per term who would study "Ethics of the Midwifery Profession," obstetrics, public health, and delivery and obstetrics ward practicum. Additionally, each student was required to handle 10 hospital and five home deliveries, for a total of 1,198 classroom and practicum hours.[85] Most students in the first year were from Jiangsu Province, where Yang Chongrui had undertaken significant consulting work to improve the area's maternal and child health services. By 1934, six rural *xian* (county)-level maternity hospitals in Jiangsu were under the supervision of graduates from this course.[86] Fourteen students were in this course in 1934–35, with 12 graduates that year.[87]

The Two-Month Refresher Course was given twice yearly "as a supplementary course for midwives who have received certificates from unregistered schools," thus bringing these women under the new midwifery requirements.[88] By the time that the First National Midwifery School was founded, there were between 45 and 50 private midwifery schools in China that had issued certificates to hundreds of women, most of whom had never had clinical instruction and had received, according to Yang, only "poor theoretical instruction."[89] This refresher course allowed these midwives to "make up for the deficiencies of their training" and ultimately apply for government registration after successful completion of the course. By 1932, this program had 14 students from five different midwifery schools.[90] The course consisted of 24 hours of instruction in delivery equipment, physiology or normal and abnormal presentations, and care of the infant and mother (see table 3.3). In addition, each student received practical experience in handling five delivery cases on average of four hours each (20 hours), plus 20 hours of antenatal clinic and 30 hours of postpartum visits (six hours per each of the five delivery cases), for a total of 94 hours of coursework and practicum.[91] This course was discontinued by 1934 and replaced by the Six-Month Graduate Course.

The First National Midwifery School also provided clerkships (internships) to its own midwifery students "to broaden the viewpoint in the future public health field, to learn the different methods of administration and teaching in other places than the Midwifery School, and to compare the financial conditions, the purposes and the results obtained in the different places."[92] The students were to spend one week each in the Director's Office, the Registration and Records Office, and the First Health Demonstration Station; and two weeks in the Beiping Child Health Institute, PUMC's Department of Obstetrics and

Table 3.3. Two-Month Refresher Course, First National Midwifery School. Reproduced from First National Midwifery School, Peiping, 1932.

Course Name	Total Hours
Duties of the midwife	2
Examination of pregnant woman	2
Equipment and supplies for delivery	2
Methods of aseptic delivery	2
Care of the newborn infant	2
Care of the postpartum mother	2
Physiology of normal presentation	2
Pathology of abnormal presentation	1
Anatomy and physiology of the female genitals	1
Midwifery	3
Care and prevention of infant's and children's diseases	1
How to deal with and prevent abnormal cases from the midwife's point of view	4
Total	24

Gynecology, and the First National Midwifery School's Dean's Office. A written summary of the previous day's experiences, together with comments and suggestions, was due each morning. While at the Director's Office, the clerks followed the Director on her inspections of the city's women's hospitals and those that housed maternity wards. The Registration and Records Office showed the clerks how to keep an efficient filing and record-keeping system, which included patients' files. This kind of documentation was crucial to modern medicine's reach in affecting community lifestyles and behaviors, as discussed by Stefani Pfeiffer in her work on the PUMC Social Services Department.[93] During the Health Demonstration Station rotation, the clerks accompanied "public health visitors" to schools, neighborhoods, and factories to spread the word about nutrition, hygiene, infectious diseases, and sanitation. They also assisted in the ante- and postpartum clinics, as well as the surgical clinic and school health clinic.

While at the Beiping Child Health Institute, the clerks attended mothercraft classes and demonstrations and supervised old-style midwives (see figures 3.1 and 3.2). They also participated in research projects and investigations and made home visits. The rotation at PUMC's Department of OB/GYN gave the clerks opportunities to observe medical obstetrical and gynecological procedures, such as salpingo-oophorectomy (removal of fallopian tubes and ovaries), hysterectomy, and cesarean section. They accompanied the attending physician on gynecology, maternity, and nursery ward rounds and attended lectures on difficult pregnancies and labor. The Dean's Office taught the students "how to [be] in charge and responsible," how to keep files and records of grades, make schedules, and run ante- and postpartum clinics—in short, how to be an effective administrator.[94] The First National Midwifery School also offered a three-week rotation in maternal and child health for fourth-year Peking Union Medical College students. They were to live at the school and observe administration, teaching, and midwifery practice. Furthermore, the PUMC clerks observed administration and technical and educational activities at the Child Health Institute, and made special trips to foundling homes and other organizations. Midwifery clerkships thus gave students practical experience of the principles taught in their lectures and coursework. These students were expected to "take their place satisfactorily in the community health organization as they must be possessed of a background which is insufficiently given only through a didactic course."[95] To be effective administrators, they learned how to run a modern clinic, health station, or school, thus extending the modern medical model outside Beijing.

RETRAINING *JIESHENGPO*

The number of modern midwives trained in China in the 1920s and 1930s was minuscule when compared to the number of old-style midwives who continued to assist the majority of births. To rapidly bring the *jieshengpo* into the modern world of childbirth, the First National Midwifery School partnered with the newly formed Beiping Midwifery Commission that had been appointed to act as an advisory committee to the Beiping Municipal Health Department after the Guomindang established its new central government in Nanjing in 1927.[96] Under this arrangement, in November 1928 the Beiping Child Health Institute began to offer courses for *jieshengpo*, the only course under local, instead of national, auspices. This program correlated teaching with community outreach and control and supervision of local midwifery practices.

The "'improved' old-style midwives were to 'serve as a screen which can detect abnormal and pathological cases and direct them to adequate medical attention.'"[97] These *jieshengpo* had originally received informal, practical instruction by learning from and observing other experienced midwives during deliveries. The old-style midwifery courses (see figure

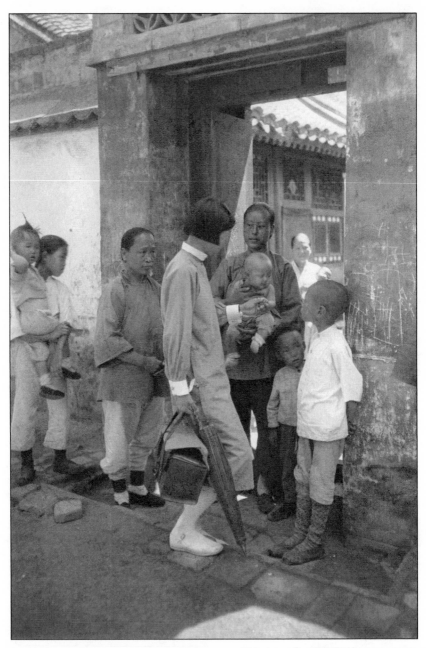

Figure 3.1.   A Mother Proudly Displays How Well Her Baby Is Growing. Courtesy of the Rockefeller Archive Center.

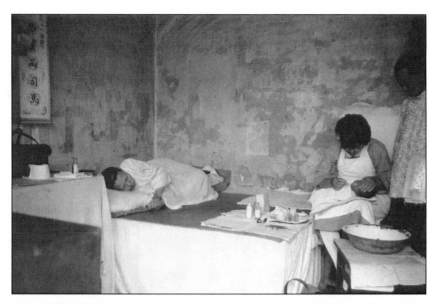

Figure 3.2. The "Kong" Makes an Excellent Table for Demonstrating to the Mother Newborn Care As It Serves Two Purposes: Mother's Bed, Baby's Toilet Table. Courtesy of the Rockefeller Archive Center.

3.3) therefore aimed to *retrain* the *jieshengpo* in aseptic normal childbirth, proper dressing of the umbilical cord, and the ability "to recognize danger signs in order to refer abnormal cases to physicians."[98] They were forbidden to use forceps, attempt to manipulate the position of the fetus in the womb, or perform any kind of invasive or surgical procedure. A supervisor was assigned to each midwifery student to "check technique and the quality of work by close supervision of the strict regulation [*sic*]," and the retrained graduates were required to submit two reports for each birth.[99] The *jieshengpo* graduates of the short retraining programs were instructed to "explain to their patients the benefit of their training to prevent puerperal fever and tetanus neonatorum and the required supervision [of labour and birth]. . . . They are obliged to urge every family to adopt and to accept the 'aseptic' method."[100]

The courses to retrain *jieshengpo* were taught by demonstration (see figure 3.4) and met six hours per week for two months and covered "cleanliness and asepsis, methods of conducting normal delivery, methods of tying and cutting the cord, methods of resuscitation, post-natal care, female anatomy and physiology."[101] According to a 1929 report by Yang Chongrui on midwifery training and supervision, the students attended lectures, demonstrations, and review sessions given by an ob-

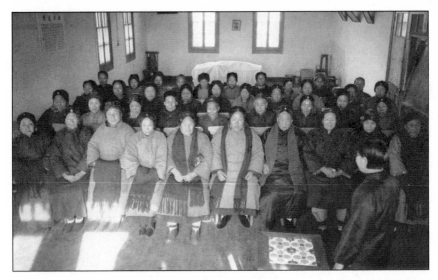

Figure 3.3. First National Midwifery School Short Course for Old-Style Midwives. Courtesy of the Rockefeller Archive Center.

stetrician or a well-trained *zhuchanshi*, consisting of 36 to 46 hours of instruction each month, divided into two- or three-hour periods.[102] The *jieshengpo* courses stressed aseptic methods of childbirth, called the "improved method," as evidenced by the final exam, which consisted of five questions. The first two were practical, and the latter two oral:

1. Prepare for delivery (washing hands?)
2. Demonstrate method of tying and dressing a cord (cleanliness used?)
3. Demonstrate care of a new born (bath & prophylactic eye treatment)
4. State care at labor—avoidance of Post partum hemorrhage, Puerperal fever
5. Differenciate [sic] between normal and abnormal labours and give care of each[103]

Although it seems that the Beiping Child Health Institute was not lacking students (each month a new class of 30 *jieshengpo* matriculated), Yang Chongrui complained of a considerable problem with attendance rates. Her report dated December 1928 stated that one-third of the students could be characterized as "fair," while one-third was "learning pretty well" and attended classes fairly regularly. However,

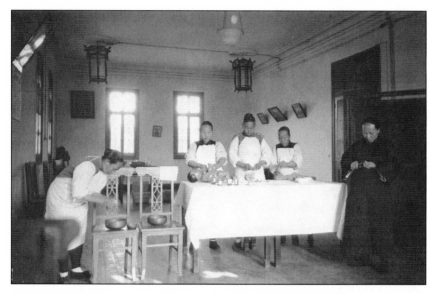

Figure 3.4.   Old-Type Midwives Teaching Demonstration, Right to Left: 1. Cut Nails; 2. Baby's Eye Drop—Silver Nitrate 1%; 3. Method of Tie Umb. Cord; 4. Method of the First Bath; 5. Method of Cleaning Hands before Delivery. *Second Annual Report*, First National Midwifery School, 1931. Courtesy of the Rockefeller Archive Center.

one-third of the group was an "entire failure" because "1) they do not attend class regularly . . . 2) they are 'too old' to see or hear as there are three students aged between 65–75, 3) they 'know too much' to learn for more [*sic*]."[104] The average age of these students was 54. The second class started on January 7, 1929, with 30 students (average age of 51), 19 of whom passed the final exam (only 26 completed the course). Yang again complained of poor attendance, this time of 35 percent, which she explained by saying that the students came from a distant area that was suffering from inclement weather. In March 1929, only 60 percent of the students (18 out of 30) were allowed to take their final exams, the remainder having missed too many classes. Seventeen out of those 18 did pass the exams, five with honors (grades over 85). By March 1929, the situation was improving somewhat, with 26–29 percent absent. In the first eight months, 106 midwives had completed the course, of which 76 passed their exams and were allowed to register with the government. By 1932, the Beiping Child Health Institute had trained 268 *jieshengpo*, as compared to only 107 modern midwives trained by the First National Midwifery School.[105]

Aside from the trouble of attending classes, the *jieshengpo* faced several other obstacles to properly carrying out their modernized work.

The first was financial. The midwives were restricted from charging high delivery fees (maximum two dollars) or refusing services to the poor. A 1929 report suggested that the Health Demonstration Area under the Beiping Department of Public Health may have provided financial aid for poor families to utilize the services of retrained *jieshengpo*. The average expenditure for materials needed for an aseptic delivery was $.30 (umbilical cord tie, liquid paraffin, alcohol, Lysol, soap, silver nitrate). According to Yang Chongrui, an average delivery fee of $1.50 per case should have been sufficient to *maintain* the old-type midwives' living standards. They were not intended to make more money as a result of their specialized training. Despite their meager earning potential, upon graduation the retrained *jieshengpo* were required to purchase a "delivery bag (basket) [which] was considered absolutely necessary for students."[106] In each graduating class, the student with the highest final exam grade received one of these as a gift from the local Health Commissioner. The delivery basket consisted of aprons, towels, sterile cord ties, scissors, medicine dropper, basin, brush, soap, Lysol, boric acid, alcohol, silver nitrate, liquid paraffin, and bottles with cork stoppers. At a cost of five dollars each, most of the midwives were unable to purchase the kit, and the school budget did not include this cost. The Beiping Child Health Institute addressed this problem with the City Health Commissioner at the January meeting of the local Midwifery Commission in January 1929, whereupon it was decided to ask for help from local officials' wives. By the end of January, the Midwifery Commission had received $430 contributed towards purchase of the delivery baskets in Beijing. The midwives paid what they could and the Commission contributed the remainder. Other local groups and individuals also donated to this two-month retraining program. According to the 1928–29 budget, in April 1928 an "earnest Buddhist" contributed $1,000 to the Beiping Department of Police toward the training of these old-style midwives.[107] Despite this gesture, most of the retrained *jieshengpo* lacked even the basic tools necessary to perform their duties. Those with the delivery bag carried a symbolic message of cleanliness and modernity, echoing the symbols of visual modernity discussed in chapter 2. Their uniform, seen in figure 3.5, is a blend of the traditional padded jacket with mandarin collar done up in white, the color of cleanliness and modernity.

The second obstacle in recreating the vocation of the *jieshengpo* relates to the retrained *jieshengpo*'s social place among other midwives. The retrained *jieshengpo* did not fit into the group of modern midwives, as the former remained illiterate and of a different social standing. Neither could they remain in their old social group among the other untrained *jieshengpo*, as now they were licensed and utilized

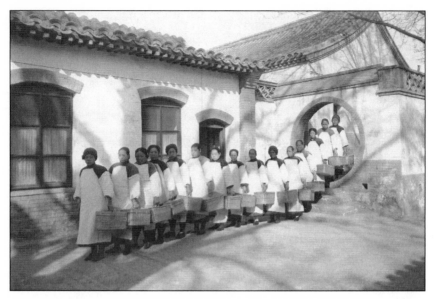

Figure 3.5. First National Midwifery School Class of Trained Old-Style Midwives. *First National Midwifery School Annual Report,* **1929. Courtesy of the Rockefeller Archive Center.**

modern childbirth methods. They existed in the fringe between the old and the new. The First National Midwifery School did not completely trust them either, and therefore a supervisor was assigned to each retrained *jieshengpo* to "check technique and the quality of work by close supervision of the strict regulation [*sic*]."[108] The graduates were also required to submit two reports for each birth: one within 24 hours and the second within two weeks after delivery. Furthermore, each midwife was instructed to call her supervisor for their first five delivery cases to ensure that the newly trained midwives carried out all they had learned in their two-month course. A record of a supervisory *zhuchanshi* named Miss Song illustrates the problems with supervision and compliance. Miss Song supervised 17 retrained *jieshengpo* in 1929. In one month there should have been 85 deliveries among the 17, but Miss Song was called only twice in one 10-day period, meaning that she supervised only 7 percent of the births. Miss Song attributed this lack of compliance to the fact that because the work was new to everyone, no one was certain how to proceed with calling the supervisor. Furthermore, there were unregistered midwives who opposed the modern midwifery techniques, and often several midwives were present at any given delivery. The unregistered and untrained midwives sometimes dissuaded the newly trained ones from calling for "modern" or "Western-style" help. However, "the attitude [sic] of family and the midwife toward the supervisor were [sic] considered to be favorable."[109] In March 1929, the supervision rate increased to 15 percent, with 13 out of 85 births under supervision.[110]

The same month, the school started a weekly conference held on Fridays with the recently graduated old-style midwives in order "to let them realize that their training was not finished [and] . . . to improve their practice by going over their cases with them."[111] The school also wanted to investigate the reasons for the old-style midwives' reluctance to be supervised, and also wished to train them in filling out the new birth reports sanctioned in March 1929 by the Beiping Health Department. In order to better track birth rates, unregistered midwives, and infant and maternal mortality, the Division of Vital Statistics of the Health Station and the Public Health Nursing Service had established a cooperative scheme to enforce birth registration. There were five conferences given on Fridays in March 1929, in which the old-style midwives discussed their cases and reports. They were further "influence[d] to stand strong for their profession."[112] These retrained *jieshengpo* were trained to go into their home communities to publicize the benefits of aseptic births in order to lower maternal and infant mortality rates. According to a 1929 monthly report, the midwives were supposed to "explain to their patients the benefit of their training to prevent puerperal fever and tetanus neo-natorum and the required supervision [of labor and birth]. . . . They are obliged to urge every family to adopt and to accept the 'aseptic' method."[113]

Retraining *jieshengpo* to become certified was difficult, not only because of their large numbers, but also because of their illiteracy and their reluctance to part with established procedures and traditions. For example, while Yang tried to develop methods for registering and controlling midwives who were reluctant to submit to supervisory and regulatory authority, as illustrated above, the midwives often simply did not report to their supervisors. Yang also struggled with instructional and supervisory methods for the illiterate *jieshengpo*. They could not file written reports, and they could not read midwifery textbooks. According to Ka-che Yip, rural health expert Li Ting'an, speaking of midwives in a rural health demonstration station,

> lamented that because of their lack of education many older midwives failed to grasp the basic concepts of modern medicine, reverting to traditional methods soon after graduating from the course. Sometimes visual reminders were used to ensure that correct proce-

dures were followed in delivery. For example, midwives were told to put two drops of medicine from a bottle with a red label (containing silver nitrate) into the eyes of newborns to prevent blindness.[114]

These problems limited the effects of the *jieshengpo*'s vocational training and the reach of the state in the processes of childbirth.

Traditional midwives performed additional important social functions outside the realm of childbirth. For centuries, they had acted as forensic examiners in legal cases that concerned women, for only women were allowed to examine other women "below the girdle" (*daixia*), as Matthew Sommer has shown in his study of late imperial Chinese law. He notes that in some chastity and rape cases of unmarried women, "magistrates ordered midwives to make pelvic examinations."[115] (Presumed to no longer be virgins, such cases concerning married women were supported only by verbal testimony of each party.) As important members of their communities, midwives did more than just deliver babies. The primary function of the old-style midwives was ritualistic, not medical, and focused on introducing the new child into its family and the wider community.[116]

The midwifery profession led a complex process that ultimately, by the end of the twentieth century, resulted in the demise of these old-style midwives with important consequences for society. Many ritual and social functions that the *jieshengpo* had provided were lost with their displacement. While the modern, educated, young, scientific *zhuchanshi* emerged as a new symbol of modern China, the old, uneducated, superstitious, "backwards" *jieshengpo* were excluded. Along with most other of the "100 professions," the *jieshengpo* were unregulated by the imperial government. With the rise of government-sponsored modern medicine in the Republican era, however, ways of thinking about birth and death changed. Whereas a *jieshengpo* negotiated community and family relationships within the home setting during the dangerous and frightening time of childbirth, the *zhuchanshi* and related personnel like doctors and nurses performed more impersonal functions in a medicalized environment for larger, national, goals. The Health Demonstration Stations in Beijing, for example, "transformed the everyday events of birth and death into specialized medical procedures."[117] Birth was removed from the traditional community and became part of the state-supported medical process. The uncommitted nature of the *zhuchanshi* exacerbated her lack of connection with her community. She moved around as needed, filling posts but rarely setting roots.

The breakdown of traditional community structures and social relations certainly occurred with state-managed childbirth. But there are other concerns that have been neglected by scholars, perhaps in an attempt to remedy the polemic nature of scientific literature on childbirth that vilified midwives against the wonders of modern medicine. In his excellent work on Beijing's public health systems in Republican China, Yang Nianqun has intimated that theoretically anyone could take the place of the midwife in aiding the parturient woman, but that only the *jieshengpo* could perform the postpartum ritual functions like the third-day bath and introducing the infant as a new member of its community.[118] While the midwives' ritual and social functions were indeed critical, Yang Nianqun underestimates the significance of their skills in managing the birth itself. The medical and biological importance of birth attendants during the processes of labor and childbirth in premodern societies should not be undervalued, especially from the point of view of the parturient. The quality of a particular *jieshengpo* or other birth helper, judged by the survival rates of mothers and infants, was known in her community, and good midwives were presumably preferred over bad ones, when there was a choice.[119] A *jieshengpo* well versed in birthing techniques could potentially ease labor pains and help deliver a child more quickly and safely. An unskilled birth attendant might indeed make labor much more difficult and dangerous—even life-threatening—by pushing, pulling, cutting, and otherwise manipulating the laboring woman and her unborn infant.

In any case, the realities of childbirth in early-twentieth-century China, or anywhere else in the world, for that matter, should not be denied. It is inappropriate to romanticize the *jieshengpo* and the happy babies, families, and communities that resulted from her expertise in ritual functions. In fact, the reality of childbirth in China during this period was problematic and often gruesome. Childbirth was dangerous. Accounts of infant craniotomy and dismemberment, prolapsed uterus, and botched abortion abound in the medical literature.[120] Rates of tetanus and puerperal sepsis were astoundingly high, and this was due primarily to the lack of medical expertise and sanitation among *jieshengpo*, areas in which modern medicine had much to offer. This is not to say that the Western model always provided a safer birth experience. An antiseptic home birth attended by a skilled midwife can be even safer than a highly regimented, physician-based hospital birth.[121] The accoutrements of modern typical birth, regardless of their facility, were markers of the profession, for example the standard uniform and delivery bag, and were used to set the modern midwife apart from the *jieshengpo*.

A NEW PROFESSION

Contemporary Western standards determine that a profession is a field that is legalized, institutionalized, and standardized.[122] According to this definition, there was no midwifery *profession* in China before the establishment of the First National Midwifery School at Peking Union Medical College. The departments of obstetrics/gynaecology and of public health at PUMC were closely modelled on the programs at Johns Hopkins University Medical School and its School of Hygiene and Public Health, the leading medical training institutions in the United States at that time. Medical training at Hopkins comprised a new, integrated approach that included lectures, clinical practice, and laboratory research. For obstetrics, that meant attending numerous births. Formerly, practical birthing experience was not part of most medical schools' curricula, and new physicians' first experience with childbirth usually occurred on the job. Johns Hopkins served as the model for medical education in the United States and was a seat of the professional medical movement. In turn PUMC became the model, with modifications, for medical schools and for the profession in China.[123]

Professional midwifery associations helped to further midwifery as a legitimate new profession in China. In the United States, physicians had displaced midwives by the 1950s largely because the latter failed to establish professional associations and educational institutions, which are essential for legitimating and institutionalizing a profession.[124] In contrast, midwifery associations in China, like other professional organizations of the time, attempted to monopolize their power by drawing distinctions between educated personnel and uneducated quacks through licensing and membership restrictions.[125] Local and national midwifery and nursing associations created forums discussing and organizing around political and social issues, published journals that promoted their profession, established and oversaw educational programs, and advocated for legal protection for professional midwives.

Like lawyers, physicians, and journalists in China, other burgeoning white-collar workers formed associations as part of a new professional, urban middle class unique to late imperial China. Professional associations' actions during this time, according to Xiaoqun Xu, were shaped by two forces: professionalization as part of modernization, as well as the "tradition of urban elite associations addressing social and political issues in the public arena."[126] Unlike many of the traditional gentry associations, however, the new professional organizations were sanctioned and supported by the Nationalist government, indicating that "professionalization was an integral part of state-society interaction."[127] William Kirby has shown how the Nationalist government utilized "an extraordinary number of party and government institutions" as part of the new *zhiye zhuyi* (ideal of professionalism) mentality in the central government.[128] Local and national governments backed professional medical associations because of the importance of public health and sanitation, especially during periods of epidemics.[129] Chinese professional associations were sanctioned by and worked closely with the Nationalist government in legislating licensing and membership restrictions, and in public health and sanitation efforts.

The midwifery and nursing associations that originated in the early 1900s are similar in many ways to the women's factory organizations and career clubs that Emily Honig, Lien Ling-ling, and others have studied in Shanghai.[130] These organizations were comprised of women, and they organized many leisure activities as well as political ones, like the Chinese Career Women's Club's fashion shows to showcase native cloth, or the drama teams of local midwifery associations that expressed public health goals and criticized "feudal thinking."[131] These organizations were stronger with regard to native-place ties, rather than encouraging or maintaining a national identity as midwife, career woman, or worker. Wen-hsin Yeh has asserted that in Shanghai, few factory workers were able to "disengage themselves from the norms and ties into which they had been born"—that native-place ties prevented workers from organizing or forming larger or different communities outside native-place identities.[132] Likewise, local midwifery professional organizations seem to be much more influential and active than the (national-level) Chinese Midwifery Association that was started by graduates of the First National Midwifery School in 1933 with the goals of "undertaking research into the science and art of midwifery, the cultivation of friendship among our fellow workers, and the promotion and development of midwifery education."[133] This organization is only mentioned once in the annual reports of the First National Midwifery School, and no other reference to its existence was found. Unlike the (national) Nurses Association of China, which was founded by foreigners in 1908 and had large membership numbers nationwide, the national Chinese Midwifery Association never seemed to find its footing in China.[134]

Local midwifery organizations could be even more influential than national ones in improving the professional and social conditions of midwives, as well as in furthering the cause of improving maternal and child health. Along with professional organizations that wielded political and social power, school organizations and their publications promoted a singular group identification. The modern midwives belonged to a new and progressive professional organization whose identity was crucial to the formation of a strong midwifery profession. Together with other members of their group, they did not see themselves as outsiders, but as an integral part of new China. This type of group identity led to the creation of a professional identity. For example, the Guangzhou Midwifery Association was a well-organized institution with over 400 members by 1947. Its stated missions were to create and regulate midwifery examinations, establish fees, represent association members in legal matters, help unemployed members find jobs, and generally improve the conditions of midwives.[135] By 1947 the Guangzhou Midwifery Association had helped to place 20 of its member midwives in hospital employment in and around Guangzhou.[136] This organization was affiliated with the Guangzhou Physicians' Association and worked with doctors and hospitals to help place midwives in both urban and rural settings. A professional affiliation such as this was invaluable in popularizing and promoting midwifery in Guangzhou. Its members published a magazine entitled *Guangzhou Municipal Midwifery Association Periodical* (*Guangzhoushi zhuchanshi gonghui tekan*) that discussed new technologies and pharmaceuticals, methods to facilitate childbirth, and licensing examinations and regulations.

Political power was crucial to the midwives' success, both via professional organizations and individually. The Guangzhou Midwifery Association magazine was a forum for promoting *professional* midwives, creating a new arena for them apart from the old-fashioned *jieshengpo*. The Association's function of representing members in alleged abortion cases and wrongful death lawsuits gave them official, legal backing. Furthermore, the organization publicized and politicized midwives during public discussions of board member election disputes that were reported in the daily newspapers.[137]

Likewise, Yang Chongrui held national and local public health political appointments which aided her goals for the professionalization of midwifery. Yang fought and won a battle with the Nurses' Association of China over the organizational control of childbirth. The Nurses' Association of China had issued a resolution "that the Nurses' Association of China cannot participate in any scheme which prepared to train non-nurses in the science of midwifery," stating that midwifery fell under the broader domain of nursing.[138] In an open letter to the medical profession in the *China Medical Journal*, Yang Chongrui publicly criticized the Nurses' Association for requiring extensive education for nurse-midwives when what China really needed, and quickly, was a large cadre of simply retrained old-style midwives led by a smaller number of professional midwives.[139] Yang argued that no industrialized nations held such high standards for their midwives. Holland, Denmark, and France all used midwives who were not nurses with very good results. Furthermore, in England and the United States pregnant women were attended by physicians. By what logic could poor, backward China, whose births numbered 12 million per year, expect to achieve standards higher than those of Europe or the United States? According to European maternal and child health criteria, one midwife could safely attend 120 to 150 deliveries per year, and China would thus need 64,000 midwives to deliver the goal of at least 80 percent of all babies. It would be impossible to give 64,000 women high-level nursing training when China's high maternal and mortality rates called for immediate action. She pled for, and won, professional recognition of *midwives*, even those with minimal training, to help improve the safety of childbirth.[140] After all, as Yang stated, "Midwifery is one of the professions."[141]

The creation of a new midwifery profession heralded new opportunities for *some* women in China to participate in nation building and modernization, while excluding others who did not conform to the new standards for modern womanhood. Professional work could be a way for women to empower themselves, setting them apart from the leisured class and the New Woman, or modern girl (*modeng nüzi*), who in the May Fourth era became the symbol of consumerist excess and frivolity.[142] The paramedical nursing and midwifery fields attracted women from middle-class families, and many attest to joining the profession in order to improve the nation. Most of the midwifery students were from the urban areas that contained midwifery schools like Shanghai and Guangzhou. In Guangzhou, a large number of midwives were from Shunde (Cantonese *Sundak*), the same district of silk weavers that Marjorie Topley and Janice Stockard researched in their studies of marriage resistance among silk weavers.[143] Shunde midwives, therefore, were from communities that encouraged, or at least did not discourage, women from attending school and working outside the home. Furthermore, as the Chinese silk industry declined, many of the spinsters may have moved into midwifery. After all, the spinster and the midwife were similar in their respective asexuality, for it was uncommon for women of either profession to marry.

As in the United States and Europe, married women in China of certain social classes did not normally pursue a profession, and most women who went into public health or medical service did not wed, or they stopped working once they did marry. In fact, one of the requirements of most medical training schools, including midwifery programs, was that their students be single, and those who wedded while in training would be dismissed. The most famous Western-trained Chinese women physicians, like Yang Chongrui, Kang Cheng, and Shi Meiyu never married, instead dedicating their lives to serving others. These women—unnatural in the Confucian sense of being single and childless, yet revered because of their dedication to their nation—were anomalies in Chinese society.[144] Reformers like Liang Qichao on one hand exhorted Chinese women to join the workforce, while others, like Chiang Kai-shek in his New Life Movement, encouraged women to fulfill traditional roles of good wife and wise mother. Some women medical professionals did have to juggle the triple burden of family member care, housework, and a professional career, regardless of their marital status, as some remained at home to care for their family members. In addition to being family caretakers, women bore the burden of being caretakers of the nation and of the nation's future population by ensuring safe and healthy births.

Unlike the factory workers in Republican Shanghai who were ostracized because of their proximity to strangers and unknown men at work, the modern midwives remained in the domestic sphere and theoretically should have been more socially accepted. However, that domestic sphere was not always held in high regard. In her brief examination of the nursing profession in China, Liu Chung-tung found the field to be a hard sell for daughters of well-to-do families.[145] Nonetheless, Ka-che Yip observed that the largest number of midwifery students in Nanchang, Jiangxi, came from middle and upper class families of doctors (36.4 percent), businessmen (26.8 percent), or educators (22 percent).[146] Although women as daughters, wives, servants, and concubines were the traditional caretakers for their own family members, it was beyond any expectation for these women to care for complete strangers due to a "lack of any equivalent of the Christian ethic in which caring could be lifted onto a plane of moral obligation," thus eliminating nursing as a respectable occupation.[147] According to the dean of PUMC's School of Nursing, Gertrude Hodgman, her "greatest challenge" was "alter[ing] the Chinese concept of nursing as an impossible profession for women."[148] Nursing in Europe and the United States had gone through its own crisis to become a valid career choice for women in the nineteenth and twentieth centuries, and midwifery in China was likely an even harder sell because of traditional notions about childbirth as polluting.[149] To help change the common perception of nurses, Hodgman traveled to middle schools throughout northern China to teach students and their families about the virtues of the nursing profession as a means to "relieve human suffering and prevent disease."[150] She noted that the "students were far more easily persuaded than their parents."[151]

The midwifery schools these students attended very deliberately presented themselves as modern, professional establishments. Their school yearbooks present a vision of coherent, progressive, and thoroughly modern institutions staffed with professionals and attended by very modern students, some replete with students' photographs in nontraditional makeup and hairdo, evidence of their modernity. The Tuqiang Advanced Midwifery School (*Tuqiang gaodeng zhuchan xuexiao*) used photography, a modern invention, to carve out an image of itself to present to the world.[152] The visages of Tuqiang's honor students in figure 3.6, clad in *qipao* with close-cropped coiffures, plucked eyebrows, and makeup differ radically from the images of traditional *jieshengpo*. The modern midwives are young, educated, and urbane. They look confident, sure of their skills and profession, though some perhaps better suited to the pages of a fashion magazine than a delivery room. As Yang Chongrui

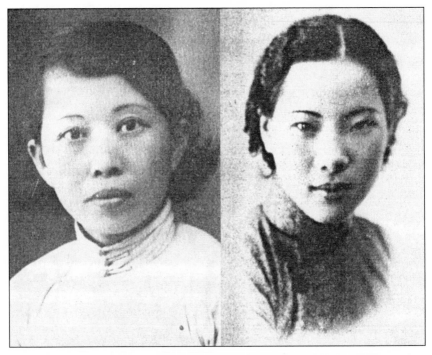

Figure 3.6. Honor Students from the Tuqiang Advanced Midwifery School's 50th Graduating Class. *Tuqiang gaodeng zhuchan xuexiao #50 jie biye tongxue lu,* **Guangzhou, 1936. Courtesy of the Guangzhou Provincial Archives.**

wrote, photographs such as these "show that an intelligent type of young Chinese woman is being attracted to the midwifery course."[153]

Students published essays, poems, and plays in these yearbooks that expressed their devotion to modern medicine and to working for a new China. These constitute the few remaining sources of the new midwives' voices. The standard language of duty and sacrifice omits personal information about the students' lives or other non-sacrificial or duty-bound motivations for joining this new profession. Hu Cao-juan, a student at Shanghai's Bethel Nursing and Obstetrics School (*Shanghai Boteli yiyuan hushi chanke xuexiao*) wrote that she decided to become a nurse to serve the people and rid China of the title "sick man of Asia."[154] Hu also expressed her hope to eliminate the reliance on unsanitary midwives and superstitious rituals that led to high infant and maternal death rates. Hu's classmate, Wang Shumin, claimed that Western medicine had a scientific foundation, whereas Chinese medicine did not. This fact made her want to study Western medicine. She later became a Christian (Bethel was a missionary enterprise) and also desired to serve God through her profession.[155]

The plays and poems have a common theme of denigrating the elder generation's ways of birthing and their reliance on religion and (unsanitary) traditional midwives to ensure safe births. One play, entitled "Old and New (*Jiu yu xin*)," by two students at the Shanghai Zhongde Professional Midwifery School, Zhu Xiaxian and Wang Yongwei, depicts a struggle between the generations.[156] The elders, Grandfather (Lao Ye) and Grandmother (Lao Taitai), both in their fifties, have called a 60-year-old midwife to attend their daughter-in-law's confinement, against the wishes of their three children in their twenties. The play opens with the eldest brother's wife in labor off stage while Lao Ye and Lao Taitai pray at their family altar to Guanyin (the Goddess of Mercy) and send for Old Midwife Wang. Their eldest daughter, Wenxin, tells them that elder brother wants his wife to deliver in a hospital, not at home attended by a dirty (*angzang*) traditional midwife. The daughters and their parents spend much of the play arguing loudly (evidenced by an overabundance of exclamation points in the text), and they express their anxiety through worried looks, wringing of hands, and shedding tears. Lao Taitai says, "The *jieshengpo* is old and experienced. How could a young girl know anything about childbirth?" Later, elder brother's wife suffers a prolonged labor and is too exhausted to even physically support herself. Younger daughter clandestinely calls for the modern midwife living next door, who performs a caesarean section and saves both mother and baby (a son, to show the facility of modern childbirth as well as its familial and national importance).

Another play in the same yearbook, called "Renewal," by Xin Dong-guang, has a similar plot with an auntie of an upper middle class family in labor. Her niece, a high school student, pleads with her mother, specified as a "good wife and wise mother" (*xianqi liangmu*) to utilize a modern midwife: "*Jieshengpo* only know how to scam money. They know nothing about cleanliness or disinfection."[157]

The script for "The Moment of Life and Death (*Shengsi guantou juben*)," by students Wang Yugang and Qu Shaoheng of Shanghai's Shengsheng Midwifery School (*Shanghai shengsheng zhuchan xuexiao*), is unceasingly direct about its intentions. The given name of the 50-year-old father, Lao Huaigu, is a play on words meaning "hold on to the past," and he predictably wants his pregnant daughter-in-law to be attended by a traditional midwife.[158] Lao Huaigu explains to his son that women have given birth with the help of traditional midwives for thousands of years, and that when a mother or infant dies in childbirth it is a matter of fate or demons. The son eventually prevails because of his wife's serious condition resulting from protracted labor. They call a modern midwife and doctor, and both lives are saved.

Like the poems and essays the midwives wrote to express their devotion to midwifery and to improving the nation, the plays utilize a standard format of tradition versus modernity, using familiar tropes like the superstitious and entrenched elder generation that attempts to alter fate by burning incense and praying to the gods. The younger generation favors science. They had learned about sanitation and cleanliness through their modern education, and they brought their knowledge home to enlighten their family members. These plays serve as guides for students to deal with relatives and friends of patients in their care who are reluctant to utilize the new midwives' training. They also present a struggle not just over childbirth, but a battle between the identity of an old, traditional China versus a new and modern nation dependent on its youth for survival. Through these yearbooks, the modern midwifery students present modern childbirth—and themselves and their schools—as a vital necessity of the new China.

Unlike the modern midwives, the retrained traditional midwives have left no such records as most of them were illiterate. Like Gail Hershatter's prostitutes of Republican Shanghai, the Republican-era *jieshengpo* have no voice. In her groundbreaking work, Hershatter utilized other types of sources written primarily by men who were devotees of the courtesans, and those varied sources provide a rich picture of the lives of those women.[159] But childbirth in China was off-limits to men, and women did not write about such a personal experience; the illiterate *jieshengpo*'s motivations and personal stories have died with them. The millions of successful and uneventful births that the *jieshengpo* attended never warranted recording. What remains are the problem cases as chronicled by Western-trained medical personnel who were called in to attend the mother or her infant after days in labor, often when it was too late to save anyone. Lawsuits and complaints by family members of the parturient about negative birth outcomes also denigrate the *jieshengpo*. An important quality of the *jieshengpo* can be ascertained even in their silence. It is certain that modern midwifery students had chosen their profession, perhaps with the persuasion of their families, but the old-style midwives had no such leisure. The *jieshengpo* were forced to comply with, or evade, the new regulations that governed them.

The employment possibilities for the newly trained midwives were varied. Retrained and registered *jieshengpo* continued working in their communities, often with supervision by modern midwives, as illustrated above. *Zhuchanshi* had more opportunities. They could work in a regular hospital, women's hospital, health station, or dispensary anywhere in the country. Graduates of the advanced course of the First National Midwifery School could teach in other midwifery programs. *Zhuchanshi* could also fill government positions in the provincial and national public health administrations. Many of these women moved from post to provincial post, whereas the old-style *jieshengpo* were firmly rooted in their local communities. For example, a graduate from Shandong of the First National Midwifery School in Beijing worked at the Beiping Municipal Maternal and Child Health Bureau (*Beiping shili gonganju baoying shiwusuo*) for one year, then at the Nanjing Central Midwifery School (the Second National Midwifery School, *Zhonghua di er zhuchan xuexiao*), then for the Fujian Provincial Nursing and Midwifery School, finally migrating to Guangdong to work for various posts in the Guangdong Provincial Public Health Administration.[160]

Modern medical personnel, including modern midwives, were often underpaid and worked under difficult conditions, especially in the early years when they worked in mission hospitals.[161] Even Chinese physicians in medical missions did not receive equal pay to Western physicians for doing the same job. The socioeconomic status of midwives, like nurses, was relatively low compared to other professions. In Shanghai in the 1930s, a trained nurse employed by the Shanghai Municipal Council earned 50 to 100 yuan per month, similar to that of a typist whose salary was 50 to 60 yuan per month.[162] A senior engineer at this time made 300 to 500 yuan per month; a minister in the Shanghai government could earn a monthly salary of around 800 yuan, while branch governmental staff made 60 to 180 yuan per month.[163]

Xu Xiaoqun has figured that Shanghai physicians could make between 300 and 3,000 yuan per month in the 1930s.[164] Modern midwives probably made a monthly salary approximate to that of a trained nurse, between 50 and 100 yuan, a relatively comfortable existence. In comparison, according to a 1930 survey of 230 families, the average monthly income among Shanghai textile workers was 31.877 yuan. A skilled worker spent on average 19.26 yuan per month on living expenses.[165] The 17 midwives on staff at the First National Midwifery School in 1932–33 made a total of $10,320, for an average individual annual salary of $607. In comparison, the four physicians on staff made a total of $7,680 ($1,920 each).[166] Thus the midwives were by no means well-paid, but they could earn a salary that allowed a comfortable existence, especially since most were unmarried and still lived at home with their parents.

Although modern midwifery was a growing field, the profession was not a common one during the Republican era. By 1934, there were 1,883 registered midwives in China and 136 licensed midwifery schools to attend the more than two million births per year.[167] The numbers of midwives and schools were woefully inadequate, though according to several contemporaries the medical profession was the fastest growing and most welcoming professional field for young women.[168] In 1933, there were 28 medical schools in China, and only two did not accept women: the Army Medical School in Nanjing and Aurora University College of Medicine, a French-run institution in Shanghai. (In an interesting contrast, the Yunnan Army Medical College in Kunming did accept women and had eight female students in 1931.)[169] Women interested in medicine were encouraged to go into the fields of public health, obstetrics/gynecology, and pediatrics, mirroring the feminization of nursing that was occurring around the same time in both China and the United States.

Well into the 1910s, most nurses and nursing students in China were male, but largely from the efforts of Peking Union Medical College the normative hospital caregiver ideal turned female.[170] This feminization is evident when comparing the number of hours required for each subject in women's colleges versus coeducational institutions. The Hackett Medical College for Women in Guangzhou required 674 hours of obstetrics and gynecology of its students, while the coeducational St. John's University College of Medicine in Shanghai listed only 96 such hours of instruction. Furthermore, Hackett's pediatrics curriculum was 252 hours versus 33 hours at St. John's.[171] Women remained in the birthing room in China, whether as traditional midwives, modern midwives, or as nurses or physicians.

Social support for midwifery students was slow in coming as well. As Paul Bailey has illustrated, there was no linear progression from house-bound Chinese woman to socially supported career woman. Several contemporaries disparaged women's "modern" schooling, asserting that if given Western-style education Chinese women would fail to fulfill their motherly and wifely duties. At least some of these new midwives and other new professionals had to contend with social ostracism for their choices.[172] Furthermore, traditionally women who became *jieshengpo* were required to have given birth themselves in order to be seen as skilled and valid. The *zhuchanshi*, on the other hand, overwhelmingly had less first-hand experience, since as students they were required to be unmarried and childless. What could they possibly know about childbirth? Patients and *jieshengpo* often "resented the young, unmarried woman . . . an inexperienced upstart" who attended and trained them.[173] Furthermore, the *zhuchanshi* wore starched white uniforms and caps, symbols of cleanliness and modernity in the West, visual representations of the *zhuchanshi*'s educational level. But in China, the color white is a sign of death and mourning, resulting in a strange dichotomy: women dressed as death who are supposed to bring life. The opposition to the new midwives continued well into the 1950s and beyond, due to distrust of the new methods and a lack of government resources to train and manage the new midwives.[174] Even in Beijing in 1931, half of all births were still attended by old-style midwives, and 25 percent by relatives or with no help from others.[175]

CONCLUSION

Yang Chongrui and the First National Midwifery School transformed the reputation of midwifery in China from an apprenticed vocation into a modern profession, and the midwifery model served as a paradigm for future maternal and child health programs under the Chinese Communist Party after 1949. Although Western and Chinese alike vilified the old-style midwife, Yang, working as a bridge between the foreign, private First National Midwifery School and the Nationalist government, renovated the mechanics of midwifery and the women who practiced it. The creation of the First National Midwifery School illustrates the melding of nation building with modern medicine. It serves as an example of the ways in which medical personnel, modernizers, and politicians used modern medicine to further China's nation-building goals. The First National Midwifery School also shows how influential one organization was in visualizing a national maternal and child health plan for China. As the national model for midwifery schools throughout China, the First National Midwifery School had government support and was overseen by the National Midwifery Board, a joint effort of the Ministries of Health and Education. This, coupled with the Nationalist efforts to regulate and control midwifery, made it a formidable opponent to old-style midwives. It is yet another example of state control over birthing bodies.

In the midst of these changes, a new profession emerged. Young, modern *zhuchanshi* replaced the old-style *jieshengpo*. In addition, the reluctance of Chinese women to patronize male physicians or attend male patients spurred the quick rise of women entering the medical professions, especially nursing, midwifery, obstetrics/gynecology, and pediatrics. The midwifery field was a new arena in which women could exercise their bodies and minds as part of a new China. Midwifery schools recruited all sorts of women to attend varying levels of midwifery courses. Bright young women could become highly skilled nurse-midwives or midwives, while old-style *jieshengpo* were shaped into (sometimes, but not always) clean and efficient *legitimate* midwives.

It is clear that Western prenatal and obstetrical care improved maternal and infant mortality rates in China. On the other hand, childbirth became a more impersonal and medicalized experience, removed from the family and larger community. This professionalization and modernization of midwifery resulted in greater state control over the body, the entire process of parturition and birth, and even childhood. Childbirth had become a serious business, no longer a function of merely reproducing the family. This new medical infrastructure affected and influenced women who entered the midwifery field as well as those who were ultimately displaced by it. On closer inspection, worldwide trends suggest that the period of male physician-dominant childbirth in the United States was an anomaly. The field of medicine is becoming increasingly feminized, and a growing proportion of obstetricians/gynecologists are women. As hospital births become more common in China, especially in urban areas, women physicians and paramedical personnel are stepping in to eliminate the role of traditional midwives. The same trends exist in the United States, as female obstetrician/gynecologists, nurses, and midwives replace male physicians as birth attendants.[176]

NOTES

1. Marion Yang, *Report of the Training and Supervision for Midwives,* February 1929, folder 371, box 45, series 601, RAC.

2. Mary Brown Bullock, *An American Transplant: The Rockefeller Foundation and Peking Union Medical College* (Berkeley: University of California Press, 1980).

3. Xiaoyang Jiang, "Cross-Cultural Philanthropy as a Gift Relationship: The Rockefeller Foundation Donors and Chinese Recipients, 1913–1921" (PhD dissertation, Bowling Green State University, 1994), 166–68.

4. Michelle Renshaw, *Accommodating the Chinese: The American Hospital in China, 1880–1920* (New York: Routledge, 2005).

5. F. Cunningham et al., *Williams Obstetrics*, 23rd ed. (Chicago: McGraw-Hill Professional, 2009).

6. Andrew Abbot, *The System of Professions: An Essay on the Division of Expert Labor* (Chicago and London: University of Chicago Press, 1988); Eliot Friedson, *Profession of Medicine: A Study of the Sociology of Applied Medicine* (New York: Dodd, Mead & Company, 1972); Magali Sarfatti Larson, *The Rise of Professionalism: A Sociological Analysis* (Berkeley and Los Angeles: University of California Press, 1977).

7. Xu, *Chinese Professionals and the Republican State: The Rise of Professional Associations in Shanghai, 1912–1937*.

8. Shemo, ""An Army of Women": The Medical Ministries of Kang Cheng and Shi Meiyu, 1873–1937."

9. John Watt, "Breaking into Public Service: The Development of Nursing in Modern China, 1870–1949," *Nursing History Review* 12 (2004): 67–96.

10. Emily Ahern, "The Power and Pollution of Chinese Women," in *Women in Chinese Society*, ed. Margery Wolf and Roxanne Witke (Stanford: Stanford University Press, 1975), 193–214; Honig, *Sisters and Strangers: Women in the Shanghai Cotton Mills, 1919–1949*.

11. Honig, *Sisters and Strangers: Women in the Shanghai Cotton Mills, 1919–1949*, 138, 170.

12. Lien, Ling-ling, "Leisure, Patriotism, and Identity: The Chinese Career Women's Club in Wartime Shanghai," in *Creating Chinese Modernity: Knowledge and Everyday Life, 1900–1940*, ed. Peter Zarrow, Studies in Modern Chinese History 4 (New York, Berne, Frankfurt am Main: Peter Lang, 2006), 213–40; Janice Stockard, *Daughters of the Canton Delta: Marriage Patterns and Economic Strategies in South China, 1860–1930* (Hong Kong: Hong Kong University Press, 1989); Honig, *Sisters and Strangers: Women in the Shanghai Cotton Mills, 1919–1949*.

13. Honig, *Sisters and Strangers: Women in the Shanghai Cotton Mills, 1919–1949*; Stockard, *Daughters of the Canton Delta: Marriage Patterns and Economic Strategies in South China, 1860–1930*; Gail Hershatter, *Dangerous Pleasures: Prostitution and Modernity in Twentieth-Century Shanghai* (Berkeley: University of California Press, 1997).

14. Caroline Beth Reeves, "The Power of Mercy: The Chinese Red Cross Society, 1900–1937" (PhD dissertation, Harvard University, 1998); Sue Ellen Gronewold, "Encountering Hope: The Door of Hope Mission in Shanghai and Taipei, 1900–1976" (PhD dissertation, Columbia University, 1996); Shemo,

""An Army of Women": The Medical Ministries of Kang Cheng and Shi Meiyu, 1873–1937."

15. Shemo, ""An Army of Women": The Medical Ministries of Kang Cheng and Shi Meiyu, 1873–1937"; Yan Renying, ed., *Dr. Yang Chongrui: 100 Year Commemoration* (*Yang Chongrui boshi: Danchen bai nian ji nian*) (Beijing: Beijing yike daxue, zhongguo xiehe yike daxue lianhe chubanshe, 1990); Guo Jianyao, *Lin Qiaozhi: China's Outstanding Female Obstetrician/Gynecologist* (*Lin Qiaozhi: Zhongguo jiechu fuchanke nu yisheng*) (Hong Kong: Xin ya wenhua shiye youxian gongsi, 1990); Huang Qinghua, *Lin Qiaozhi: Biography of China's Famous Physician* (*Lin Qiaozhi: Zhongguo zhuming kexuejia zhuanji*) (Beijing: Tuanjie chubanshe, 1997).

16. Witz, *Professions and Patriarchy*.

17. Watt, "Breaking Into Public Service: The Development of Nursing in Modern China, 1870–1949," 68.

18. Lucas, *Chinese Medical Modernization: Comparative Policy Continuities, 1930s–1980s*, 38–40.

19. Ibid.

20. Ibid., 43.

21. Bowers, *Western Medicine in a Chinese Palace: Peking Union Medical College, 1917–1951*, 31.

22. Cheng, "Going Public Through Education: Female Reformers and Girls' Schools in Late Qing Beijing."

23. For family reform in the New Culture Movement, see Glosser, *Chinese Visions of Family and State, 1915–1953*.

24. Tang, "Woman's Education in China," 23.

25. Hsu, Ou Yang, and Lew, "Education of Women in China."

26. Culp, *Articulating Citizenship: Civic Education and Student Politics in Southeastern China, 1912–1940*.

27. Tang, "Woman's Education in China," 6. The 1907 number is for girls in elementary school. The 1918–19 number includes girls in lower primary and higher primary schools, a distinction created in 1912.

28. Chinese National Association for the Advancement of Education, "Statistical Summaries of Chinese Education," *Bulletins on Chinese Education* 2 (1923): 4–5.

29. Lucas, *Chinese Medical Modernization: Comparative Policy Continuities, 1930s–1980s*, 45.

30. China Medical Commission of the Rockefeller Foundation, *Medicine in China*, 11, 103.

31. Lucas, *Chinese Medical Modernization: Comparative Policy Continuities, 1930s–1980s*, 68.

32. Choa, *"Heal the Sick" Was Their Motto: The Protestant Medical Missionaries in China*, 96.

33. Choa, *"Heal the Sick" Was Their Motto: The Protestant Medical Missionaries in China*.

34. S.M. Tao, "Medical Education of Chinese Women," *The Medical and Professional Woman's Journal* (1934): 74.

35. Tang, "Woman's Education in China," 24.

36. Ibid., 5. In addition to the adjustments noted, the system was changed to six years of elementary school, three years of junior middle school, three years of senior middle school, and four years of college.

37. Ibid., 20.

38. National Association for the Advancement of Education, "Statistical Summaries of Chinese Education," 4–5, 10–49.

39. Balme, *China and Modern Medicine: A Study in Medical Missionary Development*.

40. Yip, *Health and National Reconstruction in Nationalist China: The Development of Modern Health Services, 1928–1937*, 17.

41. John Z. Bowers, "Imperialism and Medical Education in China," *Bulletin of the History of Medicine* 48 (1974): 455–56; Weili Ye, ""Nu Liux-uesheng": The Story of American-Educated Chinese Women, 1880s–1920s," *Modern China* 20, no. 3 (1994): 343.

42. Bowers, "Imperialism and Medical Education in China," 455–56.

43. Bowers, "Imperialism and Medical Education in China."

44. Tang, "Woman's Education in China," 27–30.

45. Watt, "Breaking into Public Service: The Development of Nursing in Modern China, 1870–1949."

46. Bowers, *Western Medicine in a Chinese Palace: Peking Union Medical College, 1917–1951*, 115.

47. Ibid., 203–4.

48. Grant, "Letter to Dr. Victor Heiser."

49. John B. Grant, *Midwifery Training*, report (Peking: Peking Union Medical College, December 22, 1927), Folder 371, box 45, series 601, RG 1, RAC.

50. Ibid.

51. Grant, "Letter to Dr. Victor Heiser."

52. Ibid. Tetanus in Chinese is called *poshangfeng*, literally "wind disease" or "wind damage."

53. Ibid.

54. Ibid.

55. Chongrui Yang, "My Autobiography (*Wo de zizhuan*)," in *Dr. Yang Chongrui: 100 Year Commemoration (Yang Chongrui boshi: Danchen bai nian ji nian*), ed. Yan Renying (Beijing: Beijing yike daxue, zhongguo xiehe yike daxue lianhe chubanshe, 1990), 143–53.

56. Ibid.

57. Ibid.

58. Marion Yang and I-Chin Yuan, "Report of an Investigation on Infant Mortality and its Causes in Peiping," *Chinese Medical Journal*, no. 47 (1933): 597–604; Grant, "Letter to Dr. Victor Heiser."

59. Marion Yang, "Midwifery Training in China," *China Medical Journal* 42 (1928): 768–75.

60. The Western medical literature at this time was vehement in its criticisms of *jieshengpo*, yet even traditional Chinese medical texts also vilify them. For example, see Zi Yun (pseud.), "Childbirth Customs in My Hometown:

Beijing (Wu xiang de shengchan fengsu: Beijing)"; Yang and Yuan, "Report of an Investigation on Infant Mortality and its Causes in Peiping." Even traditional Chinese medical treatises ridiculed the *jieshengpo*. The *Treatise on Easy Childbirth (Dasheng bian)*, published in 1715, is a good example of this. J. Preston Maxwell and J.L. Liu, "Ta Sheng P'ian: A Chinese Household Manual of Obstetrics," *Annals of Medical History* 5, no. 2 (1923): 95–99; Wu, *Reproducing Women: Medicine, Metaphor and Childbirth in Late Imperial China*.

61. Yang, "My Autobiography (Wo de zizhuan)," 147.

62. Yang, "Control of Practising Midwives in China."

63. *First National Midwifery School, Peiping*, July 1, 1932, folder 373, box 45, series 601, RG1, RAC.

64. FNMS, *Sixth Annual Report, First National Midwifery School, Peiping, July 1, 1934–June 30, 1935*, Annual Report, 1935.

65. Ibid., 1.

66. FNMS, *Sixth Annual Report, First National Midwifery School, Peiping, July 1, 1934–June 30, 1935*.

67. Chung-tung Liu, "From san gu liu po to 'caring scholar': the Chinese nurse in perspective," *International Journal of Nursing Studies* 28, no. 4 (1991): 322; Watt, "Breaking into Public Service: The Development of Nursing in Modern China, 1870–1949," 86.

68. Dr. J. Preston Maxwell, *Scheme for a Six Months' Course in Midwifery for Midwives in Training*, 1926, folder 601, box 45, Series 371, RG 1, RAC.

69. Ibid.

70. FNMS, *Fifth Annual Report, First National Midwifery School, Peiping, July 1, 1933–June 30, 1934*, 4; FNMS, *Fourth Annual Report, First National Midwifery School, Peiping, July 1, 1932–June 30, 1933*, 3.

71. *First National Midwifery School, Peiping*, 5.

72. *Regulations of the First National Midwifery School*.

73. FNMS, *First Annual Report, First National Midwifery School, 1929–1931*, Annual Report, February 3, 1932.

74. This cost was derived from dividing total yearly expenditures, plus six percent of the capital expense, by the number of students during the year. FNMS, *Second Annual Report, First National Midwifery School, Peiping, July 1, 1930–June 30, 1931*, Annual Report, February 17, 1932.

75. The total cost per student divided by four.

76. *First National Midwifery School, Peiping*.

77. Yang, *Report of the Training and Supervision for Midwives*.

78. Ibid.

79. "Hygiene and Public Health: The First National Midwifery School, Peiping," *Chinese Medical Journal* 46 (1932): 32–33.

80. "Hygiene and Public Health: The First National Midwifery School, Peiping."

81. FNMS, *Second Annual Report, First National Midwifery School, Peiping, July 1, 1930–June 30, 1931*.

82. National Association for the Advancement of Education, "Statistical Summaries of Chinese Education."

83. FNMS, *Second Annual Report, First National Midwifery School, Peiping, July 1, 1930–June 30, 1931.*

84. FNMS, *Fifth Annual Report, First National Midwifery School, Peiping, July 1, 1933–June 30, 1934,* 1.

85. Ibid., ii.

86. FNMS, *Sixth Annual Report, First National Midwifery School, Peiping, July 1, 1934–June 30, 1935.*

87. Ibid.

88. *First National Midwifery School, Peiping,* 7.

89. FNMS, *Second Annual Report, First National Midwifery School, Peiping, July 1, 1930–June 30, 1931.*

90. Ibid.

91. *First National Midwifery School, Peiping,* 7.

92. FNMS, *Fifth Annual Report, First National Midwifery School, Peiping, July 1, 1933–June 30, 1934,* Appendix III: Instructions for Midwifery Clerkships, xix.

93. Stefani Pfeiffer, "Epistemology and Etiquette: Bargaining, Self-Disclosure, and the Struggle to Define the Patient Role at PUMC Hospital, 1921–1941" (presented at the Association for Asian Studies Annual Meeting, Chicago, IL, April 2, 2005).

94. FNMS, *Fifth Annual Report, First National Midwifery School, Peiping, July 1, 1933–June 30, 1934,* Appendix III: Instructions for Midwifery Clerkships, xxvii.

95. Ibid., Appendix III: Instructions for Midwifery Clerkships, xxvi.

96. Marion Yang, "Letter to Miss Mary Beard," November 7, 1930.

97. *First National Midwifery School, Peiping,* 32–33.

98. Yang, "Letter to Miss Mary Beard."

99. Yang, *Report of the Training and Supervision for Midwives.*

100. Ibid.

101. *First National Midwifery School, Peiping,* 8.

102. Yang, *Report of the Training and Supervision for Midwives.*

103. Ibid.

104. Yang, "Midwifery Training in China."

105. FNMS, *Sixth Annual Report, First National Midwifery School, Peiping, July 1, 1934–June 30, 1935.*

106. Yang, *Report of the Training and Supervision for Midwives.*

107. Ibid.

108. Ibid.

109. Ibid.

110. Ibid.

111. Ibid.

112. Yang, *Report of the Training and Supervision for Midwives.*

113. Ibid.

114. Li Ting'an, *The Problem of Rural Health in China* (*Zhongguo xiangcun weisheng wenti*) (Shanghai: Shangwu yinshuguan, 1935), 66; as cited in Yip, *Health and National Reconstruction in Nationalist China: The Development of Modern Health Services, 1928–1937,* 167.

115. Matthew Harvey Sommer, *Sex, Law, and Society in Late Imperial China* (Stanford: Stanford University Press, 2000), 83–84.

116. Yang Nianqun, "The Transformation of Space and Control of Birth and Death in Early Republican Beijing (*Minguo chunian beijing de shengsi kongzhi yu kongjian zhuanhuan*)"; Yang Nianqun, "The Establishment of Modern Health Demonstration Zones and the Regulation of Life and Death in Early Republican Beijing."

117. Yang Nianqun, "The Establishment of Modern Health Demonstration Zones and the Regulation of Life and Death in Early Republican Beijing," 91.

118. Yang Nianqun, "The Transformation of Space and Control of Birth and Death in Early Republican Beijing (*Minguo chunian beijing de shengsi kongzhi yu kongjian zhuanhuan*)," 139.

119. For a discussion of this phenomenon in the early years of the PRC, see Joshua Goldstein, "Scissors, Surveys, and Psycho-Prophylactics: Prenatal Health Care Campaigns and State Building in China, 1949–1954," *Journal of Historical Sociology* 11, no. 2 (1998): 153–83. Oftentimes, lineages were associated with particular midwifery or other medical skills. Yi-Li Wu, "Transmitted Secrets: The Doctors of the Lower Yangzi Region and Popular Gynecology in Late Imperial China" (PhD dissertation, Yale University, 1998), 340.

120. A few notable articles include Macklin, "Notes on Cases"; J. Preston Maxwell, "On Criminal Abortion in China," *Chinese Medical Journal* 16 (January 12, 1928): 1–8; J. Preston Maxwell and Amos K. Wong, "On Puerperal Mortality and Morbidity," *National Medical Journal of China* 16 (1930): 684–703; Niles, "Native Midwifery in Canton."

121. Jordan, *Birth in Four Cultures: A Crosscultural Investigation of Childbirth in Yucatan, Holland, Sweden, and the United States.*

122. Larson, *The Rise of Professionalism: A Sociological Analysis.*

123. Bullock, *An American Transplant: The Rockefeller Foundation and Peking Union Medical College.*

124. Borst, *Catching Babies: The Professionalization of Childbirth, 1870–1920*; Larson, *The Rise of Professionalism: A Sociological Analysis.*

125. Xu, *Chinese Professionals and the Republican State: The Rise of Professional Associations in Shanghai, 1912–1937.*

126. Ibid., 12.

127. Ibid., 13.

128. William C. Kirby, "Engineering China: Birth of the Developmental State, 1928–1937," in *Becoming Chinese: Passages to Modernity and Beyond*, ed. Wen-hsin Yeh (Berkeley, Los Angeles, London: University of California Press, 2000), 152–53.

129. Yip, *Health and National Reconstruction in Nationalist China: The Development of Modern Health Services, 1928–1937.*

130. Honig, *Sisters and Strangers: Women in the Shanghai Cotton Mills, 1919–1949*; Elizabeth J. Perry, *Shanghai on Strike: The Politics of Chinese Labor* (Stanford: Stanford University Press, 1993); Wen-hsin Yeh, "The Paradox of Autonomy: Nation, Revolution, and Women through the Chinese Looking Glass," in *Women in China: The Republican Period in Historical Perspective*

(Germany: LIT Verlag Munster, 2005), 40–56; Lien, Ling-ling, "Leisure, Patriotism, and Identity: The Chinese Career Women's Club in Wartime Shanghai."

131. Lien, Ling-ling, "Leisure, Patriotism, and Identity: The Chinese Career Women's Club in Wartime Shanghai," 232–33.

132. Yeh, "Shanghai Modernity: Commerce and Culture in a Republican City," 380.

133. FNMS, *Fifth Annual Report, First National Midwifery School, Peiping, July 1, 1933–June 30, 1934*, viii.

134. Yip, *Health and National Reconstruction in Nationalist China: The Development of Modern Health Services, 1928–1937*, 17, 164; Liu, "From san gu liu po to 'caring scholar': the Chinese nurse in perspective," 321–23.

135. Xie Ruiyi, "First Anniversary Report (*Yi zhounian huiwu baogao*)," *Guangzhou shi zhuchanshi gonghui tekan* (1947): 21–22.

136. Ibid., 21.

137. "Midwifery Association dispute: Pang Fu'ai issues another statement (*Zhuchanshi gonghui jiufen an: Pang Fu'ai zai fa shengming*)," *Qianduo ribao*, September 16, 1947; "Important declaration of Guangzhou Midwifery Association board member chief Pang Fu'ai (*Guangzhoushi zhuchanshi gonghui lishizhang Pang Fu'ai zhongyao shengming*)," *Daguangbao* (*Guangzhoubao*), September 13, 1947.

138. Bullock, *An American Transplant: The Rockefeller Foundation and Peking Union Medical College*, 173.

139. Yip, *Health and National Reconstruction in Nationalist China: The Development of Modern Health Services, 1928–1937*, 165–67; Marion Yang, "The Training of Midwives," *China Medical Journal* 42 (1928): 554.

140. Marion Yang, "Letter to the Editor," *China Medical Journal* 42 (1928): 554.

141. Yang, *Report of the Training and Supervision for Midwives*.

142. Lien, Ling-ling, "Leisure, Patriotism, and Identity: The Chinese Career Women's Club in Wartime Shanghai," 215, 233.

143. Stockard, *Daughters of the Canton Delta: Marriage Patterns and Economic Strategies in South China, 1860–1930*; Marjorie Topley, "Marriage Resistance in Rural Kwangtung," in *Women in Chinese Society*, ed. Margery Wolf and Roxane Witke (Stanford: Stanford University Press, 1975), 67–88.

144. Ye, ""Nu Liuxuesheng": The Story of American-Educated Chinese Women, 1880s–1920s." 338–39.

145. Liu, "From san gu liu po to 'caring scholar': the Chinese nurse in perspective."

146. Yip, *Health and National Reconstruction in Nationalist China: The Development of Modern Health Services, 1928–1937*, 167.

147. Liu, "From san gu liu po to 'caring scholar': the Chinese nurse in perspective," 320.

148. Gertrude Hodgman, personal communication, as quoted in Bowers, *Western Medicine in a Chinese Palace: Peking Union Medical College, 1917–1951*, 208.

149. Robert Dingwall, Anne Marie Rafferty, and Charles Webster, *An Introduction to the Social History of Nursing* (London: Routledge, 1988), chapter two, "Revolution in Nursing." On the pollution of childbirth in China, see Ahern, "The Power and Pollution of Chinese Women."

150. Gertrude Hodgman, personal communication, as quoted in Bowers, *Western Medicine in a Chinese Palace: Peking Union Medical College, 1917–1951*, 208.

151. Ibid.

152. Tuqiang Advanced Midwifery School, *Record of the 50th Graduating Class of Tuqiang Advanced Midwifery School (Tuqiang gaodeng zhuchan xuexiao #50 jie biye tongxue lu)* (Guangzhou: Dongya zhongxi yinwuju, 1936).

153. Yang, "Control of Practising Midwives in China."

154. Caojuan Hu, "Why I Want to Study Nursing (*Wo wei shenme yao xue hushi*)," in *Bethel Annual (Boteli niankan)* (Shanghai: Shanghai Boteli yiyuan hushi chanke xuexiao bian zuan, 1936), 4–5.

155. Shumin Wang, "My Reflections on Entering Bethel Obstetrics School (*Wo ru Boteli chanke xuexiao de ganxiang*)," in *Bethel Annual (Boteli niankan)* (Shanghai: Shanghai Boteli yiyuan hushi chanke xuexiao bian zuan, 1936), 16–17.

156. Zhongde Professional Midwifery School Association (*Zhongde gaoji zhuchan zhuanye xuexiao weiyuanhui*), ed., *Zhongde Professional Midwifery School 15th Anniversary Commemorative Publication (Zhongde gaoji zhuchan zhuanye xuexiao 15 zhounian jinian kan)* (Shanghai, 1940).

157. Ibid., 25–30.

158. Wang Yugang and Qu Shaoheng, "Script for The Moment of Life and Death (*Sheng si guantou juben*)," in *Shengsheng Midwifery School Yearbook* (Shanghai: Shengsheng Midwifery School, 1935), 49–64.

159. Hershatter, *Dangerous Pleasures: Prostitution and Modernity in Twentieth-Century Shanghai.*

160. Xie Ruiyi, "First Anniversary Report (*Yi zhounian huiwu baogao*)."

161. Rong Wangxi, "The Life of a Nurse in the Old Days (*Jiu shehui hushi de shenghuo*)," in *Hua County Gazetteer (Huaxian wenshi ziliao)*, vol. 5 (Henan sheng, Huaxian: Zhengxie huaxian weiyuanhui wenshi ziliao yanjiu weiyuanhui bian, 1989), 100–103.

162. Yun Qin, "Hygiene and Fetal Education during Pregnancy (*Renshen de weisheng yu taijiao*)."

163. Ibid.

164. Xu, *Chinese Professionals and the Republican State: The Rise of Professional Associations in Shanghai, 1912–1937*, 57.

165. Sheng Jun, *Index of Living Cost in Shanghai* (Shanghai: The National Tariff Commission, 1930).

166. *First National Midwifery School, Peiping.*

167. FNMS, *Fifth Annual Report, First National Midwifery School, Peiping, July 1, 1933–June 30, 1934.*

168. Tao, "Medical Education of Chinese Women"; Lee T'ao, "Some Statistics on Medical Schools in China for 1932–1933," *Chinese Medical Journal* 47 (1933): 1029–1039.

169. Tao, "Medical Education of Chinese Women," 1034.

170. Tatchell, "The Training of Male Nurses."

171. Tao, "Medical Education of Chinese Women," 1034.

172. Paul Bailey, "'Unharnessed Fillies': Discourse on the 'Modern' Female Student in Early Twentieth-Century China," in *Wu sheng zhi sheng (III): Zhongguo de funü yu wenhua 1600–1950* (*Voices amid Silence [III]: Women and the Culture in Modern China 1600–1950*), ed. Lo Jiu-jung and Lu Miaw-fen, vol. 3 (Taibei shi: Zhongyang yanjiuyuan jindaishi yanjiusuo chuban, 2003), 327–57.

173. Chen and Bunge, *Medicine in Rural China: A Personal Account*, 91.

174. Goldstein, "Scissors, Surveys, and Psycho-Prophylactics: Prenatal Health Care Campaigns and State Building in China, 1949–1954," 177–78.

175. Grant, *Midwifery Training*.

176. According to surveys by the American Congress of Obstetricians and Gynecologists, the proportion of female obstetrician/gynecologists increased from 21% in 1991 to 39% in 2003. "Profile of Ob-Gyn Practice" (American Congress of Obstetricians and Gynecologists, 2003), http://www.acog.org/from_home/departments/practice/ProfileofOb-gynPractice1991–2003.pdf; W.F. Rayburn et al., "Trends in the Academic Workforce of Obstetrics and Gynecology," *Obstetrics and Gynecology* 115 (2010): 141–46.

4

National Reproduction in Republican China

The Guangdong Police Department sees that there cannot help but be a close connection between the good of the people and the management and regulation . . . of all Western doctors, obstetrists [chankesheng], pharmacists, pharmacies, Western hospitals, the Red Cross Society, etc.[1]

State control over private lives progressively increased in twentieth-century China. Its implications are notable in state involvement in the realm of reproduction, exemplified by the stringent family planning policies of the 1970s onward. Government policies concerning reproduction illustrate the ease in which individual or family jurisdiction over oneself and one's body can be gradually, or suddenly, stripped away and replaced by state mandate. Reproduction in Republican China became both a private and public affair rooted in one's family and community, and a social one that is intertwined with the well-being of the nation.[2] Many scholars have shown that during revolution, war, and nationalist movements, all of which were occurring in Republican China, women's bodies may become a site of nation-building or nation-preserving strategies.[3] As Haleh Afshar and Katherine Verdery have shown for Eastern Europe and Iran, respectively, the modernizing state explicitly calls upon women to bear children as their "national duty," to become "honorable mothers" to strengthen the nation and maintain the culture.[4] In all cases, women are the targets of these nationalistic cultural policies, partly because it is women who do the reproducing, but also because targeting males may threaten cultural gender distinctions of virile men and passive, malleable women.

China's governmental control over "births and bodies" did not originate with the Chinese Communist Party in the 1980s, although most of the literature on reproduction in China focuses on this period.[5] It began instead in the 1920s with legislation supporting state-managed childbirth. The Guomindang attempted to alter women's social roles by implementing laws and encouraging modern childbirth practices. The highly medicalized and state-sponsored birth model has remained standard in urban China. Western philanthropists were crucial to this transformation of birth into a state-controlled arena. Their medical resources, methods, policies, and infrastructure were transferred to China as the Guomindang lacked the organization, the funds, or the personnel to implement their wide-ranging initiatives.

The fetish of modernity in the early twentieth century extended into many areas and claimed its authority in science. When the Guomindang established a central government and moved the capital to Nanjing in 1927, its focus on reconstructing China included scientific fields like transportation and engineering, wastewater and sewage sanitation, and food production and distribution.[6] Likewise, cultural alterations like family reform, racial determinism, and child rearing claimed scientific backing.[7] Reproduction legislation had long-lasting effects on women in China, and indeed on the entire population, as childbirth affects everyone. All are connected to birth by personal experience, and a person's birth environment can affect his or her health throughout one's lifetime.

This examination of Guomindang midwifery legislation at the national, provincial, and municipal levels illustrates the extensive plans for reforming childbirth nationwide. By the 1920s the Guomindang firmly advocated, without always implementing, midwifery reform at all levels. However, if one sees only the public health and reproduction laws passed in the 1920s and 1930s in China, the picture is overwhelmingly positive. The reality was quite bleak, as lack of funding and resources, along with political and social turmoil, prevented many of these reforms from being carried out. This dichotomy illustrates the fracture between ideal and reality, and cautions against drawing inappropriate conclusions from the available historical materials. The reality is that the Guomindang did not have the central organization, planning, or political control to effect the changes that some of its leaders wanted to make. Legislation reforming and regulating childbirth was written and passed, though the necessary organs to enforce the new policies were not. Thus, for example, while traditional, unregistered midwives were deemed illegal in 1913, enforcement of that law was impossible. On the other hand, China's "age of openness" and limited governmental reach allowed those with foresight, such as Yang Chongrui and Liu Ruiheng, to create very grand visions about China's future.[8] The study of legislation, while providing a poor reflection of reality, does show very clearly the intention of the Guomindang government: the continued emphasis on reforming reproduction. This emphasis has remained a primary occupation of the Chinese government since this period.

The initial impetus for reforming reproduction came from foreign medical missionaries, thus the relationship between the Guomindang and the foreign philanthropists, as well as the importance of Western-trained Chinese personnel, is of utmost importance in creating the new vision of reproduction. The most significant efforts at midwifery reform took place in treaty ports and urban centers like Guangzhou, Shanghai, and Beijing. These cities had established or were building the infrastructure and administration necessary to realize these reforms, as examined in chapter 1. Urban centers were subject to significant foreign influence in the realm of public health and medicine. Many other municipalities and provincial governments incorporated midwifery training and regulation into their modernization plans with direction and instruction, though not always funding, from the central government. The cities of Kunming and Tianjin, and the provinces of Fujian, Jiangxi, Gansu, and Ningxia all established midwifery programs by the 1930s, though many of these programs and plans were generally not as intensive or as successful as those in Shanghai, Beijing, or Guangzhou.[9] Their efforts were hindered by poor tax collection and allocation, as well as the financial burden placed on them by the central Guomindang government.[10]

GUOMINDANG MIDWIFERY LEGISLATION

Varied attempts to regulate midwives existed as early as the late Ming dynasty, although efforts at systematic control increased from the 1910s onward.[11] 1913 marks the first Republican national legislation outlawing traditional midwives and enforcing training, registration, and regulation of modern ones.[12] The Guomindang was founded in Guangzhou in 1912, and that was the first city to establish a modern public health program. Early efforts at midwifery reform illustrate the government's intention to regulate reproduction at such an early stage in its founding. Home of Canton Hospital (founded in 1835), Guangzhou also trained some of the first modern midwives. While traditionally a treaty-port city, Guangzhou was displaced by Hong Kong as a major foreign settlement by the early twentieth century.

In 1934, there were an estimated 410 foreigners in Guangzhou, as compared to 69,797 foreigners in Shanghai in 1932.[13] Yet many of the native Chinese who were in charge of the Guangzhou city government were trained abroad. Guangzhou's first mayor, Sun Fo (served 1921–22, 1923–24, and 1926–27), the son of Sun Yat-sen, studied municipal administration at the University of California at Berkeley. All of the six bureau chiefs under Sun Fo had studied abroad: two in Japan, one in Europe, and three in the United States.[14] Furthermore, Guangzhou was the headquarters of the Guomindang intermittently in the 1910s and 1920s, so many of the city's progressive public health policies may be attributed to Guomindang ideals of a strong, centralized, modern government. When the Guomindang established a national government in Nanjing, these programs were expanded to the national level and were intended to reach into the rural areas.

In 1913, the year after the Guomindang was founded there, Guangdong Province passed a set of regulations controlling midwives (see table 4.1). These early laws strictly prohibited unlicensed midwives from practicing midwifery in Guangzhou for payment. In order to obtain a license, the midwife had to complete a training program and pay a registration fee. These were harsh laws for a period in which there were few trained midwives and extremely limited opportunities for midwifery training, not to mention the impossibility of enforcing such rules. As we have seen, midwifery was not a respectable profession in most areas during this period, and it was difficult to persuade women to enter the limited number of training programs. Most women and their families had no access to trained midwives or physicians because the majority of these health workers were employed in urban areas and in hospitals. Many families did not have the resources to pay for their services even if they desired them. In theory, this left the pregnant women of China in a bind. Although legislation from this time does not specifically ban the hiring of untrained midwives (aside from government employment), it follows that if traditional midwives were prohibited from practicing, then pregnant women could not retain them. Of course, most parturient women and practitioners during this time operated outside the radar of the authorities. Nevertheless, these early local laws restricting untrained midwives did not offer any solutions to the problem of who should attend labor and childbirth, as there were very few modern midwives relative to the number of births.

Attention to public health quickly moved from the local to the national level when the Guomindang gained nominal control over China in 1927. Modernizing efforts included forming a central government

Table 4.1.   Police Department Announcement of Proposed Regulations for Registered Western Doctors, Obstetrists, Pharmacists, Prescriptions, Western Hospitals and the Red Cross. Guangdong Provincial Government, 1913.

1. Midwives graduated from a specialized midwifery school must register with the Municipal Police Department;

2. Midwives must not call themselves "doctor" [yisheng] but had to call themselves "obstetrist" [chankesheng];

3. Midwives must not use medicine or any means to cause abortion. Aside from being brought to trial, the accused midwife will also have her licensed [sic] revoked by the Police Department;

4. During birth, the midwife may not threaten or coerce the parturient woman or her family members to use unnecessary tools resulting in injury to mother or child. If accused, after strict investigation the midwife will be brought to trial and her license revoked;

5. During a difficult birth, the midwife must not dismember [sui, lit. break to pieces] the infant. If there is no choice and the midwife must use this method, the midwife must call in a licensed physician;

6. If after a birth there is blood poisoning [xueduzheng], the midwife must report it to the Police Department, and the midwife cannot deliver another infant for two weeks in order to stop the spread of the disease;

7. The midwife license costs 5 yuan; and

8. Unlicensed midwives must meet the following conditions:

   a. The government cannot use unlicensed midwives;

   b. Unlicensed midwives may not put up a sign on their own ["put up a shingle," meaning that they may not open an office or clinic];

   c. Unlicensed midwives may not obtain fees for their services;

   d. Unlicensed midwives cannot testify in court for medical lawsuits.

staffed with optimistic members who had a new "ideal of professionalism" that "only recently had asserted itself in municipal and provincial affairs" in New Policies reforms from the later years of the Qing dynasty.[15] The new government in Nanjing aimed to "control China's progress from the center," resulting in an "extraordinary number of party and government institutions founded in 1927–28," including new ministries of health and of education.[16] Restructuring policies built on Sun Yat-sen's "Industrial Plan" were published in 1921 and focused on national reconstruction with the goal of the "integrated economic development of a unified China."[17] The reforms targeted the transportation system and manufacturing sector, and also aimed to shape the very character of China's citizens.

In the 1920s, ideas about public health expanded from the occasional street cleaning and night soil campaigns to crusades for individual health and hygiene and "acceptable social behavior."[18] These plans would fundamentally change the daily lives of Chinese. For example, a movement existed to use Western eating and serving utensils instead of chopsticks to halt the spread of tuberculosis.[19] Such reforms reached their peak during the New Life Movement examined below. Although the main focus of China's newly established Ministry of Health was communicable disease prevention and sanitation, maternal and child health was a significant component. According to Vice-minister of Health and later Director of the National Health Administration Liu Ruiheng, "the important bearing of maternal and infant health on the health of the future citizens and the present entire absence of adequate facilities in midwifery practice make this question a matter that demands immediate attention."[20] Nationalist policies aimed to regulate and educate midwives, mothers, and family members within the broader context of improving China's public health.

WESTERN PHILANTHROPY AND PUBLIC HEALTH

However noble their intentions, Guomindang support of health projects was minimal and the Ministry of Health was weak. Western philanthropic organizations like the League of Nations-Health Organization (LON-HO) and the Rockefeller Foundation's International Health Division helped to fill the need for improved medical care and public health policy by providing consulting support, cash, and personnel. These two organizations formed a partnership in the 1920s in order to tackle public health problems left in the devastating wake of World War I.[21] They focused on disease prevention founded on improved nutrition and hygiene from the program developed at Johns Hopkins University School of Public Health in Baltimore. The Rockefeller Foundation initially started with hookworm and yellow fever eradication campaigns in the southern United States, but this soon extended to public health endeavors on every continent.[22]

In 1926, LON-HO undertook a preliminary investigation in several European countries and found that most infant mortality was caused by poor prenatal or obstetrical care. According to a 1931 LON-HO report, infant mortality (figured as deaths under one year of age) accounted for one-tenth of all deaths worldwide.[23] Because the main causes of maternal and infant mortality were easily preventable with prenatal care and aseptic birth techniques, maternal and child health fell under the domain of preventive medicine, and thus one of the main concentrations of the global health movement was lowering infant and maternal mortality rates. Both LON-HO and the Rockefeller Foundation promoted maternal and infant health around the globe, including breastfeeding, pre- and postnatal education, and "maternal hygiene" campaigns.[24] The Rockefeller Foundation formed the China Medical Board to improve health in China as part of a larger project to improve health worldwide.

The Rockefeller Foundation's China Medical Board was the primary architect of China's model hospital and medical school, Peking Union Medical College (PUMC).[25] All told, between 1913 and 1949, the China Medical Board poured US$45 million into health care in China, funneled directly or indirectly through Peking Union Medical College;[26] PUMC's physical plant alone cost more than $7.5 million.[27] The China Medical Board enforced a hierarchy of medical schools and itself acted as the authority on medical training throughout China. The organization classified preexisting medical schools, colleges, and training programs according to the quality of their curricula, faculty and staff, and facilities. Most of the schools were deemed inadequate, even those run by Western missionaries. The Japanese schools were especially criticized.[28] The China Medical Board's importance in funding medicine and public health in China is especially evident because once the resources from the Rockefeller Foundation ceased, the Nationalist government funding was unable to properly maintain Peking Union Medical College. By the late 1930s, the government was rife with factionalism within its ranks, and much of its attention and money had turned towards other matters like the Japanese and communist threats. The school was closed in 1942, eventually to reopen again as China Union Medical College under the People's Republic of China after 1949.[29]

Improving public health had been one of the key goals of Peking Union Medical College since its inception. Of the first four divisions of the school—communicable diseases, general sanitation, vital statistics, and medical services—three were related to public health. The school quickly grew to include other specialized fields (medicine, including pediatrics, dermatology and syphilology, and neurology; surgery; OB/GYN; roentgenology [radiology]; urology; anesthetics; orthopedics; and ophthalmology), as well as the Training School for Nurses. The nursing school opened in 1920 with three students and placed its emphasis on nursing education, rather than just serving as a supplier of nursing services to hospitals. In 1924, as part of its legitimizing and professionalizing efforts to be incorporated into the university, the training school changed its name to the School of Nursing, and the leader of the school gained the title of dean. Half of the 39 students the school had graduated by 1932 were working in midwifery or public health.[30]

Peking Union Medical College served as a training ground for some of the most influential public health personnel in China. Chen Zhiqian, a graduate of PUMC, was simultaneously appointed in 1936 the superintendent of both the Peking First Health Demonstration Station and the Dingxian Rural Health Station, two organizations discussed later in this chapter. Liu Ruiheng, former director of PUMC hospital, was China's Vice-Minister of Health, Minister of Health from 1928 to 1931, and Director of the National Health Administration-Central Field Health Station from 1931 to 1937. Yang Chongrui was head of the National Midwifery Board and director of the First National Midwifery School from 1929 to 1936. Many other graduates filled government posts throughout the country.

After the Guomindang established its capital in Nanjing in 1927, Chiang Kai-shek commonly allotted ministry posts as political favors, creating a serious lack of cohesion and consistency at the highest levels of government. Hung-mao Tien illustrated that the Ministry of the Interior had a total of 12 ministers between 1927 and 1938, many of whom cared little for their administrative duties.[31] Several of these appointed political protégés and military leaders held simultaneous posts, thus reinforcing the problem of inadequacy and disinterest in policy making and implementation.[32] According to Chen Zhiqian, Chiang Kai-shek gave control of the newly formed Ministry of Health to "a warlord as a token of appreciation for his support of the party."[33] The government leaders were not interested in the ministry, so the new warlord minister turned to Peking Union Medical College to staff his agency and to help devise national health policy.[34]

In the 1930s Peking Union Medical College administrators grew concerned about Guomindang pressure on physicians to leave the school to take up government posts. After PUMC graduate Liu Ruiheng became Minister of Health, he eagerly "reach[ed] out for all of [PUMC's] men who can be diverted into Government service."[35] China Medical Board director Henry Houghton in 1937 expressed "fears about the pressure that is being put upon our senior Chinese staff members to leave here for the educational service of the Government in Central China."[36] Liu Ruiheng and the China Medical Board's Dr. John B. Grant "guided the establishment of new municipal and province-level health administrations, placing many former students in these agencies as well."[37] Through these activities PUMC graduates, in conjunction with the China Medical Board, greatly influenced the Nationalist health administration and indeed formulated much of the government's public health policy.

CHINA'S NATIONAL MIDWIFERY BOARD

As part of the Nationalist government's mandate to emphasize public health "for the sake of the nation," government officials undertook a concentrated effort to develop maternal and child health programs.[38] In 1929, the ministries of health and education jointly established the National Midwifery Board (Zhuchan jiaoyu weiyuanhui) "to promote midwifery education in the country."[39] Also in 1929, the Ministry of Health's first Five-Year Plan aimed to provide preventive and clinical maternal and child health care in cities and rural areas. This plan focused on building a health administration unit and training facilities. It included the creation of the Central Field Health Station (Weisheng shiyan chu) in Nanjing, a central hygiene institute with research labs and a drug production unit. The Five-Year Plan created strategies to train old-style and modern midwives and public health nurses, as well as to provide a nationwide maternal and child health care network.

The National Midwifery Board included in its ranks several graduates of Peking Union Medical College. Its nine members included two representatives each from the Ministries of Health and of Education, to hold office for two-year terms. In 1932 the board was comprised of the following: from the Ministry of Health, Dr. Liu Ruiheng and Dr. L.C. Yen (Chief of the Department of Medical Administration); from the Ministry of Education, Mr. Wu Lai Chua (Vice Minister of Education) and Dr. Shilu Hong (Physiologist); and Honorary Members Madam Feng Yuxiang (wife of a progressive "Christian General"),[40] Madame Chiang Kai-shek, Dr. F.C. Yen (Dean of Central University Medical School), Dr. Sun Keh-chi (Obstetrician, Red Cross hospital, Shanghai) and Dr. Yang Chongrui (Obstetrician, Peking Union Medical College).[41] The board met twice yearly and focused on sponsoring and developing midwifery programs, writing legislation and training curricula, and overseeing registration of midwives and training institutions.[42] Through funding to hospitals and medical schools, the state thus promoted the professionalization of midwives, the dissemination of "modern" models of parenthood, as well as "scientific" anatomical charts of wombs and fetuses for teaching the new methods.[43] The first task of the National Midwifery Board was to standardize midwifery training, and thus the

First National Midwifery School was established in Beijing in 1929 at PUMC as the national model training program with Dr. Yang Chongrui as director. It was affiliated with PUMC's departments of public health, nursing, and obstetrics and gynecology.

The First National Midwifery School acted as the official arm of the National Midwifery Board in planning, implementing, and staffing new midwifery schools, hospitals, and maternal and child health programs across China. Yang Chongrui and John B. Grant both consulted on and lobbied for public health programs nationwide and helped to establish several other important institutions. Furthermore, First National Midwifery School staff members were often sent to fledgling programs in rural and urban areas to help administer midwifery schools and maternal and child health initiatives. By 1934, all of the First National Midwifery School's senior staff had been sent elsewhere to work. Four midwives and one physician went to the Central Midwifery School in Nanjing; one physician and one midwife were sent to take charge of the Shaanxi Provincial Midwifery School in Xi'an; one physician and two midwives went to the Jiangxi Provincial Midwifery School in Nanchang; and one physician and one midwife went to Lanzhou, Gansu, to open a provincial midwifery school there.[44]

The National Midwifery Board attempted to propagate midwifery reform across the country through First National Midwifery School personnel. In the 1930s, several organizations around the country requested advice and personnel from the school. In 1932–33, Yang Chongrui took five leaves of absence for a total of 50 days to go on such advising trips.[45] These included Dingxian, the YWCAs of Wuchang (Hubei Province) and Wujiang (Anhui Province), Yenching University's Department of Sociology, the Local Gentry Association of Yutian (Hebei Province), the Taixian government (Jiangsu Province), the Nanjing municipal government, and the Zhejiang and Jiangsu provincial governments. Yang made preliminary investigations of local conditions in each of these areas and drew up tentative plans for improving these locales' maternal and child health. Between September 1933 and May 1934 alone, she made technical assistance visits to Shanghai (September 29–October 8), Zhenjiang and Taixian (Jiangsu Province, October 30–November 2), Nanzhang and Hankou (Jiangxi Province, November 25–December 8), Zhangzhou (March 10), and Xi'an (Shaanxi Province, May 13–31). She also gave technical assistance to numerous other fledgling maternal and child health programs around the country like Gaoqiao Public Health Model Village in Shanghai.[46] Yang was both an advocate and a representative of the Nationalist government as head of the First National Midwifery School and member of the National

Midwifery Board. She worked to extend the influence of modern maternal and child health throughout China.

After the First National Midwifery School in Beijing got under way, in 1933 the Central Hospital in Nanjing and the Nanjing Municipal Health Station jointly opened the second national-level midwife training institution, the Nanjing Central Midwifery School (also called the Second National Midwifery School), one year after the Central School of Nursing was established in that city. This school was supported by the Guomindang as part of their efforts to remake Nanjing into a modern city. Yang Chongrui left her post as head of the First National Midwifery School in 1931 to help establish Central in its new half-million dollar building, and she acted as director there for an initial three-month period.[47] Six affiliated antenatal clinics were established around Nanjing to provide practical field experience for Central Midwifery School students. The school opened in 1932 and offered a two-year course, with 41 students enrolled in 1934.[48] Selected personnel were to receive special training from the First National Midwifery School and Peking Union Medical College's Departments of Hygiene and Public Health and of Obstetrics/Gynecology. By 1934, many of the First National Midwifery School's senior personnel were sent to the Central Midwifery School to work.[49] The Central School of Nursing (*Zhongyang hushi xuexiao*, changed in 1935 to *zhongyang gaoji hushi zhuanye xuexiao*) was established in Nanjing in 1932 and also included public health and midwifery courses in which 91 students were enrolled in 1935. In fact, the entire second year of course work was devoted to pregnancy, birth, and postpartum management.[50] The overarching aim of these projects was to have a citywide maternal and child health service in Nanjing within 10 years.

PROVINCIAL MIDWIFERY PROGRAMS

By 1936, several provinces with considerable input from the First National Midwifery School and its affiliates had set up some type of public health administration or hospital that promoted public health. However, as Hung-mao Tien has shown, provincial governments in the Republican period were not any more successful than the national government in affecting meaningful social change or modernization. He notes that problems with tax accounting and collection, coupled with demands for funds from the central government, effectively prevented the provinces from making substantial improvements in infrastructure or on social issues.[51] Nevertheless, Hunan, Gansu, Ningxia,

Qinghai, and Zhejiang all established provincial public health experimental stations (*sheng weisheng shiyanchu*), Jiangxi created a provincial public health department (*sheng weisheng chu*), and Shanxi formed a public health committee (*weisheng weiyuanhui*) by the 1930s. In addition, Jiangsu, Henan, and Guangxi all established provincial hospitals that promoted public health throughout the province.[52]

Several provinces also established official provincial midwifery schools in the 1930s, and many more supported private institutions. According to Liu Ruiheng's 1937 report on the National Health Administration, the National Health Administration and the Central Field Health Station in Nanjing helped to establish provincial midwifery schools in the late 1930s in Fujian, Jiangxi, Gansu, and Ningxia.[53] The 1943 Records of the Yunnan Administration (*Yunnan xingzheng jishi*) states that the National Health Administration also assisted Kunming in establishing a provincial midwifery school as early as 1933.[54] Zhejiang had begun a provincial midwifery school attached to the provincial hospital (*Zhejiang shengli zhuchan xuexiao*) under the provincial civil administration department (*minzhengting*) in 1928, and it was approved by the Department of Education in 1931. During that year, the hospital delivered 296 infants.[55] Furthermore, in 1933 Hubei Province opened a provincial nursing school in the provincial hospital, a midwifery school (*zhuchan xuexiao*), and an old-style midwife training program (*chanpo xunlianban*) under the provincial public security department (*gonganju*).[56]

The following year Jiangsu and Hunan opened not proper schools but provincial maternity hospitals, by 1935 Shanxi had its own midwifery school and maternity hospital,[57] and in 1933–34 the First National Midwifery School provided technical assistance to the Shaanxi Provincial Midwifery School in Xi'an.[58] Jiangsu's commoners' maternity hospital (*pingmin chanyuan*), part of its larger provincial hospital, was administered by the Jiangsu provincial public health affairs department (*Jiangsu sheng hui weisheng shiwusuo*) under the public security department. When the maternity hospital opened in 1932, there were six beds with three patients, and deliveries numbered about 15 per month, including home deliveries.[59] Plans were in effect in 1932 to establish 10 maternity homes with antenatal and postnatal supervision in 10 different counties within two years in Jiangsu Province. Their goal, aside from the obvious one of improving maternal and child health in rural locales, was to open up areas in which the Jiangsu Provincial Midwifery School graduates could obtain practical experience. The Jiangsu provincial government also began training old-type midwives in May 1932, the instructors of whom were graduates of the

First National Midwifery School.[60] Hunan's maternity hospital (*Hunan chanyuan*), administered by its civil administration office, was the "central organization established to 'move forward' and manage the whole province's midwifery work" (*tuijin ju guanli quan sheng zhuchan gongzuo zhi zhongxin jiguan*).[61]

It is unclear whether all of these schools and hospitals had the support or assistance of the National Health Administration and likewise, the National Midwifery Board, which illustrates the disarray and deficiency of some early twentieth-century Chinese government documents. The scattered and spotty records that do exist point to a massive nationwide campaign to quickly and dramatically change normative childbirth in China to a modern model. On paper, the plans are astounding. In reality, government reach did not achieve these far-ranging schemes. Although the National Health Administration existed to govern public health, and the National Midwifery Board to oversee maternal and child health projects, due to China's unstable political and social conditions, reporting to these governing bodies was either inconsistent or nonexistent. It seems as though many provincial governments jumped on the public health bandwagon in the 1930s, but the extent and efficacy of their programs was usually lacking due to funding and administration problems. Liu Ruiheng's 1937 report to LON-HO states that nine out of 18 provinces had established provincial health services, with three in stages of advanced planning. In the same report Liu also noted that traditional Chinese medical practitioners still attended over 65 percent of patients, and 26 percent of sick people were estimated to die without treatment each year. Furthermore, it was difficult to persuade qualified doctors to live in remote rural areas, battle traditional beliefs, and compete with traditional Chinese medical practitioners. There were also the continuing shortages of funding and resources, corruption, and lack of transportation for medical supplies and people. [62]

RURAL MIDWIFERY PROGRAMS

Rural programs were also beset with financial and staffing problems. The First National Midwifery School assisted Dingxian and Qinghe, two model mass education movement districts that received foreign support and provided technical assistance to rural areas around the country. In a plea for funding, Yang Chongrui wrote:

> It has been felt that, considering the present state of China, we give too thorough training to maternity and child health officers and

workers. However, if we consider our large rural population (85%), our economic education and transportation, it becomes necessary to set up strong units in the rural centers that they may handle both physiological and pathological conditions. We can not progress by referring the pathological cases to urban hospitals.[63]

Thus the national Department of Public Health's Five-Year Plan drawn up in 1934 stated that every *xian* (county) in every province would have public health facilities within five years.[64] With help from the League of Nations-Health Organization member Dr. Berislav Borçic, a tiered model was established for rural areas, based on one he had created for Yugoslavia.[65] Eventually every rural *xian* was to have a public health clinic with a 30–50 bed hospital, a diagnostic laboratory, and a health administration office. Each *xian* health station was staffed by one physician, two nurses, and one midwife, with a monthly budget of 200–300 yuan.

Part of each health station's mission was to carry out maternal and child health and midwifery work, oversee school health, and propagate and disseminate public health methods and information. Plans stated that the hospital should staff five to seven nurses and two *zhuchanshi*, along with a head doctor, laboratory and public health workers, and administrative personnel.[66] Below the *xian*, health stations (*weishengsuo*) were established for each 50,000 people and subordinate "health substations" (*weisheng fensuo*) in each *xian* or administrative village. The substations each had a nurse trained in public health and with midwifery experience who could handle "routine maternity and health problems, school hygiene, vaccination, and general first-aid emergencies."[67] The monthly budget of 50–70 yuan was to cover outpatient treatment; smallpox and other vaccinations; school health programs; maternal and child health work and midwifery; reporting births, deaths, moves, and marriages; and propagating public health.[68] The Five-Year Plan also declared that each *xian* should have maternal and child health facilities and training programs (*xunlianban*) for old-style midwives. In fact, these goals were included in the first year of the Five-Year Plan, second only to opening 25-bed hospitals in each county. Year one also included provisions for public health programs in schools, as well as unspecified methods to "propagate public health" (*weisheng xuanchuan*).[69]

At the village level, by the end of the first Five-Year Plan each *cun* (village) or group of *cun* was to establish a 25-bed hospital with internal medicine, surgery, and obstetrics/gynecology departments. The head of the hospital should be a medical doctor and was charged with attending patients, including pregnant women and newborns, as well as overseeing the district public health work. Each *cun* was to have a local "village health assistant" (*xiezhu yishi*) and a district dispensary with old-style midwives trained in modern methods whose duties were to assist childbirth and report births and deaths to their district dispensaries (*zhiliaosuo*).[70] The head nurse in charge of the district dispensary had as her duties to treat minor venereal illnesses (*qing xing jibing*), promote maternal and child health (*fuying weisheng*), train old-style midwives (*chanpo jiesheng*), give preventive injections (inoculations, *yufang zhushe*), promote public health, supervise and help in the work of rural relief workers and old-style midwives, and gather the *cun*'s birth and death reports.[71]

The budgets for the district dispensaries and hospitals were small and depended upon provincial and county funding, which was often insufficient. The budgeted start-up costs for each 25-bed *xian* hospital totaled 3,275 yuan, and operating expenses were allowed 1,430 yuan per month, give or take depending upon the county's size and financial situation. District dispensaries were budgeted 850 yuan for start-up costs and operating expenses of 253 yuan per month, also depending on the district's size and financial conditions.[72] The first Three-Year Plan for the Chinese National Health Administration (1931–34) called for local and national governments to pay for all medical services in the *xian* until local cooperative health insurance plans were established.[73] However, due to lack of funds, only Jiangsu, Zhejiang, Jiangxi, Guangxi, and Henan had counties with such facilities by 1935.[74]

Places where public health programs gained purchase were in locales that had the support of local government agencies in conjunction with foreign funding, reinforcing this important relationship. The experimental counties of Jiangningxian (*Jiangning zizhi shiyan xian*), Dingxian, and the Central Field Health Station were supported by the Milbank Memorial Fund and the China Medical Board.[75] These *xian* incorporated rural health centers staffed with midwives and nurses whose duties included pre- and postnatal care and submitting birth and death reports. By 1933 Jiangning had a "health demonstration area" (*weisheng shiyan qu*) and a public health clinic (*weishengyuan*) five miles outside of Nanjing that was established to test the medical education policy of creating model *xian*-level rural health centers.[76] In 1934, Jiangningxian's public health center, clinic, stations, and substations aided in 221 births (*jiesheng*), inspected 5,154 households (*jiating fangshi*), and treated 2,394 pregnant women (*chanfu huli*) and 1,694 children (*ying'er huli*).[77]

The Dingxian Mass Education Movement was established in 1929 by James Yen (Yan Yangchu) and funded by the Milbank Memorial

Fund, individual philanthropists, and the Rockefeller Foundation's China Medical Board and Peking Union Medical College.[78] Dingxian is in Hebei Province, 60 miles from the nearest medical school and modern hospital in Baoding, which is 100 miles southwest of Beijing. Like Jiangningxian, its health system was also based on the *xian* model. At its peak, between 1929 and 1937, it had a 50-bed hospital and an administrative office in the *xian* center, 15 subcenter health stations, and local health workers in 150 villages. Its subcenter stations were staffed by a physician and a nurse, usually graduates from the medical school in Baoding who had completed extra public health training at the *xian*-level hospital. Eventually each village within the subcenters was to have voluntary "village health workers" or "medical helpers" (*zhuliyuan*).[79]

Funded in part by the Rockefeller Foundation's International Health Division, the Central Field Health Station outside Nanjing was run by Liu Ruiheng and modeled on Jiangningxian. Between 1929 and 1934, the International Health Division gave a total of Mex$82,000 for capital and annual running expenses.[80] The National Health Administration-Central Field Health Station sponsored public health campaigns via central broadcasting stations in Nanjing, health exhibits, public lectures, pamphlets, posters, lantern slides, and mobile medical units. The station also continued to train public health workers, doctors, nurses, midwives, school hygienists, paramedics, and sanitation workers.[81]

From 1929 to 1936, the Department of Maternity and Child Health of the Central Field Health Station graduated 189 individuals, nearly 90 percent of whom worked in a public health or similar institution in 16 different provinces. Many of them took positions as instructors or deans of midwifery schools.[82] In 1932, the Chinese Ministry of Education and the National Midwifery Board planned to start a class at the Central Field Health Station for instructors and administrators at all types of midwifery schools. The National Health Administration offered a grant-in-aid "with the stipulation that graduates from this course were obliged to return to their own schools for at least two years."[83] Between 1932 and 1936, 40 students graduated from this course. Furthermore, the maternal and child health division of the Central Field Health Station offered a teachers' course for midwives. Sixteen students from 14 different institutions participated in 1936. After their one-year term, they all returned to their home institutions "as future leaders and teachers in these communities."[84] The maternal and child health division of the Central Field Health Station had big plans: to train 100,000 maternity and child health workers (one for every 4,000 persons), 1,000 maternal and child health supervisors, 400 maternal and child health medical officers, and 10 maternal and child health medical organizers. The division also wanted to establish teaching and demonstration centers in Nanjing, Shanghai, and Beijing, as well as numerous rural and provincial centers.[85]

Aside from the more well-known and successful rural model health counties like Jiangningxian, Dingxian, and the Central Field Health Station, there were numerous other *xian*-level public health stations and hospitals, all of which had a maternal and child health division listed in their organizational charts, and most offering some sort of maternal and child health care and/or training. Most received personnel and funding from Western philanthropies in China. For example, the Tai County Hospital (*Taixian xianli yiyuan*) had two *zhuchanshi* and one nurse, and in 1933 opened a commoners' maternity hospital (*pingmin chanyuan*), the first rural maternity hospital of its kind in China. These were the result of a technical assistance visit by Yang Chongrui and the work of two First National Midwifery School midwives sent to help improve rural maternal and child health in Taixian.[86] In 1933, the hospital had four beds plus a separate delivery room and a nursery, in which were delivered nearly 20 babies. Its three midwives on staff gave prenatal checkups to 31 pregnant women, gave postnatal nursing care to 179 people, 31 infant check-ups, and nursing care to 951 infants.[87] Similarly, Hezexian had two nurses and one midwife who attended more than 250 births per month and gave pre- and postnatal checkups.[88] Six rural health districts within Jiangxi Province gave a total of 131 lectures and talks on modern childbirth.[89]

The public health program of the Qinghe experimental district (*Qinghe shiyanqu*) was a project of the Harvard University-sponsored Yenching University Department of Sociology and the Beiping City Police Department's Number One Public Health Station (*Beipingshi gong'anju di yi weisheng shiwusuo*).[90] It was established in July 1931 in Wanpingxian of Hebei Province, an area that included 40 villages with a total population of 32,000. The Public Health Station sent one doctor each Saturday to Qinghe to carry out public health and dispensary work. In August of the same year, they formally established a health station (*shiwusuo*), and a year later, because they "deeply believed in the importance of rural public health" (*shenjue weisheng gongzuo zai xiangcun zhi zhongyao*), expanded the organization and established another station.

In 1932, Yenching's Sociology Department entered into a cooperative agreement with the First National Midwifery School to open a rural maternity and child health service in Qinghe similar to the one in Dingxian.[91] This agreement provided rural practical service opportunities for First National Midwifery School students and graduates and aimed to improve Qinghe's maternal and child health. The FNMS provided technical direction and supervision of the service but did not assume financial responsibility. A graduate of FNMS's two-year course took charge of midwifery work and strove to advance maternal and child health (*fuying weisheng*). Most of her work consisted of monthly home visits to talk to families about the importance of maternal and child health, and many services were carried out in the patients' homes. In 1932–33, the staff midwife made 1,052 home education visits, 740 routine ante- and postnatal visits, and 41 home deliveries.[92] The clinic saw 228 new cases in 1932–33 and 401 new cases in 1933–34. In addition, there were 78 deliveries that year, four of which were referred to a hospital.[93] The delivery fee was $4 if the family was able to pay; otherwise, the service was free. In 1933–34, the service received $106.50 for deliveries. The district also included eight Mothers' Clubs (*muqin hui*) organized throughout the district that taught women modern childcare methods.[94] In 1932–33, there were 51 club meetings with a total attendance of 896 participants.[95]

In 1932–33, Qinghe began training old-style midwives. The outline for teaching midwifery prepared by the staff of the Qinghe rural maternal and child health service was published in a manual at the request of the Ministry of Education in 1934 and distributed to vocational schools throughout China.[96] In April 1935, the rural maternal and child health service began to give training to a group of women aged 25 to 35 who were selected by village leaders as "Maternity and Child Health Helpers." Upon completion of training, each helper would work in her own village and be supported by her own people. This would be a model for other rural villages throughout China.[97]

Education of the local people was often the goal in these rural areas because women were reluctant to utilize young, unmarried women dressed in mourning whites. Many programs were not wildly successful. Huaxian, Shanxi Province, had developed a significant maternal and child health education program, but the workers had found that maternal and child health work was difficult because of lack of knowledge among local women. Therefore, its main goal was educating the populace and publicizing maternal and child health methods and local facilities.[98] In February 1936, a survey of 1,000 mothers found that of the 1,000, 42 now elderly women had in their earlier years given birth to a total of 292 children. Of these, miscarriage and stillbirth had taken 25 of the infants, and tetanus another 51. In order to help prevent tetanus, the rural health station distributed 15 sets of clean umbilical cord-wrapping gauze with instructions for its use. Furthermore, this health station saw a total of 16 people in its women's and children's clinic (*fuying menzhen*), delivered only two babies, gave 14 pre- and postnatal nursing checkups, visited/inspected 170 homes, and distributed 200 fliers.[99]

Training old-style midwives in these rural areas was especially difficult. Chen Zhiqian, chief of the Xiaozhuang Rural Health Demonstration Program and superintendent of the Dingxian Rural Health Station, noted that his midwifery programs in these two locations were not popular and had to be dismantled because of resistance to new childbirth methods and reluctance to rely on young, unmarried, and childless midwives.[100] Chen resorted to training younger relatives of the old midwives instead, "who, as a member of their [*sic*] own family, would receive the older woman's support in her new role . . . and eliminate the problem of jealousy."[101] However, this program also was short-lived because its organizers could not get enough women to undertake the work, due in part to other household and occupational duties.[102]

Because of the problems rural families had in accepting young, new midwives, Chen Zhiqian instituted a program for the rural mothers to learn aseptic childcare techniques and receive pre- and postnatal home visits. He and his colleagues also "persuaded a continually growing number of women to deliver their babies at the district center under qualified care."[103] Chen remarked that although the mortality "figures reflected a lamentably low health level, we were making progress. The rates of puerperal sepsis, tetanus neonatorum, and problems related to childbirth and early infancy in general were declining."[104] The 1934 figures for Dingxian show infant mortality at 185.2 per 1,000 live births; death among people under five years old was 44.5 percent (partly because of epidemics of dysentery and scarlet fever that year). The death rate among children under two years of age was 200 per 100,000.[105] Although efforts at midwife training were not succeeding, health education programs aimed at mothers were positively impacting the health of mothers and infants.

MUNICIPAL AND PRIVATE PROGRAMS

The city governments of Beijing, Shanghai, Guangzhou, and Nanjing established midwifery training and registration programs as part of model sanitation districts (*weisheng mofan qu*) or experimental public health districts (*weisheng shiyan chu*), which included substantial midwifery education and maternal and child health projects. These public health projects were popular in the 1930s and garnered support from local notables and government officials, as Ruth Rogaski and Kerry

MacPherson have shown in their respective studies of public health projects in Tianjin and Shanghai.[106] However, their studies only briefly consider midwife training and related programs, although maternal and child health was often a key part of public health plans. In addition to the midwife training programs and the nursing schools that invariably included midwife training, public health nurses (*gonggong weisheng hushi*) and public health doctors (*gonggong weisheng yishi*) also received instruction in modern pregnancy, childbirth, and postpartum care.

In 1925, Peking Union Medical College's Dr. John B. Grant persuaded the municipal police department in Beijing to open the Beiping First Health Demonstration Station, a sort of laboratory established jointly by PUMC and the municipal government to conduct research and to train public health personnel, which became a model for cities across China.[107] The station also served as a data collection point for detailed birth and death statistics. Peking Union Medical College contributed 60 percent and the Beiping municipality (under the police department, which oversaw public health) 40 percent of the budget.[108] The station had three divisions: medical services, general sanitation, and vital statistics/communicable diseases, and a full staff of six physicians (including one director appointed by PUMC), 17 nurses (including midwives), three sanitary inspectors, one dental hygienist, one pharmacist, one secretary, and three clerks. Its purpose was twofold: to teach public health and preventive medicine to nursing and medical students, "and to cooperate with local agencies in demonstration programs in community health practices." [109] Its staff also conducted epidemiological studies and attempted to adapt "modern public health practices to local conditions."[110] Furthermore, station staff participated in a school health program whereby medical personnel examined school children and taught them basic modern public health methods like brushing teeth and washing hands. They administered free inoculations, especially for smallpox. In 1928, their efforts included 25,660 home visits by nurses, 78,870 sanitary inspections, 57,787 curative treatments (which included 44,575 for trachoma alone), and 1,148 death investigations.[111]

In 1932, the Health Demonstration Station entered into a formal agreement of cooperation with the Peking Union Medical College Department of Obstetrics. The agreement provided for a maternity service run by the Health Demonstration Station to give practical experience to PUMC's medical obstetrics students. The Department of Obstetrics was to provide a staff member and one student to oversee one antenatal and one postpartum clinic. Each patient at the antenatal clinic was to receive a leaflet (in Chinese) stating that at the onset of labor a male or female doctor would be sent with a public health visitor to attend the birth. When a patient went into labor, her case was referred to the Health Station and then relayed to the information desk at the hospital, which would then summon the physician and public health visitor on call. The Obstetrics Department was to provide all necessary instruments for such deliveries outside the hospital, and it also provided free ambulance service to those unable to pay for it. All records were kept in Chinese at the Health Demonstration Station, with a duplicate record housed at PUMC in case a patient was to be admitted to the hospital. The public health visitor was responsible for all postnatal care and reporting the cases to the physician in charge.[112]

A Second Health Demonstration Station was established in October 1933 by the Department of Hygiene and Public Health of the Beiping National Medical College, in cooperation with the Municipal Health Department. The First National Midwifery School organized and supervised the station's maternal and child health clinic with one part-time physician and one full-time midwife assigned to this work. Between 1933 and 1934, total attendance at the second clinic was 779, with 53 deliveries, two of which were referred to hospital.[113]

In Shanghai, midwifery and maternal and child health formed a substantial part of the city's public health efforts. In 1928, the Greater Shanghai Bureau of Public Health was established in 1928 as an administrative unit of the municipal government. Its program included sanitation, control of communicable diseases, vital statistics, and "public health education, which includes personal health talks, public lectures, demonstrations, health movements, health motion picture shows, health posters, circulars, newspapers and reprints, etc."[114] The bureau also organized a medical service to promote mental and physical health, including medical services from birth to death: "maternity and infant hygiene, pre-school health, school health, health of the workers, medical clinics, hospital facilities, and registration of hospitals, physicians, midwives and nurses, etc."[115] Between 1933 and 1934, the number of deliveries made by the bureau's personnel nearly doubled, from 234 to 426. The postnatal clinic service also expanded dramatically, from 39 visits in 1933 to 451 in 1934. The municipal public health bureau distributed over one million public health fliers and pamphlets in this period and examined more than 40,000 school children.[116]

The Shanghai Health Commissioner in 1933 had plans to establish one health center in each of the 16 police districts, some of which would also have infirmaries. Two primary public health centers started in Shanghai in the 1920s were at the Gaoqiao and Zhabei districts. The Gaoqiao Village Public Health Model District

(*Gaoqiao xiangcun weisheng mofan qu*) was begun in 1927 under the jurisdiction of the Shanghai Municipal Public Health Bureau. Its staff of two full-time and two part-time physicians, three public health nurses, two midwives, and one sanitary inspector provided public health care and education to a rural population of 38,000 with an annual budget of $18,000.[117] In addition to public health and sanitation campaigns, Gaoqiao had a trained midwife (*zhuchanshi*) for normal deliveries (*zhengchangchan*) and a doctor (*yisheng*) for difficult deliveries (*nanchan*). The district also advocated pre- and postnatal care for the masses (*minzhong*). According to its 1936 annual report, the public health station's midwives delivered more than 30 percent of the district's babies.[118] The ever-present Yang Chongrui gave technical assistance to Gaoqiao's maternal and child health efforts in 1933. Zhabei district focused on improving maternal and child health under the Shanghai Child Welfare Association established in 1933 under the auspices of the bureaus of Social Affairs, Public Health, and Education. It became a branch association of the National Child Welfare Association, a private organization founded in 1927 primarily from foreign contributions.[119]

Municipal government support of midwifery training was also present in 1930s Guangzhou. Part of the Guangzhou government's extremely progressive Three-Year Plan passed in 1933 included the establishment of municipal nurse training programs, a municipal maternity hostel "for the common people," and an eventual maternity hospital. It also listed provisions for improving the municipal midwifery school and establishing city-wide nursing and midwifery graduation examinations. Each year of the Three-Year Plan enforced nurse training among girls in municipal schools (while all boys were to receive military training).[120]

As the seat of the central government, as discussed above, the Central Field Health Station and the Nanjing Central Midwifery School were national-level programs sponsored by the National Midwifery Board and the national government. In addition, the National Departments of Internal Affairs and Public Health, along with the National Economic Board (*quanguo jingji weiyuanhui*) and the Public Health Experimental Station (*weisheng shiyanchu*) established a city-level public health personnel training program (*gonggong weisheng renyuan xunlianban*) to improve public health knowledge among trained doctors and nurses in Nanjing municipality.[121] The first six-month course for doctors began in 1933 with 16 students and included 16 hours each of maternal and child health courses and practicum. There were 18 students the following year. The public health nurse program began the same year with 23 students, and the 1934 course had 30 students. It included 36 hours of obstetrics instruction and 216 hours of obstetrics practicum.[122]

As well as government-sponsored programs, private midwifery training schools sprang up, as hospital affiliates and independently, throughout China in the 1930s, as introduced in chapter 1. In 1934, there were 52 such private programs in China that were registered with the government, in addition to 10 private provincial training schools, and countless others that operated under the radar of the authorities.[123] Private midwifery training programs were established throughout China on both large and small scales. Some of the largest and most well-known of these were run by medical missionary outfits or other foreign medical organizations. Others were established by local Chinese who had, or claimed to have had, medical training abroad or in one of the Western medical schools in China.

One example out of the dozens of registered private midwifery schools is Xiangya (Hsiang-ya) Medical College's School of Midwifery, opened in 1928 in Changsha, Hunan, a project of the Yale-China Association mentioned in chapter 1.[124] The first school of its kind in Hunan Province, it received a monthly grant of $1,000 from the provincial government. The two-year course aimed to supply the local community with trained midwives. In 1930 there were 30 students. By this time, there was also a prenatal clinic and free beds in the maternity ward for the poor. The school established an affiliated clinic at its local YWCA to encourage hospital admissions with the aim of decreasing maternal and infant mortality rates. Further public health work included health campaigns, students' clinic, vaccination training classes, and free inoculations.[125]

Shortly thereafter, the Department of Education approved the private Hangzhou Guangji Hospital Midwifery School (*Hangzhou guangji yiyuan fushe zhuchan xuexiao*) and the Shanghai Zhongde Professional Midwifery School (*Shanghai zhongde gaoji zhuchan zhuanye xuexiao*) in 1931 and 1933, respectively. Several other schools were also established in the 1930s: the Beiping Municipal Private Welfare High Ranking Midwifery School (*Beijingshi sili gongyi gaoji zhuchan zhuanye xuexiao*), the Guangdong Provincial High Grade Nursing and Midwifery Professional School (*Guangdong gaoji hushi zhuchan zhuanye xuexiao*), the Republic of China Private High Ranking Midwifery School (*Sili minguo gaoji zhuchan zhuanye xuexiao*), the Shanghai Private Tongde Midwifery School (*Shanghai sili gongde zhuchan xuexiao*), and the Tuqiang Advanced Midwifery School in Guangzhou (*Tuqiang gaodeng zhuchan xuexiao*).

CONTRACEPTION SERVICES

Safe access to contraception, including abortion, was the goal of some influential modern medical personnel by the 1920s, spurred in part by Margaret Sanger's visits in 1922 and 1936, and the prevailing ideas about eugenics and population control necessary to prevent China's further decline.[126] The Chinese Medical Association resolved in 1935 to "officially recognize contraception as part of public health activity in the field of maternity," largely to stem the prevalence of criminal abortion performed by traditional midwives, healers, and physicians.[127] Abortion was criminalized in Republican China though still regularly practiced.[128] Dr. J. Preston Maxwell outlined several astounding cases of failed abortion and problems resulting from abortion attempts, in an article in *The China Medical Journal*. The women who sought help from Peking Union Medical College had attempted various methods to induce abortion, including taking oral herbal concoctions, inserting a chopstick into the cervix, placement of a tampon soaked in a known abortifacient in the vagina, external manipulation of the abdomen and uterus, and "ecbolic acupuncture," whereby a very long needle is inserted into one or more of the acupuncture points on the abdomen. According to Dr. Maxwell, "At the 'Life Origin Position' a needle can be inserted to a depth of 3 to 6 inches, dependent on the health of the patient and thickness of the abdominal wall" to induce fetal expulsion.[129] The obstetrics and gynaecology department at Peking Union Medical College had received several patients who, upon x-ray, were found to have such a device lodged in the abdominal cavity. Some had developed peritonitis and profuse bleeding following the procedure, leading to their admission to PUMC. Others had massive vaginal scarring from a resulting infection that often left these women infertile.

Contraception supporters proclaimed that birth control clinics would provide maternity care; birth spacing and planning; sex education; and knowledge, prevention, and treatment of sexually transmitted diseases, therefore improving the health of mothers and their offspring. Dr. W. Neubauer promoted the theory of "social gynaecology" as "the backbone of the whole moving structure of society and it is through them that the health of the Chinese mother can be secured."[130] Illegal abortions, one of the primary forms of contraception, were life-threatening or debilitating to the mother, as were unchecked multiple pregnancies and births. Other crippling disabilities could ensue from repeated closely spaced births, such as prolapsed uterus, perineal tears, infertility, painful scarring, and vesico-vaginal fistulas, in which a hole is present between the bladder and the vaginal wall, resulting in constant urine leakage.

The Peiping (Beijing) Committee on Maternal Health was formed in 1930 under Dr. Yang Chongrui with the specific purpose of limiting the number of children born in China and decreasing the number of unwanted children.[131] Its goals were "to increase individual happiness through economic, social, and eugenic improvements," to diminish social and personal misery, and "to avert danger of over-population of China." [132] Yang Chongrui again recalled China's alarming infant and maternal mortality rates that she linked not only to poor hygiene and lack of modern medicine, but also to overpopulation.[133] The committee's first Five-Year Plan on Birth Control aimed to decrease unnecessary maternal deaths and to promote mental, physical, and spiritual social standards by way of literature distribution and counseling of pregnant women. The committee sponsored a weekly birth control clinic in Beijing that saw 99 cases between 1930 and 1933, mainly from the middle and upper classes. A few years later, in 1936 a national Committee on Contraception was formed, also staffed by Dr. Yang Chongrui along with several other physicians, in conjunction with the Shanghai Birth Control League.[134] The committee helped to establish and support contraceptive clinics in several major cities, asserting that "Birth Control is an established thing in all progressive nations of the world and China is not going to be a progressive nation without it."[135] Unfortunately for the birth control commission, Chinese women rarely visited the clinic to limit or space their pregnancies. Instead, most sought help for their infertility or failure to give birth to sons.[136]

STANDARDIZING CHILDBIRTH

Clearly, midwifery and childbirth education, both public and private, greatly expanded in China during the 1930s. As more people opened hospitals and more patients patronized these institutions, regulation posed a problem. According to the Nationalist government's plan to grow and expand public health, all hospitals and medical schools had to be registered and conform to particular standards. Numerous small maternity hospitals and schools emerged, especially in urban areas like Shanghai and Guangzhou. They were often run by individuals with dubious educational backgrounds and credentials, and they took in paying students to train them in modern midwifery techniques. By law, all of these hospitals had to be inspected and regulated and registered with the municipal government, as did all of their staff. In 1934–35, six midwifery schools in Beijing alone were closed down by the municipal public health authorities.[137] Countless others continued to operate illegally because of lack of oversight at the governmental level. The varied and erratic maternal and child health programs point to a lack of uniformity or conformity with national standards for public health programs.

However, the Nationalist government attempted to legislate and regulate childbirth and the modern and traditional midwives. In provincial, municipal, and rural settings, agents of the state collected birth and death statistics, encouraged prenatal and postnatal care, and urged women to deliver their children in a modern setting with modern methods. Likewise, during the 1920s and 1930s, Chinese government officials and medical professionals began to exert more control over the training and licensing of midwives. Midwifery was incorporated into the ranks of the medical personnel being trained in modern medicine as part of modernization and nation-building efforts. Old-style midwives—elderly, uneducated, and apprenticed—were replaced by young, literate, and modern midwives. Government officials and modernizers created and supported modern childbirth and the midwifery profession, creating changes in women's participation in childbirth as both professionals and as patients. The regulation and standardization of medical care and education grew in intensity as the Nationalist era progressed, culminating in the New Life Movement and its attempted hyper-control of all aspects of personal and private lives.

The Guomindang focused on eliminating traditional midwives and legitimizing the modern midwives, beginning with its founding in Guangzhou with its midwifery restrictions in 1913 and continuing throughout the Nanjing decade. The Nationalist government, through the National Midwifery Board, enacted a series of national laws governing midwives beginning in 1928. These laws restricted old-style midwives from practicing, created and enforced midwife licensing and registration, and standardized midwifery school curriculum and exams nationwide. Because childbirth was so important to the nation's health, politicians, modernizers, and medical personnel in the 1920s and 1930s attacked and vilified the *jieshengpo* on several fronts: these women were unsanitary, superstitious, dangerous, backward, and *uncontrollable*, all characteristics that the Guomindang attempted to thwart.[138] Modern midwives were sanitary, scientific, safe, modern, and more easily controlled by the state. To support this shift in childbirth practices, the Guomindang enacted stringent legal reforms to control traditional *jieshengpo* and to support the trained *zhuchanshi*.

The *jieshengpo* were deviant and had to be confined, whereas the *zhuchanshi* were acceptable participants in nation building as the foundation for healthy births.[139] In effect, the Nationalist government designated who could and could not legitimately participate in the modern state.

As agents of the state, one of the main duties of the retrained and modern midwives was the registration of births. Thus midwives became some of the earliest actors in the broader national programs of population regulation and control. Furthermore, childbirth was for most of the population the first contact Chinese had with either modern medicine or state regulation of birth and death. The government's public health efforts also proved a good starting place for midwives' entry into civil service. Many *zhuchanshi* were recruited to serve as instructors in public health programs like the Guangzhou Public Health Officer Training Institute of the 1930s.

Guomindang midwifery regulations explicitly outlined the differences between traditional and modern midwives. *Jieshengpo* had to be between 30 and 60 *sui*,[140] with intact eyes, ears, limbs, and mental capacity, and free of infectious disease in order to obtain a license to practice midwifery. By 1929, un-retrained *jieshengpo* were forbidden to practice at all.[141] Chinese *jieshengpo* had to have graduated from a medical school or a midwife training school in order to practice midwifery. This law eliminated the ability of nearly all old-style midwives to practice legally, for short courses in midwife training were only in their infancy at this time in limited locations. Furthermore, in order to practice legally, the midwife was required to obtain a license from the government that stipulated she had undergone additional training. (Midwives already practicing before this law was instituted had six months to obtain a license.)

In contrast, national standardized entrance requirements limited modern midwifery (*zhuchanshi*) candidates to females between 20 and 30 *sui* who were graduates of a junior middle school or those having similar qualifications. The number of students admitted could not exceed twice the number of available maternity beds in the school's affiliated hospital. To enter the First National Midwifery School's two-year midwifery program, which constituted national entrance requirements, all candidates had to be unmarried, between 20 and 30 *sui*, of "good character and in good health," middle school graduates with primary school courses in Chinese and basic science who had successfully passed the First National Midwifery School entrance examinations.[142] To obtain a national license to practice midwifery, the *zhuchanshi* had to be mentally stable, at least 20 *sui*, and hold a diploma from a registered two-year midwifery school.[143] By definition according to the national regulations, midwives formed two distinct groups of women: uneducated old women whose physical and mental health were in question; and young, modern, educated female elites.

This construction of *jieshengpo* versus *zhuchanshi* was artificial, as there was undoubtedly much overlap between the two groups in practice. A rare glimpse into the life of a Chinese midwife, Maxine Hong Kingston's memoir of growing up as a first generation Chinese-American in California recounts stories of her mother's life in Guangzhou before emigrating to the United States. A graduate of Hackett Medical College, Kingston's mother mixed traditional ideas about sickness and health with her modern medical training.[144] Regardless of training or background, the midwives' common goal was to deliver healthy infants, but the state only recognized the official status of the modern midwives.

Both of these types of midwives—the modern and the traditional—were still subordinate to physicians, as shown by the numerous regulations prohibiting midwives from using instruments like forceps; requiring that they call on a physician for difficult cases or when any intervention, such as version, was necessary; and forbidding all midwives from calling themselves "doctor" (*yisheng*).[145] The occupational distinctions were not solely based on gender, however, with female midwives subordinate to male physicians. At this time, many women in China were entering the medical field as physicians, including Yang Chongrui herself, though most female medical students went into the typically female-gendered fields of obstetrics, gynecology, and pediatrics. Unlike in the United States where (primarily male) physicians rapidly displaced midwives in the early twentieth century, no one in China ever advocated that men take over the role of birth helper. No one suggested eliminating female attendants from the birth environment. Childbirth remained women's responsibility, but one that must be regulated by the government.

The National Midwifery Board also regulated midwifery schools and training programs. In 1931, the national government ordered "all midwifery schools to register with the National Midwifery Board and for students to take examinations and obtain a license before going into practice."[146] At the third meeting of the National Midwifery Board in 1932, its members issued a declaration outlining methods and enforcement of midwifery school licensing. All midwifery schools—national, provincial, private, and rural—and their affiliated hospitals seeking national registration were subjected to a joint inspection by local educational and health officers. The inspectors had to complete a standardized form listing information such as the school's size, personnel, number of students, operating expenses, physical plant and equipment, along with "reputation of the school in the locality" and "among the medical circle."[147] Successfully qualified and registered schools were required to conform to the national standardized entrance requirements and midwifery curriculum set by the National Midwifery Board. [148] All schools had to offer a two-year course with the curriculum shown in table 4.2. The maternity ward practice grouped together no more than three students to take care of delivery and the postnatal mother and baby for at least 25 deliveries. The students were required to submit detailed notes about their maternity ward experiences.[149]

The body of knowledge that was given to the newly minted modern midwives was regulated and controlled, an essential part of any profession. The midwives had to carefully document the labor and delivery routines that were standardized by the National Midwifery Board. From the first time the midwife examined her patient, detailed records were kept on cervical dilation, contractions, blood pressure, temperature, fetal activity, and postnatal care like tying the umbilical cord and administering silver nitrate eye drops to curb eye infection. But childbirth is anything but routine; each is a very personal and individual experience, and every woman's birth is different. The standardization of modern medicine, however, eases the fears of childbirth by claiming the ability to control it. The routinization of labor and delivery, taken directly from the American hospital of the 1930s, was meant to control a very uncontrollable situation. Recording and standardizing every step of labor and birth gives a semblance of being in charge of a life-threatening situation, as medical science was meant to explain and control life and death. By eliminating or reducing the risk of human error and carelessness, and by quantifying events (timing contractions, signifying the three stages of labor, measuring cervical dilation), modern medicine purports to make birth safe and controllable. The *jieshengpo* as a group had no such standardized birth routines, and traditional midwifery practices varied widely even within the same city or town. The *jieshengpo* were retrained to follow a standard birth model and to refer deviant cases to Western physicians to monitor and control. There was no place for the un-retrained *jieshengpo* in the new regulated birth environment.

The New Life Movement was the culmination of the striving for an elusive and unyielding modernity, as bodily comportment and physical appearance were elevated to representations of progress. This movement was a revolutionary attempt to create loyalty and

Table 4.2. Standardized Curriculum for Two-Year Midwifery Training, as Set by the National Midwifery Board. Reproduced from FNMS, *Sixth Annual Report*, viii.

Semester	Subjects	Number of Hours Per Week
1st	Anatomy	4
	Physiology	3
	Nursing	1
	Bacteriology	2
	Materia Medica	2
	On Duty	20
	Practice in Maternity Ward	12
2nd	Anatomy	4
	Physiology	3
	Urinalysis	1
	Midwifery	4
	Care & Feeding of Children	2
	First Aid	1
	On Duty	17
	Practice in Maternity Ward	12
3rd	Midwifery	4
	Gynecology	2
	Care & Feeding of Children	2
	Clinic	2
	Class Demonstration	4
	On Duty	10
	Practice in Maternity Ward	22
4th	Abnormal Midwifery	2
	Dietetics	1
	Dermatology	1
	Practice in Maternity Ward, etc.	10
	On Duty	30

obedience to the new Chinese state, to create public awareness and a mass movement to generate a new, modern China. It was launched by the Guomindang in 1934 with the goals of reforming China's spiritual and material life through improvements in hygiene and behavior. [150] The movement began by focusing on improving public health and good manners, prohibiting spitting and urinating in public. It then grew to encompass larger social problems like gambling and opium smoking, among other things, as well as an endeavor to encourage native over foreign goods. The New Life Movement was a revolutionary attempt to create loyalty and obedience to the new Chinese state, to create public awareness and a mass movement to generate a new, modern China. Education reform that had begun earlier in the Republican period became retrenched and conservative, stressing neo-Confucian values with the state as the provider of social advances. According to Robert Culp, the Guomindang advocated "social equality within a modern, industrialized society" by "rework[ing] Confucian models of hierarchy and the family-based society to encourage unity and social order."[151]

The movement's stance toward women was a complicated one fraught with contradictions. Girls' education emphasized a new and modern version of the traditional "good wife and wise mother."[152] On one hand, the New Life Movement sought to eradicate what many viewed as degenerate "modern" girls who wore makeup and Western clothes and bought foreign products.[153] On the other, women played a crucial role in the public health and hygiene campaigns and were encouraged to enter into medical and public health fields, turning their bodies into sites of contestation. The images of midwifery students in school yearbooks of this period portray women with permanent waves and bobbed hair, makeup, Western clothes, and plucked eyebrows, the very characteristics that the New Life Movement attempted to eradicate in favor of a more modest and traditional manifestation. [154] It is unclear how the New Life Movement reconciled the conflicting notions of the ideal traditional, conservative woman responsible for child rearing with the modern, educated woman so necessary to help revitalize the nation. While the Guomindang during the Nanjing decade turned towards conservatism, they also utilized women to help build the nation, a very forward-looking concept.

A major goal of the movement was to improve the health of the Chinese people and, in turn, create a healthier China. Footbinding and breast binding were both illegal under the Guomindang, and in 1934 the importance of woman's "healthy beauty," as opposed to the traditional ideal of "fragile beauty," was "promoted by the state as the new norm of femininity."[155] The movement advocated physical education for men and women. In fact, Peking Union Medical College's First National Midwifery School built a "playground" in which its students could play basketball and other sports. The Guomindang's and the

New Life Movement's focus on individual health for the benefit of the nation began with the fetus and the emphasis on fetal education, or *taijiao*. Chapter 2 discussed how this concept was popular in the 1930s as a scientific method to ensure healthy, intelligent offspring, resulting in the publication of numerous articles and books on the subject.[156] These works dealt with appropriate foods, clothing, and environment for the mother and extended into the care of the newborn. Furthermore, women could join "mothercraft" classes and Mothers' Clubs sponsored by local hospitals to learn the most up-to-date and modern methods of child rearing. The health of the nation was crucial for building a strong society, and this began at conception. According to many scientists and public health modernizers, without live, healthy infants, the population would deteriorate.[157] This deterioration could only be stopped by standardizing and regulating childbirth.

CONCLUSION

The sterile birth environment that the *zhuchanshi* advocated—white sheets and towels, clean hands, and sterilized equipment, routine procedures—certainly reduced maternal and infant mortality. In Beijing between 1929 and 1930, the infant mortality rate at the First National Midwifery School hospital was 12 percent, maternal mortality three percent; though these statistics should be read very carefully as they were gathered and reported by a school with a goal of validating its existence.[158] The nationwide average maternal and infant mortality rate at this time is estimated at 50 to 70 percent.[159] In the rural areas too, successful programs did lower the high maternal, infant, and child mortality rates. The 1934 figures for Dingxian show the death rate among children under two years of age as 200 per 100,000.[160] In 1948, the infant mortality rate in areas served by modern midwives was an estimated 11 percent, and maternal mortality was estimated by some to be an astoundingly low .4 percent.[161] In comparison, the overall infant mortality rate in China in the early 1950s was 20 percent.[162]

However, even at the height of midwife training in the 1930s, the majority of women still utilized old-style midwives. Yang Chongrui asserted that in Beijing, the center of midwifery training during the Guomindang era, 50 percent of all births were attended by untrained midwives and 25 percent by the parturient woman's relatives or the parturient woman herself.[163] This means that new midwives reached only 25 percent of Beijing's childbearing population in the peak years of China's modern midwifery campaigns. Certainly in the countryside the number of modern midwife-assisted births was infinitesimal. Furthermore, although the number of registered trained midwives did grow considerably during this time, from 1883 in 1934 to 6000 in 1948, this number was in no way sufficient to manage and treat all of China's women of childbearing age.[164]

The effects of state-controlled childbirth were not all positive, nor are they very clear-cut. Mortality rates in areas served by modern midwives in the Nationalist era did indeed decline, and they are one important indicator of quality of life. Quality of birth is also important, as is independence from oppression and coercion regarding reproductive choices. But did Chinese women have any more freedom under the traditional patriarchal system in the realm of childbirth, when women gave birth alone in the barn or attended by midwives their mothers-in-law retained? Or was the traditional oppressor just replaced by the faceless state with assistance from hegemonic and unquestionable modern medicine? While the *jieshengpo* primarily dealt with the birth process and neonatal period, in contrast state governance over birth supremely began before conception with the choice of a eugenically sound marital partner, and continued with *taijiao*. The *zhuchanshi*'s responsibilities began as soon as the pregnancy was discovered and included numerous documented prenatal visits. Modernized, state-run care extended over the life of the fetus and neonate and continued well beyond birth and into the child's first few years, after which period school nurses would take over the charting, measuring, and inoculation duties. Modern midwifery as a new profession also reflected the importance of motherhood and childbirth *vis a vis* the nation. Mothers were important actors in the new nation as the source of China's optimistically healthier population.

Despite the lack of compliance and commitment on the part of patients and administrators, Guomindang midwifery reform was part of the larger effort to extend state control over its people by bringing previously private matters into the public sphere. This included regulating the family as well as the newly emerging midwifery profession. The midwifery laws of the Guomindang era removed childbirth from the community to the state-run arena as midwives managed and recorded births on behalf of the nation. Thus the Guomindang sought to extend its control into the private lives of its citizens, much more so than China's imperial governments had attempted in the past. The state took over the family authority that had previously been held by the elder generations. These policies were accepted because many modernizers believed that China needed a strong state in order to survive. This control was best accomplished through science and law.[165] Public health programs, including modern midwifery, aimed to improve the people's health through science. The modern midwives filled a crucial slot in the development of a larger modern medical assembly, with one of their main duties being the registration of births. In this way, they became some of the earliest actors in the broader national programs of population regulation and control. Furthermore, this bureaucratization helped to solidify the midwives' place as legitimate constituents in the new nation.

The Guomindang's plans for reforming childbirth were, on paper, extraordinary, though the reality never matched the intended results. Laws, schools, and public health centers all point to a dedication to improving the health of women and children for the benefit of the entire population, yet many of these plans never came to fruition because of the dearth of allocated resources and personnel, coupled with reliance on Western philanthropists to create and maintain relevant programs. The Guomindang was indeed sincere in its efforts to formulate a new model of childbirth in order to improve the health of its citizenry, but problems related to fiscal and political instability prevented its success. The state apparatus and funding for public health were weak, and the Guomindang had larger problems looming other than improving and controlling reproduction. There was no consensus at the top levels of government on how best to remedy China's many ills.

In fact, the few dedicated physicians and public health professionals—Yang Chongrui, Liu Ruiheng, Chen Zhiqian, Li Ting'an—along with their foreign benefactors, were the true driving force for childbirth reform during the Nationalist era. Although they succeeded in creating government health programs and legislation that regulated childbirth, and building urban and rural midwifery training programs and centers in several urban and rural locations, these actors engaged in childbirth reform were never able to create unified or wide-reaching changes, regardless of their overarching vision. Without government backing, their best intentions on paper disintegrated without financial and political commitment. Nonetheless, the model of state reproduction in China stands, despite these early setbacks, and is the precursor to stronger and more successful management of births in subsequent regimes in China.

NOTES

1. Guangdong Provincial Government Police Department, *Police Department announcement*, vol. 23.

2. Yang Nianqun, "The Transformation of Space and Control of Birth and Death in Early Republican Beijing (*Minguo chunian beijing de shengsi kongzhi yu kongjian zhuanhuan*)." Individual liberty is a post-Enlightenment Western concept that may or may not have its place in China; in any case, it is important not to assume popular desire among the Chinese for such individual freedoms.

3. Tamar Mayer, "Gender Ironies of Nationalism: Setting the Stage," in *Gender Ironies of Nationalism: Sexing the Nation*, ed. Tamar Mayer (London and New York: Routledge, 2000), 1–22; Nira Yuval-Davis, "Women and the Biological Reproduction of "the Nation"," *Women's Studies International Forum* 19, no. 1 (1996): 17–24.

4. Katherine Verdery, "From Parent-State to Family Patriarchs: Gender and Nation in Contemporary Eastern Europe," *East European Politics and Societies* 8, no. 2 (1994): 225–55; Haleh Afshar, "Women and Reproduction in Iran," in *Woman-Nation-State*, ed. N. Yuval-Davis and F. Anthias (New York: St. Martin's Press, 1989), 110–25.

5. Susan Greenhalgh, "Controlling Births and Bodies in Village China," *American Ethnologist* 21, no. 1 (1994): 3–30. AnElissa Lucas relates continuities between Republican and Communist China's public health programs in Lucas, *Chinese Medical Modernization: Comparative Policy Continuities, 1930s–1980s*.

6. Kirby, "Engineering China: Birth of the Developmental State, 1928–1937."

7. Glosser, *Chinese Visions of Family and State, 1915–1953*.

8. Dikötter, *The Age of Openness: China before Mao*.

9. J. Heng Liu, "National Health Organization," in *The China Christian Yearbook, 1936–37*, ed. Frank Rawlinson (Glendale, CA: The Arthur H. Clark Co., 1937), 336–55; Yun Long, ed., *Administrative Records of Kunming (Kunming xingzheng jishi)*, vol. 22 (Kunming: Yunnan zezhengting yinshua, 1943).

10. Tien, *Government and Politics in Kuomintang China 1927–1937*, 170–74.

11. Angela Ki-che Leung, "Women Practicing Medicine in Premodern China," in *Chinese Women in the Imperial Past: New Perspectives*, ed. Harriet T. Zurndorfer (Leiden: Brill, 1999), 101–34.

12. Neizhengbu nianjian bianzuan weiyuanhui, *Yearbook of Internal Affairs (Neizheng nianjian)*, 4: G206–211; Zaitong Zhang and Cheng Rijin, *Selected Republican-Era Medical and Public Health Legislation (Minguo yiyao weisheng fagui xuanbian, 1912–1948)*.

13. Anon, *All about Shanghai and Environs: A Standard Guidebook, Historical and Contemporary Facts and Statistics* (Shanghai: The University Press, 1934); Lee, *Modern Canton*, Appendix 6.

14. Winston Hsieh, "The Ideas and Ideals of a Warlord: Ch'en Chiung-Ming (1978–1933)," *Papers on China: Harvard University Committee on Regional Studies* 16 (1962): 219.

15. Kirby, "Engineering China: Birth of the Developmental State, 1928–1937," 152.

16. Ibid., 152–53.

17. Ibid., 138.

18. Yip, *Health and National Reconstruction in Nationalist China: The Development of Modern Health Services, 1928–1937*, 102.

19. Yip, *Health and National Reconstruction in Nationalist China: The Development of Modern Health Services, 1928–1937*, 102; Lei, "Habituate Individuality: Framing of Tuberculosis and Its Material Solutions in Republican China."

20. J. Heng Liu, "The Chinese Ministry of Health," *National Medical Journal of China* 15 (1929): 145.

21. Alison Bashford, "Global Biopolitics and the History of World Health," *History of the Human Sciences* 19, no. 1 (2006): 67–88.

22. Brown, *Rockefeller Medicine Men: Medicine and Capitalism in America*.

23. League of Nations Health Organization, *Health* (Geneva, Switzerland: League of Nations Health Organization Information Section, 1931).

24. Bashford, "Global Biopolitics and the History of World Health."

25. Brown, *Rockefeller Medicine Men: Medicine and Capitalism in America*; Bullock, *An American Transplant: The Rockefeller Foundation and Peking Union Medical College*.

26. Jiang, "Cross-cultural Philanthropy as a Gift Relationship: The Rockefeller Foundation Donors and Chinese Recipients, 1913–1921," 162.

27. Bowers, *Western Medicine in a Chinese Palace: Peking Union Medical College, 1917–1951*, 59.

28. China Medical Commission of the Rockefeller Foundation, *Medicine in China*.

29. Bullock, *An American Transplant: The Rockefeller Foundation and Peking Union Medical College*, 190–93, 215.

30. Bowers, *Western Medicine in a Chinese Palace: Peking Union Medical College, 1917–1951*, 208.

31. Tien, *Government and Politics in Kuomintang China 1927–1937*, 23.

32. Ibid., 23–24.

33. Chen and Bunge, *Medicine in Rural China: A Personal Account*, 61.

34. Ibid.

35. Henry S Houghton, "Letter to E.C. Lobenstein," October 11, 1937, folder 669, box 94, RG IV2B9, RAC.

36. Ibid.

37. Chen and Bunge, *Medicine in Rural China: A Personal Account*, 61.

38. Yip, *Health and National Reconstruction in Nationalist China: The Development of Modern Health Services, 1928–1937*, 26.

39. Liu, "The Chinese Ministry of Health," 139; Neizhengbu nianjian bianzuan weiyuanhui, *Yearbook of Internal Affairs (Neizheng nianjian)*, vol. 4, vol. 4, G303–4.

40. Mrs. Feng Yuxiang had opened a midwifery school in Kaifeng, Henan, in 1927 or 1928, which had "taught her the necessity for trained personnel." John B. Grant, *Letter to Victor Heiser*, 1928.

41. FNMS, *First Annual Report, First National Midwifery School, 1929–1931*, iii.

42. Zaitong Zhang and Cheng Rijin, *Selected Republican-Era Medical and Public Health Legislation (Minguo yiyao weisheng fagui xuanbian, 1912–1948)*, 79–81.

43. Liu, "National Health Organization"; Liu, "The Chinese Ministry of Health," 140.

44. FNMS, *Sixth Annual Report, First National Midwifery School, Peiping, July 1, 1934–June 30, 1935*.

45. FNMS, *Fifth Annual Report, First National Midwifery School, Peiping, July 1, 1933–June 30, 1934*, 3.

46. FNMS, *Sixth Annual Report, First National Midwifery School, Peiping, July 1, 1934–June 30, 1935*.

47. Neizhengbu nianjian bianzuan weiyuanhui, *Yearbook of Internal Affairs (Neizheng nianjian)*, 4: 206–7.

48. Neizhengbu nianjian bianzuan weiyuanhui, *Yearbook of Internal Affairs (Neizheng nianjian)*, 4: 208–9; Yip, *Health and National Reconstruction in Nationalist China: The Development of Modern Health Services, 1928–1937*, 166. Yip gives the opening date of the Central Midwifery School as 1933, but I have used the 1936 *Neizheng nianjian* date of 1932.

49. FNMS, *Sixth Annual Report, First National Midwifery School, Peiping, July 1, 1934–June 30, 1935*, 2.

50. Neizhengbu nianjian bianzuan weiyuanhui, *Yearbook of Internal Affairs (Neizheng nianjian)*, 4: G201–3; Liu, "National Health Organization," 338.

51. Tien, *Government and Politics in Kuomintang China 1927–1937*, 170–74.

52. Neizhengbu nianjian bianzuan weiyuanhui, *Yearbook of Internal Affairs (Neizheng nianjian)*, 4: G4.

53. Liu, "National Health Organization."

54. Yun Long, *Administrative Records of Kunming (Kunming xingzheng jishi)*, vol. 22. The school was started in 1928 but, according to the report, did not receive National Midwifery Board assistance until 1934.

55. FNMS, *Second Annual Report, First National Midwifery School, Peiping, July 1, 1930–June 30, 1931*, 24.

56. Liu, "National Health Organization."

57. Jiaying Shen, "Report on the School and Lying-in Hospital (Ben xiao chanyuan liang zhou shixi zhi jingkuang)," *Shanxi shengli zhuchan xuexiao niankan* (1935): 91–92.

58. FNMS, *Sixth Annual Report, First National Midwifery School, Peiping, July 1, 1934–June 30, 1935*.

59. Ibid., Appendix III, xix.

60. FNMS, *Fourth Annual Report, First National Midwifery School, Peiping, July 1, 1932–June 30, 1933*, Appendix I: Suggested Plans for Places Surveyed, xi–xiii.

61. Neizhengbu nianjian bianzuan weiyuanhui, *Yearbook of Internal Affairs (Neizheng nianjian)*, 4: G226.

62. Lucas, *Chinese Medical Modernization: Comparative Policy Continuities, 1930s–1980s*, 88–89; Ruiheng Liu, *Report Given at the 1937 League of*

Nations-Health Organization Intergovernmental Conference of Far Eastern Countries on Rural Hygiene (Geneva, Switzerland: League of Nations Health Organization, 1937).

63. Marion Yang, "Letter to Dr. W.A. Sawyer," January 21, 1937, folder 374, box 45, series 601, RG 1, RAC.

64. Neizhengbu nianjian bianzuan weiyuanhui, *Yearbook of Internal Affairs (Neizheng nianjian)*, vol. 4.

65. Lucas, *Chinese Medical Modernization: Comparative Policy Continuities, 1930s–1980s*, 239.

66. Neizhengbu nianjian bianzuan weiyuanhui, *Yearbook of Internal Affairs (Neizheng nianjian)*, vol. 4.

67. Lucas, *Chinese Medical Modernization: Comparative Policy Continuities, 1930s–1980s*, 72–73.

68. Lucas, *Chinese Medical Modernization: Comparative Policy Continuities, 1930s–1980s*, 72; Neizhengbu nianjian bianzuan weiyuanhui, *Yearbook of Internal Affairs (Neizheng nianjian)*, 4: 218.

69. Neizhengbu nianjian bianzuan weiyuanhui, *Yearbook of Internal Affairs (Neizheng nianjian)*, 4: 218–19.

70. Lucas, *Chinese Medical Modernization: Comparative Policy Continuities, 1930s–1980s*, 72–74.

71. Neizhengbu nianjian bianzuan weiyuanhui, *Yearbook of Internal Affairs (Neizheng nianjian)*, 4: 218–19.

72. Ibid.

73. Lucas, *Chinese Medical Modernization: Comparative Policy Continuities, 1930s - 1980s*, 72–73.

74. Neizhengbu nianjian bianzuan weiyuanhui, *Yearbook of Internal Affairs (Neizheng nianjian)*, 4: 219.

75. Yip, *Health and National Reconstruction in Nationalist China: The Development of Modern Health Services, 1928–1937*, 167.

76. Neizhengbu nianjian bianzuan weiyuanhui, *Yearbook of Internal Affairs (Neizheng nianjian)*, 4: 218–19.

77. Ibid.

78. Hayford, *To the People: James Yen and Village China*; Lucas, *Chinese Medical Modernization: Comparative Policy Continuities, 1930s–1980s*.

79. Lucas, *Chinese Medical Modernization: Comparative Policy Continuities, 1930s–1980s*, 72–74.

80. Ibid., 86–87.

81. Ibid.

82. Yang, "Letter to Dr. W.A. Sawyer."

83. Ibid.

84. Ibid.

85. Ibid.

86. FNMS, *Fifth Annual Report, First National Midwifery School, Peiping, July 1, 1933 - June 30, 1934*.

87. Neizhengbu nianjian bianzuan weiyuanhui, *Yearbook of Internal Affairs (Neizheng nianjian)*, 4: G227–28.

88. Ibid., 4: G230–31.

89. Ibid., 4: G234.

90. FNMS, *Fifth Annual Report, First National Midwifery School, Peiping, July 1, 1933–June 30, 1934.*

91. Ibid.

92. Ibid.

93. FNMS, *Sixth Annual Report, First National Midwifery School, Peiping, July 1, 1934–June 30, 1935.*

94. Neizhengbu nianjian bianzuan weiyuanhui, *Yearbook of Internal Affairs (Neizheng nianjian)*, 4: G222–23.

95. FNMS, *Fifth Annual Report, First National Midwifery School, Peiping, July 1, 1933 - June 30, 1934.*

96. FNMS, *Sixth Annual Report, First National Midwifery School, Peiping, July 1, 1934–June 30, 1935.*

97. Ibid.

98. Neizhengbu nianjian bianzuan weiyuanhui, *Yearbook of Internal Affairs (Neizheng nianjian)*, 4: G231–32.

99. Ibid.

100. Chen and Bunge, *Medicine in Rural China: A Personal Account*, 90–91.

101. Ibid.

102. Ibid.

103. Ibid., 91.

104. Ibid., 87.

105. Ibid.

106. MacPherson, *A Wilderness of Marshes: The Origins of Public Health in Shanghai, 1843–1943*; Rogaski, "Hygienic Modernity in Tianjin."

107. Campbell, "Public Health Efforts in China Before and After 1949 and their Effects on Mortality," 18.

108. Bowers, *Western Medicine in a Chinese Palace: Peking Union Medical College, 1917–1951*, 117.

109. Ibid.

110. Ibid.

111. Ibid.

112. *Minutes of the Peiping Union Medical College Committee on the Hospital*, Plan of Cooperation Between the Department of Obstetrics and the Health Station, November 22, 1932, folder 669, box 94, RG IV2B9, RAC.

113. Ibid.

114. H.G.W. Woodhead, ed., *The China Yearbook 1935* (Shanghai: The North China Daily News and Herald, Ltd., 1935), 291–92.

115. Ibid., 292.

116. Ibid.

117. FNMS, *Sixth Annual Report, First National Midwifery School, Peiping, July 1, 1934–June 30, 1935.*

118. Neizhengbu nianjian bianzuan weiyuanhui, *Yearbook of Internal Affairs (Neizheng nianjian)*, 4: G223–24.

119. Ibid.

120. Lee, *Modern Canton*, especially Appendix III, 153–68.

121. Neizhengbu nianjian bianzuan weiyuanhui, *Yearbook of Internal Affairs (Neizheng nianjian)*, 4: G211–13.

122. Ibid.

123. Yip, *Health and National Reconstruction in Nationalist China: The Development of Modern Health Services, 1928–1937*, 166.

124. Wang, *A Report of Hsiang-Ya Medical College & Hospital*.

125. Ibid.

126. Dikötter, *Imperfect Conceptions: Medical Knowledge, Birth Defects, and Eugenics in China*.

127. W. Neubauer, "Social Gynaecology in China," *Chinese Medical Journal* 51 (June 1937): 825–32.

128. H.D. Lamson, "Educated Women and Birth Control in China," *China Medical Journal* 44, no. 11 (1930): 1100–1109; Herbert D. Lamson, "Family Limitation among Educated Chinese Married Women: A Study of the Practice and Attitudes of 120 Women," *Chinese Medical Journal* 47 (1933): 493–503; Maxwell, "On Criminal Abortion in China."

129. Maxwell, "On Criminal Abortion in China," 3. For abortion in late imperial China, see Francesca Bray, *Technology and Gender: Fabrics of Power in Late Imperial China* (Berkeley and Los Angeles: University of California Press, 1997).

130. Neubauer, "Social Gynaecology in China," 832.

131. Marion Yang, "Birth Control in Peiping: First Report of the Peiping Committee on Maternal Health," *Chinese Medical Journal* 48 (1934): 787.

132. T'ao, "Some Statistics on Medical Schools in China for 1932–1933," 1029–39; FNMS, *Third Annual Report, First National Midwifery School, Peiping, July 1, 1931–June 30, 1932*, Annual Report, August 1, 1932.

133. Yang, "Birth Control in Peiping: First Report of the Peiping Committee on Maternal Health."

134. Amos Wong, "Committee on Contraception," *Chinese Medical Journal* 51 (1937): 770–71.

135. Ibid.

136. Lamson, "Educated Women and Birth Control in China."

137. FNMS, *Sixth Annual Report, First National Midwifery School, Peiping, July 1, 1934–June 30, 1935*.

138. For example, see Chen Jianshan, *Fetal Education (Taijiao)*, vol. 75; Liu, "The Chinese Ministry of Health"; Zi Yun (pseud.), "Childbirth customs in my hometown: Beijing (*Wu xiang de shengchan fengsu: Beijing*)."

139. Zwia Lipkin, *Useless to the State: "Social Problems" and Social Engineering in Nationalist Nanjing, 1927–1937* (Cambridge, MA: Harvard University Asia Center, 2006).

140. Chinese traditionally calculate age according to the lunar calendar, so that each person turns one year older on the Chinese Lunar New Year, which falls in January or February. Furthermore, a person is considered to be one year old at birth, thus adding one or two years to one's age as figured according to

Western calculations. For example, a 20-*sui* person according to Chinese calculations is either 18 or 19 years old by Western calculations.

141. Zaitong Zhang and Cheng Rijin, *Selected Republican-Era Medical and Public Health Legislation (Minguo yiyao weisheng fagui xuanbian, 1912–1948)*.

142. *Regulations of the First National Midwifery School.*

143. Zaitong Zhang and Cheng Rijin, *Selected Republican-Era Medical and Public Health Legislation (Minguo yiyao weisheng fagui xuanbian, 1912–1948)*.

144. Maxine Hong Kingston, *Woman Warrior: Memoirs of a Girlhood among Ghosts* (Vintage, 1976), especially Chapter Three.

145. Neizhengbu nianjian bianzuan weiyuanhui, *Yearbook of Internal Affairs (Neizheng nianjian)*, vol. 4; Zaitong Zhang and Cheng Rijin, *Selected Republican-Era Medical and Public Health Legislation (Minguo yiyao weisheng fagui xuanbian, 1912–1948)*.

146. FNMS, *First Annual Report, First National Midwifery School, 1929–1931*, 11.

147. Neizhengbu nianjian bianzuan weiyuanhui, *Yearbook of Internal Affairs (Neizheng nianjian)*, 4:208.

148. Ibid.

149. FNMS, *Sixth Annual Report, First National Midwifery School, Peiping, July 1, 1934–June 30, 1935*, Appendix III: Report on the Visit to Shanghai, September 30–October 8, 1933, viii.

150. Arif Dirlik, "The Ideological Foundations of the New Life Movement: A Study in Counterrevolution," *Journal of Asian Studies* 34, no. 4 (1975): 945–980.

151. Culp, *Articulating Citizenship: Civic Education and Student Politics in Southeastern China, 1912–1940*, 152.

152. Lien, Ling-ling, "Searching for the "New Womanhood": Career Women in Shanghai, 1912–1945" (University of California at Irvine, 2001), 114–28.

153. Hsiao-pei Yen, "Body Politics, Modernity and National Salvation: The Modern Girl and the New Life Movement," *Asian Studies Review* 29 (2005): 165–186.

154. Ibid.

155. Ibid.

156. Chen Jianshan, *Fetal Education (Taijiao)*, vol. 75; Yun Qin, "Hygiene and Fetal Education during Pregnancy (Renshen de weisheng yu taijiao)"; Zhu Wenyin, "Fetal Education and Eugenics (Taijiao yu youshengxue)," *Ladies' Journal (Funü zazhi)* 17, no. 8 (1931): 11–19; Also see Dikötter, *Sex, Culture and Modernity in China: Medical Science and the Construction of Sexual Identities in the Early Republican Period*; Stevens, "Making Female Sexuality in Republican China: Women's Bodies in the Discourses of Hygiene, Education, and Literature."

157. For example, see Yun Qin, "Hygiene and Fetal Education during Pregnancy (Renshen de weisheng yu taijiao)"; Zhu Wenyin, "Fetal Education and Eugenics (Taijiao yu youshengxue)."

158. FNMS, *First Annual Report, First National Midwifery School, 1929–1931*, iii.

159. Xiao Wenwen, "The History of Modern Obstetrics in Western Medicine in China (i)," (*Zhonghua yishi zazhi*) *Chinese Journal of Medical History* 25, no. 4 (1995): 204–210; Maxwell and Wong, "On Puerperal Mortality and Morbidity."

160. Chen and Bunge, *Medicine in Rural China: A Personal Account,* 90–91.

161. Chen and Bunge, *Medicine in Rural China: A Personal Account.*

162. Information Office of the State Council of the People's Republic of China, "Children's Health and Care," *White Papers of the Government,* April 1996, http://www.china.org.cn/e-white/children/c-3.htm.

163. Grant, *Midwifery Training.*

164. Marion Yang, "Letter to Dr. Frank E. Whitacre," June 8, 1948.

165. Glosser, *Chinese Visions of Family and State, 1915–1953.*

Epilogue: Reproduction in Twentieth-Century China

Many of the changes in reproduction introduced during the Republican period continued or intensified throughout the twentieth century. These advances included the professionalization of a once-apprenticed midwifery vocation, increasing state involvement in previously private endeavors like reproduction, the growing medicalization of childbirth, and considerable upheavals in gender roles with regard to occupation, family life, and parenthood. This epilogue reconsiders these changes following the end of the Republican period. It is in the light of the twentieth century that the drama of changing theories and practices of reproduction open toward future transformations.

In wartime China, from 1937 to 1949, the Chinese Communist Party (CCP) made fledgling efforts to positively affect reproductive health in areas under its control, while the Guomindang spent much of its resources fighting the communists. After the founding of the People's Republic, from the 1950s through the 1970s the CCP retreated from earlier Guomindang restrictions on traditional midwives and instead strongly supported their training in aseptic methods. Simultaneously, the CCP continued mass campaigns to shape individual and collective action regarding reproduction.[1] During the market reforms of the 1980s onward and the accompanying decentralization of medical and health care, the Chinese government increasingly turned its attention to population policies in the realm of reproduction.[2]

Throughout these political shifts, reproduction became, and remains, a social concern that is intertwined with the well-being of the modern nation. The trajectory of reproductive health reforms in twentieth-century China illustrates the clear national priority given to improve maternal and child health, regardless of the form of government in control at a given time, and certainly with disregard to available financial and occupational resources. The continuities between the modern Guomindang model of reproduction and the modern twenty-first century one are striking.

WARTIME CHINA, 1937–1949

The Japanese invasion of northern China in 1931 affected the already tenuous hold that the Guomindang had over China and effectively put an end to any wide-ranging plans for public health reform. The subsequent Second Sino-Japanese War (1937–1945) and civil war with the Chinese Communist Party (1945–1949) further hindered Guomindang efforts at implementing the policies they had earlier created. Schools and hospitals were closed or severely restricted and much of the medical personnel in all fields, including obstetrics and midwifery, were sent to help the war effort elsewhere. Nonetheless, scattered sources show that during the tumultuous period between 1931 and 1949, the First National Midwifery School and some Guomindang ministries continued to function in the midst of the political disturbance. Even more remarkable is the evidence of reproductive health programs in Chinese Communist Party-controlled rural areas such as Shanxi-Gansu-Ningxia (Shan-Gan-Ning) and Yan'an.

The First National Midwifery School operated at a reduced capacity beginning in 1933, with 70 percent of the staff and 85 percent of the students remaining to study in Beijing after the Mukden Incident.[3] The school later eliminated its winter entrance examination because of a decrease in the number of applicants and in 1938 had only 36 undergraduates enrolled and graduated only five students, half the number of the year before.[4] Its staff also had problems placing new graduates as hospitals, schools, and clinics closed or were occupied by Japanese forces. Plans to further develop graduate-level midwifery instruction for government maternal and child officers were postponed, partly because of staff changes within Peking Union Medical College's Department of Obstetrics, and also because most medical personnel worked towards saving lives and treating wounds of civilians and soldiers injured during the war.[5] After 1937, the First National Midwifery School was cut off from the central government, and because part of its funding came from the national Ministry of Health it was questionable whether or not the school would continue to operate. A small group of PUMC staff organized an interim trustee body and registered the school with the local educational authorities, authorizing the use of the reserve fund and requesting an emergency appropriation from the China Medical Board and the Rockefeller Foundation's International Health Division. They also cabled Dr. Yang Chongrui, who immediately cut short her trip to Europe to return to Beijing. However, on September 24, 1937, the acting head of the FNMS, a Dr. Chow, received a letter from the Nanjing government "instructing her to close the School and to transfer the staff to Wuchang" in Hubei Province, temporary home of the Nationalist government after Nanjing fell to the Japanese.[6] Various departments of the Peking Union Medical College were closed or moved during the war, and after 1949 the school was nationalized. The First National Midwifery School was disbanded.[7]

While the Guomindang struggled unsuccessfully to regain control of China, in some areas controlled by the Chinese Communist Party, midwifery training and childbirth reforms were part of a wider project to improve the health of rural inhabitants and gain support for the CCP. Since its establishment the CCP implemented, or attempted to implement, intensive maternal and health projects to "creat[e] an image of a government which cared for the welfare of the people," leading to popular support for the Communists.[8] Health policies in Chinese Communist Party-controlled areas like Shan-Gan-Ning and Yan'an were a crucial part of their success. Between 1936 and 1949, maternal and child health were important components of health policies in the Shan-Gan-Ning border region, which encompassed 35,000 square miles and had a population of 1.5 million people. Pregnant and post-partum women received extra rations of meat, cooking oil, salt, and vegetables, and newborns were allotted "35 feet of spun cloth and five catties of raw cotton."[9] The CCP utilized traditional Chinese medicine combined with training in aseptic births, even providing free midwifery training for both existing traditional and new midwives in "people's schools" (*minban*), cooperative training programs administered by the people, with goal of having "a midwife in every village."[10] The CCP in rural Yan'an also began to utilize and support traditional Chinese practitioners, opposing the "evil, imperialist" Western medicine.[11] Mao Zedong in 1944 asserted,

> We must call on the masses to arise in struggle against their own illiteracy, superstitions and unhygienic habits. . . .This approach is even more necessary in the field of medicine. . . . Our task is to unite with all intellectuals, artists and doctors of the old type who can be useful, to help them, convert them and transform them.[12]

The nationalization of midwifery was thus institutionalized.

However, as Karen Minden and Kim Taylor both have noted, necessity, not only ideology, drove the movement to utilize traditional Chinese medical practitioners, as there were not enough modern physicians to serve this large rural area. The CCP set up short-term training programs for paramedical personnel, primarily traditional midwives or "young peasant boys" to establish medical cooperatives in their villages.[13] One of the primary goals of the CCP rural health movement was to reduce infant mortality by training midwives in aseptic techniques, and by encouraging pregnant women to utilize trained midwives as their birth helpers. Wartime efforts to improve public health may have given the CCP an even greater basis on which to build its medical system, in terms of working with limited resources in a fragmented and unstable situation.

THE EARLY PEOPLE'S REPUBLIC, 1949–1980

After the founding of the People's Republic in 1949, improving maternal and infant health was made a national priority, though it was not at the top of the CCP's long list of improvements for the new nation. Combined with "promot[ing] the people's physical culture," advancing maternal and infant health was the forty-eighth principle of the 1949 Chinese People's Political Consultative Conference.[14] The reproductive health programs of the CCP appear remarkably effective on paper with drastic drops in infant and maternal mortality rates. According to Dr. Lin Qiaozhi, China's maternal and child health policies resulted in lower maternal and infant mortality rates nationwide, as by 1959 approximately 60 percent of rural births were attended by trained health workers; that number was 95 percent in large cities.[15] While these numbers are impossible to verify, even exaggerated numbers indicate the fundamental national importance of improved maternal and child health.

The CCP worked with the national All-China Women's Federation and the Ministry of Health to establish a xian-based public health system, a continuation of policies begun during the Nationalist era.[16] Like housing and food allotment, health care was controlled by one's work unit (danwei) under the Chinese communist system, and in rural areas was managed largely by Barefoot Doctors who covered many aspects of public health including immunization, sanitation, and maternal and child health.[17] The leaders of this system recruited maternal and child health activists and began a two-tier method of midwife training, similar to Yang Chongrui's training structure, with education of new, younger midwives as well as the retraining of traditional ones. The CCP, however, did not consider the traditional midwives to be as negative an influence as the Guomindang had. Instead, as in their rural outposts the CCP encouraged utilizing the experience and knowledge of the traditional midwives combined with the "new birth method" in order to improve the health of the population.[18] This designated "new birth method" was a series of aseptic procedures largely for home births that included washing hands, tying and packing the umbilical cord, and administering silver nitrate eye drops to prevent eye infections. The new method was in fact not new at all, having begun in the 1920s at the First National Midwifery School.

The new childbirth methods in the early People's Republic were largely resisted by the midwives themselves and the public they were meant to serve, as Gail Hershatter has shown in her interviews of rural women in Shaanxi Province in the 1990s.[19] Hershatter argues that a focus on policy only reveals part of the story of childbirth reform in China. Reliance on state rhetoric alone does not account for the actualities of childbirth during this time period. Accordingly, Li Xiaojiang has collected interviews of rural women in Henan and Yunnan provinces, many of them of minority ethnicities, which illustrate both the broad diversity of birth practices as well as the limited reach of the state.[20] Individual practices, beliefs, actions, superstitions, customs, and so on must be considered through an investigation of women's memories.[21] Despite the state rhetoric and the policies aimed at reforming midwives, few women utilized the state's orthodox procedures. A three-year study completed in 1953 showed only five to ten percent of women availed themselves of the new birth method.[22] Other complaints charged that discussing personal issues like childbirth in public was offensive and crazy.[23] Even among the midwifery students, the detailed clinical diagrams of internal and external organs induced embarrassment and disgust.[24]

The curriculum and pedagogy of these courses is strikingly similar to those used by First National Midwifery School instruction of the old-style midwife retraining programs. Thirty years apart, the courses focused on simple aseptic birth techniques, using shock and awe tactics of gruesome birth stories and maternal and infant mortality statistics among traditional births.[25] The CCP government had difficulties persuading women to enter into public service as nurses and midwives. While the official rhetoric heralded these selfless women as actors in the new nation, in actuality the state pushed production for women as factory workers and toilers rather than as helpers in the path of reproduction.[26] As in the Republican era, national policies and local practices diverged considerably under the CCP.

While the commercialization of reproduction technology may have halted during the early years of the People's Republic as citizens were compelled to produce, not consume, under a pseudo-communist state, women were still urged to utilize information on the new birth method, as well as pre- and postnatal care and feminine hygiene. Issues of magazines like *New Women of China* (*Xin zhongguo funü*), the official publication of the All-China Women's Federation, carried stories about the modern birth method and invectives on the dangers of uncontrollable and dangerous traditional childbirth. This publication also conveyed news and information about campaigns aimed at improving the health of the population, like International Children's Day celebrations and a 1950 anti-tetanus exhibition in Beijing in which a banner was hung compelling its viewers to "Struggle to raise the Chinese population." [27]

The CCP thus targeted women, as the Guomindang had done in decades prior, in campaigns to encourage national motherhood that, according to Joshua Goldstein, "inject[ed] political incentives into domestic chores," making family life a national priority.[28] During the 1950s and 1960s, women were urged to be good housewives and good mothers so that their husbands could in turn become more effective workers and producers.[29] The good wife created healthy offspring and a clean and peaceful home, both of which contributed to her husband's productivity. Mao Zedong's pronatalist campaigns during the 1950s and 1960s seem to contradict the simultaneous calls for female labor and their liberation from the shackles of patriarchal households and onerous housework.[30]

Arguably the most striking program in the years immediately following the founding of the PRC was the promulgation of the Soviet "psychoprophylactic painless childbirth method" that was to free women from the pain of childbirth without the use of chemical anesthesia or analgesia.[31] This procedure is similar to the ideology-driven "cosmologically resonant" childbirth advocated by Qing-era physicians, as examined by Yi-Li Wu and discussed in the introduction to this book.[32] In each practice, childbirth is stressed as a natural event that is only complicated or painful due to fear, intervention, or inappropriate beliefs or actions. Whether following the cosmologically resonant pattern or the psychoprophylactic method, the parturient is supposed to allow nature to take its course without meddling in the process. As cosmologically resonant childbirth was the epitome of harmony within the universe, the most important ideology of the time, the psychoprophylactic method was indeed the ultimate expression of political ideology: women's freedom from oppression as bestowed by Mao Zedong and the CCP. According to a contemporary, "The women of the era of Mao Zedong not only have been freed from the shackles of feudalism, but also the pain of giving birth has been eliminated. This good fortune could only be attained under the leadership of Chairman Mao and the Chinese Communist Party."[33] While on one hand the Party "liberated" women by granting them legal equality in the workplace and in the home, in reality these efforts fell short in many areas, not least with the promise of pain-free childbirth.[34]

Maternal and child health policies during this period mark a continuation of human biology as managed by the state in China, the creation of a framework for more extensive efforts of population management, whether for increasing, decreasing, or generally improving its health.[35] Early CCP campaigns aimed for compliance with the new policies, beginning with the "one pregnancy, one live birth; one live birth, one healthy child" movement in the 1950s, and in the early 1970s the "late, spaced, and few" policy.[36] These campaigns, driven by alarming statistics on China's high maternal and infant mortality rates, "conceptualized birth on a national scale" and constituted a "precondition for population control." [37] Joshua Goldstein maintains that the publication and dissemination of maternal and health statistics "link[ed] birth to concepts of population, labor force, and national defense."[38] In this way in the early People's Republic reproduction practices were politically and ideologically nationalized through medical discourse.

THE LEGACY OF REPRODUCTIVE HEALTH, 1980–2000s

Under the leadership of Deng Xiaoping in the 1980s, China gradually began to dismantle its state-controlled medical system and increasingly turned its attention to population planning, reinforcing its most strenuous policies concerning reproduction and birth control.[39] Stories abound concerning the atrocities committed by zealous public health officials in the 1980s and 1990s: late-term abortions, forced sterilizations, secret pregnancies, and orphanages overflowing with baby girls. Numerous scholars have examined these policies and their effects in detail.[40] China's population policies, however, did not begin with the Chinese Communist Party; instead, the foundation for controlling births and reproductive health was laid thirty years prior in the Republican period, so that we may speak of continuities over the twentieth century with regard to increasing state control, medicalization, and consumerism in the realm of reproduction.

The emphasis on midwifery beginning in Republican China was a major social and cultural change, for it created a new professional avenue for women to enter at a time when such opportunities were limited. The profession of midwifery also allowed women to engage in China's nation-building processes and, in fact, many women from the First National Midwifery School served in either or both of the Nationalist and the Chinese Communist Party governments.[41] However, the continuing medicalization of childbirth in China is marked by a significant decline in the use of traditional midwives and the increasing educational requirements of modern birth attendants, similar to the state-run and police-managed midwifery models in late Meiji Japan and colonial Taiwan.[42] Modern midwives started to displace traditional midwives in China beginning in the 1920s, and the latter suffered extreme legal discrimination at the hands of the Guomindang, though the laws restricting traditional midwives were sparsely enforced.

In China in the twenty-first century, as medical training has improved, the *zhuchanshi* have given way to physicians (*yisheng*) and nurses (*hushi*). The Chinese government discontinued midwifery training in 1993 along with the recommendation of hospital confinement for all births.[43] The elimination of midwifery education was also due in part to China's increasing number of trained medical practitioners and a corresponding limited number of occupational opportunities for them. Midwives therefore were replaced by obstetric physicians and labor and delivery room nurses.[44] According to a 2004 *People's Daily* article, 76 percent of all Chinese women deliver babies in hospitals or clinics, which leaves little room for an aging population of untrained midwives to practice.[45] In the largest urban centers like Shanghai, nearly all women go to hospitals to have their babies.[46]

Today, the few *jieshengpo* that exist in China are in many cases associated with back-alley practices of dealing with unwanted pregnancies. But these old-style midwives are not the same as they were around the turn of the last millennium: today many use the "new birth method" or at least partial aseptic techniques to deliver babies at home. Nonetheless, they continue to be vilified as unsanitary and superstitious. In 2002, Ministry of Public Health Official Fu Wei attributed China's high maternal mortality rate to traditional midwifery malpractice.[47] China's 1995 Law on Maternal and Infant Health Care allocated more money to build rural health care facilities across China; as more and more clinics are established in rural areas, *jieshengpo* are being displaced by modern personnel. Nurses, or nurse-midwives who have received additional training in obstetrics, assist in all urban hospital and clinic births, with physicians making decisions on medical interventions like caesarean sections.

The market and population reforms of the 1980s and 1990s that led to a growing middle class and a shrinking number of familial offspring have spurred an even greater rise in the consumption of scientific parenting paraphernalia like handbooks, clothing, and food than what occurred in the Republican era. Books on *taijiao* and modern motherhood fill the shelves of China's bookstores. Consumption and scientific parenting as related to child rearing clearly build on Republican-era practices, but the goods and services available for the modern family have expanded exponentially. After a visit to a fertility clinic to ensure an heir, the Chinese family in the twenty-first century then spends much of its resources on that single offspring.[48] Doulas, or lay birth attendants, have become popular among the affluent in cities like Shanghai, creating a new vocation for the retired or phased-out midwives and giving parturient women personalized assistance in the labor delivery room.[49] Commercial *zuo yuezi* centers offer facilities for private care during the one-month postpartum confinement period, or a family may hire a *yuesao* (confinement nurse) to attend the new mother in her own home, changing diapers, looking after the mother, and performing household tasks while the mother rests.[50]

A quick look at the advertisements aimed at the growing affluent sections of urban China illustrates the exploding array of services and products available to parents: high-end clothing stores, play centers, and amusement parks for the adornment and entertainment of the child; "scientific" foods like concentrated chicken essence and dairy products considered to boost brain power and physical growth; and the proliferation of expensive private schools and professional tutors guaranteed to provide the best route to university. The best and most modern goods and services are available for a generation of "little emperors." [51]

CONTINUITIES: PAST AND PRESENT

Modern reproduction remains a national imperative in China since it was first publicized as such in the 1920s. Women were markers of China's political weakness in the early part of the twentieth century, and, for reformers like Liang Qichao, the key to China's advancement and modernization.[52] Women's roles as "mothers of citizens" gained popularity in China from the 1920s onward as intellectuals struggled to define the modern woman.[53] Reformers and politicians exhorted women to learn the most modern methods of selecting a suitable marriage partner; of prenatal care, childbirth, and child rearing; and of enlightened nuclear family life.

Modern medical childbirth did indeed lower maternal and infant mortality rates in China because of the easily attained goal of maintaining an aseptic, or at least relatively clean, birth environment. Old-style midwives, when instructed to wash hands and all utensils before handling the mother or newborn, could quickly reduce the risk of infant tetanus and puerperal sepsis infections. The maternal and infant mortality rates in China after modernization of childbirth are much lower than in the days of the *jieshengpo*. Before the Republican period, and in areas without modern medical resources, infant mortality was estimated in the range of 250–300 per 1,000 births, and maternal mortality at 15 per 1,000 births.[54] In 1948, the infant mortality rate in areas served by modern midwives was an estimated 114 per 1,000 births, and maternal mortality was 4 per 1,000 births. In 2000, infant mortality was 32 per 100,000 births, and the maternal mortality rate in China was 70 per 100,000 births.[55] Maternal and infant mortality has declined markedly. However, the system in China, as in the West, is not perfect, even after decades of public maternal and child health work.

Reproduction potentially defines and limits women, and it is therefore a pillar in arguments concerning women's personal, political, and economic rights.[56] Women in China have been liberated in many ways physically and socially. They have legal status as individuals instead of as property to be bought or sold, footbinding has ended, and women are free to marry and divorce and to work outside the home. Despite the real improvements in women's daily lives since the 1920s, their role in reproduction has important continuities with the past. Women are responsible for reproduction and contraception and continue to be the targets of state policies with regard to childbirth. In the Maoist era of the 1950s through the 1970s, they were often targets of pronatalist legislation that restricted or banned contraception, and Barefoot Doctors were trained in contraception as well as aseptic delivery and traditional Chinese herbal preparations.[57]

Women remain targets of social and political objectives relating to reproduction. Since the mid-1970s, women bear the burden of limiting reproduction for the sake of the nation.[58] Population growth has replaced women's backwardness "as a major indicator of national crisis, mandating that the population must be contained even at great cost to women individually and collectively," for it is women, not men, who are responsible for birth control.[59] Simultaneously, women are expected to fulfill the utmost example of filial piety by propagating the family line. In fact, as Lisa Handwerker has shown, the prevailing idea in the 1990s was the "all must have one child" model.[60] Legislation in 1980 and 1988 protecting women's labor during menstruation, pregnancy, delivery, nursing and, later, menopause, enforces the primacy of women's reproductive capabilities.[61] Reproduction continues to be a social responsibility. Men and women are faced with mandatory marriage and reproduction regardless of conflicting desires to remain single or childless.

The intensification of the Republican trend toward medicalization of childbirth can make women feel helpless, uncomfortable, and degraded because of largely unnecessary routine procedures.[62] According to a 2001 study, hospital births in four Shanghai hospitals (including one outlying rural county hospital) were highly medicalized, with women receiving routine episiotomies, rectal examinations, supine position, and pubic shaving. All of these routine procedures are considered unnecessary or excessive according to current medical theory. At the same time, fewer than 27 percent of women received pain relief in the form of acupuncture, epidural analgesia, abdominal massage, or intravenous diazepam or pethidine, though more than half of the women reported that their pain was "intolerable."[63] Caesarean rates in China are very high in urban areas, with approximately 60 percent of women in Shanghai and Beijing requesting the procedure for various reasons: belief that the caesarean is safer, fear of a painful vaginal birth without analgesia or anesthesia; and the desire to recover their physique more quickly, to maintain the quality of their sex lives, or to choose an auspicious birth date.[64] Hospitals are eager to perform caesarean sections because of higher profits.[65] These developments have continued regardless of whether they produced better outcomes; medicalized hospital births have not necessarily resulted in lowered maternal and infant mortality rates. However, a medical birth is a valorized modern one, as noted by the prevalence of ultrasound machines even in rural areas where basic equipment like infant scales are missing. Such machines are often used before performing illegal sex-selective abortions.[66]

As late as 2002, the Chinese government was still attempting to "dramatically improve the health of pregnant women and children" based on a "health-for-all" World Health Organization initiative.[67] The modernization of childbirth in China is widespread in urban areas, but China's poorest regions still do not have affordable maternal health care. Only in 2004, Qinghai Province began a pilot program to provide low-cost or free maternal health services for its impoverished herder women.[68] There have been significant advances, but still the mortality rates are relatively high, especially in underprivileged regions. The challenge to provide health care to all of China's women and children has not been completed. What was begun in fits and starts by a few medical missionaries grew into a national program with an overarching vision. The hierarchy of medical training begun in the 1920s and 1930s with places like the First National Midwifery School and Dingxian was the model for the CCP public health program. This model was originally designed to reach as many people as possible as quickly as possible by training a few highly qualified individuals who would give abbreviated training to even more people. Barefoot Doctors—both male and female—would refer the difficult cases to more qualified technicians or physicians. The process of changing the normative birth model continues, as the Chinese government in the twenty-first century is still working to improve maternal and child health care in many rural areas, and public health professionals aim to limit the high cesarean rates common in some Chinese cities.[69] Yang Chongrui was correct in her assessment of China's needs—that the country was too vast and underdeveloped to simply impose a Western public health model. Nearly 80 years later, though China's maternal and child health care has markedly improved, Yang's vision of maternal and child health care for all is still incomplete.

NOTES

1. Goldstein, "Scissors, Surveys, and Psycho-Prophylactics: Prenatal Health Care Campaigns and State Building in China, 1949–1954," 153.

2. Tyrene White, "The Origins of China's Birth Planning Policy," in *Engendering China: Women, Culture, and the State*, ed. Christina Gilmartin et al. (Cambridge: Harvard University Press, 1994), 250–78.

3. On September 18, 1931, a section of Japanese-owned railroad was blown up, ostensibly by Chinese dissidents, in Mukden, Manchuria. This served as the pretext for Japan's annexation of Manchuria and led to increasing hostilities between the two countries. FNMS, *Fifth Annual Report, First National Midwifery School, Peiping, July 1, 1933–June 30, 1934*, 2.

4. I.C. Yuan, "Letter to Dr. John B. Grant," March 21, 1939.

5. Yuan, "Letter to Dr. John B. Grant"; Bullock, *An American Transplant: The Rockefeller Foundation and Peking Union Medical College*, 190–202.

6. Houghton, "Letter to E.C. Lobenstein."

7. Bullock, *An American Transplant: The Rockefeller Foundation and Peking Union Medical College*, 207–8; Fu Hui, "First National Midwifery School and Director Yang Chongrui (*Guoli di yi zhuchan xuexiao yu Yang Chongrui xiaozhang*)," in *Wenshi ziliao xuan bian*, 30 (Beijing: Beijing shi haidian qu weiyuanhui, 1986).

8. Karen Minden, "The Development of Early Chinese Communist Health Policy: Health Care in the Border Region, 1936–1949," *American Journal of Chinese Medicine* VII, no. 4 (1979): 310.

9. Ibid., 303.

10. Ibid., 306–7.

11. Taylor, *Chinese Medicine in Early Communist China, 1945–63: A Medicine of Revolution.*

12. Mao Zedong, "On the United Front in Cultural Work," in *Selected Readings* (Peking: Foreign Language Press, 1967), 185–86; as quoted in Minden, "The Development of Early Chinese Communist Health Policy: Health Care in the Border Region, 1936–1949," 304–5.

13. Minden, "The Development of Early Chinese Communist Health Policy: Health Care in the Border Region, 1936–1949," 305.

14. Goldstein, "Scissors, Surveys, and Psycho-Prophylactics: Prenatal Health Care Campaigns and State Building in China, 1949–1954," 157.

15. Khati Lim (Lin Qiaozhi), "Obstetrics and Gynecology in the Past Ten Years," *Chinese Medical Journal* 79, no. 5 (November 1959): 375–83.

16. Goldstein, "Scissors, Surveys, and Psycho-Prophylactics: Prenatal Health Care Campaigns and State Building in China, 1949–1954," 153.

17. Pi-chao Chen, "Birth Control Methods and Organization in China," in *China's One-Child Family Policy*, ed. Elisabeth Croll, Delia Davin, and Penny Kane (New York: St. Martin's Press, 1985), 136.

18. Goldstein, "Scissors, Surveys, and Psycho-Prophylactics: Prenatal Health Care Campaigns and State Building in China, 1949–1954," 166; Hershatter, "Birthing Stories: Rural Midwives in 1950s China."

19. Hershatter, "Birthing Stories: Rural Midwives in 1950s China."

20. Li Xiaojiang, ed., *Birth: Tradition and Modernization* (*Shengyu: Chuangtong yu xiandaihua*) (Henan: Henan renmin chubanshe, 1997).

21. Hershatter, "Birthing Stories: Rural Midwives in 1950s China."

22. All-China Women's Federation, Department of Child Welfare (*Zhonghua quanguo minzhu funü lianhe hui, ertong fuli bu*), "Universal Outreach on New Knowledge about Childbirth Methods and Childcare (*Xuanchuan puji xinfa jiesheng he you'er zhishi*)," *New Woman of China* (*Xin zhongguo funü*) (June 1953): 6; as cited in Goldstein, "Scissors, Surveys, and Psycho-Prophylactics: Prenatal Health Care Campaigns and State Building in China, 1949–1954," 166.

23. Goldstein, "Scissors, Surveys, and Psycho-Prophylactics: Prenatal Health Care Campaigns and State Building in China, 1949–1954," 168.

24. Ibid., 162n37.

25. Zhu Dan, "How to Manage Midwife Training (*Zenyang ban jiesheng xunlianban*)," *New Woman of China* (*Xin zhongguo funü*) (November 1949): 9; as cited in Goldstein, "Scissors, Surveys, and Psycho-Prophylactics: Prenatal Health Care Campaigns and State Building in China, 1949–1954," 162–63.

26. Goldstein, "Scissors, Surveys, and Psycho-Prophylactics: Prenatal Health Care Campaigns and State Building in China, 1949–1954," 158.

27. Ibid., 163.

28. Ibid., 159.

29. Ibid.

30. Kimberley Ens Manning, "The Gendered Politics of Woman-work: Rethinking Radicalism in the Great Leap Forward," *Modern China* 32, no. 3 (2006): 349–84.

31. Goldstein, "Scissors, Surveys, and Psycho-Prophylactics: Prenatal Health Care Campaigns and State Building in China, 1949–1954," 174–76.

32. Wu, *Reproducing Women: Medicine, Metaphor and Childbirth in Late Imperial China*, especially chapter 5, "Born Like a Lamb": The Discourse of Cosmologically Resonant Childbirth.

33. Wang Xiuhua, "The Prophylactic Painless Childbirth Method Brings Good Fortune to Mothers," from *New China Provides Welfare to Mothers and Children*, as cited in Goldstein, "Scissors, Surveys, and Psycho-Prophylactics: Prenatal Health Care Campaigns and State Building in China, 1949–1954," 176 n89.

34. Manning, "The Gendered Politics of Woman-work: Rethinking Radicalism in the Great Leap Forward"; Kay Ann Johnson, *Women, the Family, and Peasant Revolution in China* (Chicago: University of Chicago Press, 1983).

35. Goldstein, "Scissors, Surveys, and Psycho-Prophylactics: Prenatal Health Care Campaigns and State Building in China, 1949–1954," 161, 169, 173.

36. Delia Davin, "The Single-Child Family Policy in the Countryside," in *China's One-Child Family Policy*, ed. Elisabeth Croll, Delia Davin, and Penny Kane (New York: St. Martin's Press, 1985), 43; Chen, "Birth Control Methods and Organization in China," 15.

37. Goldstein, "Scissors, Surveys, and Psycho-Prophylactics: Prenatal Health Care Campaigns and State Building in China, 1949–1954," 178.

38. Ibid., 163.

39. White, "The Origins of China's Birth Planning Policy."

40. Some notable works are Handwerker, "The Hen That Can't Lay an Egg (*Bu Xia Dan de Mu Ji*): Conceptions of Infertility in Modern China"; Susan Greenhalgh, *Just One Child: Science and Policy in Deng's China* (Berkeley: University of California Press, 2008); Anagnost, "A Surfeit of Bodies: Population and the Rationality of the State in Post-Mao China."

41. Dr. Yang Chongrui and Dr. Lin Qiaozhi are two of the most well-known examples of First National Midwifery School staff who continued to work with the CCP. In fact, Lin Qiaozhi was instrumental in creating the CCP's birth planning policies. Yan Renying, *Dr. Yang Chongrui: 100 Year Commemoration (Yang Chongrui boshi: Danchen bai nian ji nian)*; Guo Jianyao, *Lin Qiaozhi: China's Outstanding Female Obstetrician/Gynecologist (Lin Qiaozhi: Zhongguo jiechu fuchanke nu yisheng)*.

42. Brigitte Steger, "From Impurity to Hygiene: The Role of Midwives in the Modernisation of Japan," *Japan Forum* 6, no. 2 (1994): 175–187; Chien-Ming Yu, "Midwives During the Japanese Occupation," in *Research on Women in Modern Chinese History*, vol. 1 (Taipei: Academia Sinica, Institute of Modern History Publications, 1993), 49–89.

43. Cheung, "The 'Doula-Midwives' in Shanghai," 74.

44. Ibid.

45. "Low-Cost Midwifery Offered to Qinghai Women," *China Daily Online,* November 2, 2004, http://china.org.cn/english/2004/Nov/110984.htm.

46. Qian et al., "Evidence-Based Obstetrics in Four Hospitals in China: An Observational Study to Explore Clinical Practice, Women's Preferences and Provider's Views."

47. "Midwifery Phased out in China's Rural Areas," *People's Daily Online,* September 30, 2002, http://english.people.com.cn/200209/30/eng20020930_104171.shtml#; Travis Anna Harvey, "The Jie Sheng Po of China," *Midwifery Today* 66 (2003): 53–54.

48. Handwerker, "The Hen That Can't Lay an Egg (*Bu Xia Dan de Mu Ji*): Conceptions of Infertility in Modern China."

49. Cheung, "The 'Doula-Midwives' in Shanghai."

50. Cheung et al., "'Zuoyuezi' after Caesarean in China: An Interview Survey."

51. Jun, *Feeding China's Little Emperors: Food, Children, and Social Change.*

52. Gail Hershatter, *Women in China's Long Twentieth Century* (Berkeley and Los Angeles: University of California Press, 2007), 87.

53. Judge, "Citizens or Mothers of Citizens? Gender and the Meaning of Modern Chinese Citizenship"; Cheng, "Going Public Through Education: Female Reformers and Girls' Schools in Late Qing Beijing," 111.

54. Yang, "Midwifery Training in China."

55. "China Vows Health Care for 900 Million," *China Daily Online,* June 11, 2002, http://china.org.cn/english/China/34280.htm. As a comparison, UNICEF reports the United States infant mortality rate in 2004 was 7 per 1,000 births; maternal mortality was 17 per 100,000. Japan's rates were 3/1,000 infant mortality and 10/100,000 maternal mortality for the same dates. See http://www.unicef.org/infobycountry. The higher maternal mortality in the U.S. is due in part to racial disparities in health care and advanced maternal age. African-American women are nearly four times as likely to die from pregnancy-related conditions as are white women, the most common causes of death being hemorrhage, embolism, and pregnancy-induced hypertension. If monitored and treated, the risk of death from these conditions is reduced. Furthermore, more women are having children at later ages, and the risk of maternal mortality rises after age 30. D. Hollander, "Maternal Mortality Exceeds U.S. Goal; Age and Racial Differences are Marked," *Perspectives on Sexual and Reproductive Health* 35, no. 4 (2003): 189–90.

56. For a thorough journalistic, if alarming, exposition of global reproductive rights in the twenty-first century, see Michelle Goldberg, *The Means of Reproduction: Sex, Power, and the Future of the World* (New York: The Penguin Press, 2009).

57. *A Barefoot Doctor's Manual (Translation of a Chinese Instruction to Certain Chinese Health Personnel)* (U.S. Department of Health, Education, and Welfare, Public Health Service, National Institutes of Health: Geographic Health Studies Program of the John E. Fogarty International Center for Advanced Study in the Health Sciences, 1974), 176–83; White, "The Origins of China's Birth Planning Policy."

58. Greenhalgh, "Controlling Births and Bodies in Village China."

59. Hershatter, *Women in China's Long Twentieth Century*, 97.

60. Handwerker, "The Hen That Can't Lay an Egg (*Bu Xia Dan de Mu Ji*): Conceptions of Infertility in Modern China."

61. Margaret Y.K. Woo, "Chinese Women Workers: The Delicate Balance between Protection and Equality," in *Engendering China: Women, Culture, and the State*, ed. Christina Gilmartin et al. (Cambridge, MA: Harvard University Press, 1994), 281.

62. Qian et al., "Evidence-Based Obstetrics in Four Hospitals in China: An Observational Study to Explore Clinical Practice, Women's Preferences and Provider's Views"; Barbara Ehrenreich and Deirdre English, *For Her Own Good: 150 Years of the Experts' Advice to Women* (New York: Doubleday, 1978); Adrienne Rich, *Of Woman Born: Motherhood as Experience and Institution* (New York: Bantam Books, 1977).

63. Qian et al., "Evidence-Based Obstetrics in Four Hospitals in China: An Observational Study to Explore Clinical Practice, Women's Preferences and Provider's Views."

64. Cheung et al., "'Zuoyuezi' after Caesarean in China: An Interview Survey," 27.

65. In Beijing in 2004, a caesarean birth cost 6,000 yuan, or US$750, versus 2,400 yuan (US$300 in 2004) for a vaginal birth. "Beijing Reports Higher Caesarian Birth Rate." *Xinhua News Agency*, May 1, 2006.

66. Zhuochun Wu et al., "Maternal care in rural China: A case study from Anhui province," *BMC Health Services Research* 8, no. 55 (March 10, 2008), www.biomedcentral.com/1472–6963/8/55, accessed September 5, 2010; Qian et al., "Evidence-Based Obstetrics in Four Hospitals in China: An Observational Study to Explore Clinical Practice, Women's Preferences and Provider's Views."

67. "China Vows Health Care for 900 Million."

68. "Low-cost Midwifery Offered to Qinghai Women."

69. Zhuochun Wu et al., "Maternal Care in Rural China: A Case Study from Anhui Province"; "Midwifery Phased out in China's Rural Areas"; "Beijing Reports Higher Caesarian Birth Rate."

Appendix: Translation of "Good Methods for Protecting Newborns and Infants"

1. Eyes. For newborns and infants one must mix hot water with boric acid to form a paste and apply to eyes with cotton.
2. Umbilical cord. Every day one must clean the umbilical cord with boric acid, apply lotion and change cotton dressing.
3. Bathing. After umbilical cord falls off, give infant bath in hot water that has gradually cooled to warm once daily, and use suitable cloth to dry off.
4. Breastfeeding. When nursing a newborn use clean white cloth or cotton to lightly clean [nipple].
5. Food. The first day newborn is able to drink, give boiled water every two hours during the day and every four hours at night to give the infant's stomach a rest. You should not nurse when ill or if you become pregnant for it is easy to have a miscarriage.
6. Atmosphere. In the infant's room, no matter whether summer or winter, day or night, you should open the window to allow fresh air.
7. Sleep. In order to allow for a natural rest when sleeping, the infant should not be hemmed in or shaken.
8. Illness. If the infant becomes sick or has diarrhea, stop giving food and give only liquids. Give small amounts of cold [previously] boiled water and take to hospital.
9. Flies. Flies are a vehicle for disease. If they land on cups and plates, they can carry infectious diseases on their feet if you are not careful.

Reproduced from Changsha Mother and Child Assistance Organization, folder 254, box 16, RG 4, RAC.

Bibliography

Abbot, Andrew. *The System of Professions: An Essay on the Division of Expert Labor*. Chicago and London: University of Chicago Press, 1988.

Afshar, Haleh. "Women and Reproduction in Iran." In *Woman-Nation-State*, edited by N. Yuval-Davis and F. Anthias, 110–25. New York: St. Martin's Press, 1989.

Ahern, Emily. "The Power and Pollution of Chinese Women." In *Women in Chinese Society*, edited by Margery Wolf and Roxanne Witke, 193–214. Stanford: Stanford University Press, 1975.

All-China Women's Federation, Department of Child Welfare (*Zhonghua quanguo minzhu funu lianhe hui, ertong fuli bu*). "Universal Outreach on New Knowledge about Childbirth Methods and Childcare (*Xuanchuan puji xinfa jiesheng he you'er zhishi*)." *New Woman of China* (*Xin zhongguo funu*) (June 1953): 6.

Anagnost, Ann. "A Surfeit of Bodies: Population and the Rationality of the State in Post-Mao China." In *Conceiving the New World Order: The Global Politics of Reproduction*, edited by Faye D. Ginsburg and Rayna Rapp, 22–41. Berkeley: University of California Press, 1995.

Andrews, Bridie. "Judging Western Medicine by Chinese Values: Zhang Xichun and His Work." In *Association for Asian Studies Annual Conference*. Chicago, IL, 2001.

———. "Tailoring Tradition: The Impact of Modern Medicine on Traditional Chinese Medicine, 1887–1937." In *Notions et perceptions du changement en Chine*, edited by Viviane Alleton and Alexeï Volkov, 149–66. Paris: Collège du France Institute des Hautes Études Chinoises, 1994.

Anon. *All about Shanghai and Environs: A Standard Guidebook, Historical and Contemporary Facts and Statistics*. Shanghai: The University Press, 1934.

Arnold, David. *Colonizing the Body: State Medicine and Epidemic Disease in 19th-Century India*. Berkeley: University of California Press, 1993.

Bailey, Paul. "'Unharnessed Fillies': Discourse on the 'Modern' Female Student in Early Twentieth-Century China." In *Wu sheng zhi sheng (III): Zhongguo de funü yu wenhua 1600–1950 (Voices amid Silence (III): Women and the Culture in Modern China 1600–1950)*, edited by Lo Jiu-jung and Lu Miaw-fen, 3: 327–57. Taibei shi: Zhongyang yanjiuyuan jindaishi yanjiusuo chuban, 2003.

Bakalar, Nicholas. "U.S. Still Struggling with Infant Mortality." *New York Times*, April 7, 2009.

Balme, Harold. *China and Modern Medicine: A Study in Medical Missionary Development.* London: United Council for Missionary Education, 1921.

A Barefoot Doctor's Manual (Translation of a Chinese Instruction to Certain Chinese Health Personnel). U.S. Department of Health, Education, and Welfare, Public Health Service, National Institutes of Health: Geographic Health Studies Program of the John E. Fogarty International Center for Advanced Study in the Health Sciences, 1974.

Barlow, Tani. "Wanting Some: Commodity Desire and the Eugenic Modern Girl." In *Women in China: The Republican Period in Historical Perspective*, 312–50. Germany: LIT Verlag Munster, 2005.

Bashford, Alison. "Global Biopolitics and the History of World Health." *History of the Human Sciences* 19, no. 1 (2006): 67–88.

Beahan, Charlotte. "Feminism and Nationalism in the Chinese Women's Press, 1902–1911." *Modern China* 1, no. 4 (1975): 379–416.

"Beijing Reports Higher Caesarian Birth Rate." *Xinhua News Agency*, May 1, 2006.

Benedict, Carol. *Bubonic Plague in Nineteenth-Century China.* Stanford: Stanford University Press, 1996.

Berry, Robert J., Zhu Li, J. David Erickson, Song Li, Cynthia A. Moore, Hong Wang, Jacqueline Gindler, Shi-Xin Hong, and Adolfo Correa. "Prevention of Neural-Tube Defects with Folic Acid in China." *New England Journal of Medicine* 341, no. 20 (November 11, 1999): 1485–90.

Bixby, Josephine. "Obstetric Cases." *The China Medical Missionary Journal* 14, no. 3 (July 1900): 160–62.

Borst, Charlotte G. *Catching Babies: The Professionalization of Childbirth, 1870–1920.* Cambridge, MA: Harvard University Press, 1995.

Borthwick, Sally. "Changing Concepts of the Role of Women from the Late Qing to the May Fourth Period." In *Ideal and Reality: Social and Political Change in Modern China, 1860–1949*, edited by David Pong and Edmund S.K. Fung, 63–91. Lanham, New York, London: University Press of America, 1985.

Bowers, John Z. "Imperialism and Medical Education in China." *Bulletin of the History of Medicine* 48 (1974): 449–64.

———. *Western Medicine in a Chinese Palace: Peking Union Medical College, 1917–1951.* New York: The Josiah Macy, Jr. Foundation, 1972.

Bray, Francesca. "A Deathly Disorder: Understanding Women's Health in Late Imperial China." In *Knowledge and the Scholarly Medical Traditions*, edited by Don Bates, 235–50. Cambridge: Cambridge University Press, 1995.

———. *Technology and Gender: Fabrics of Power in Late Imperial China.* Berkeley and Los Angeles: University of California Press, 1997.

Britton, R.S. *The Chinese Periodical Press, 1800–1912.* Taipei: Chengwen, 1966.

Brown, E. Richard. "Public Health in Imperialism: Early Rockefeller Programs at Home and Abroad." *American Journal of Public Health* 66 (1976): 897–903.

———. *Rockefeller Medicine Men: Medicine and Capitalism in America.* Berkeley: University of California Press, 1981.

Browning, Dr. "Notes of Cases." *China Medical Missionary Journal* 6, no. 2 (1892): 82–85.

Bryson, Mary F. *John Kenneth Mackenzie, Medical Missionary to China.* New York: Fleming H. Revell Company, 1891.

Bullock, Mary Brown. *An American Transplant: The Rockefeller Foundation and Peking Union Medical College.* Berkeley: University of California Press, 1980.

Cadbury, William Warder, and Mary Hoxie Jones. *At the Point of a Lancet: One Hundred Years of the Canton Hospital, 1835–1935.* Shanghai: Kelly and Walsh, Limited, 1935.

"Caesarean Section (Pou fu chu er)." *Dianshizhai Pictorial (Dianshizhai huabao)*, 1892.

Campbell, Cameron. "Public Health Efforts in China Before and After 1949 and their Effects on Mortality." *Social Science History* 21, no. 2 (Summer 1997): 179–218.

Chen Jianshan. *Fetal Education (Taijiao).* Vol. 75. 1st ed. Universal Library. Shanghai: Shangwu yinshuguan, 1925.

Chen, C.C. (Chen Zhiqian), and Frederica M. Bunge. *Medicine in Rural China: A Personal Account.* Berkeley: University of California Press, 1989.

Chen, Pi-chao. "Birth Control Methods and Organization in China." In *China's One-Child Family Policy*, edited by Elisabeth Croll, Delia Davin, and Penny Kane, 135–48. New York: St. Martin's Press, 1985.

Cheng, Weikun. "Going Public Through Education: Female Reformers and Girls' Schools in Late Qing Beijing." *Late Imperial China* 21, no. 1 (2000): 107–44.

Cheung, N.F. "The 'Doula-Midwives' in Shanghai." *Evidence Based Midwifery* 3 (2005): 73–79.

Cheung, Ngai-en, Rosemary Mander, Linan Cheng, Vivian Yan Chen, Xiu Qun Yang, Hong Ping Qian, and Jie Yan Qian. "'Zuoyuezi' after Caesarean in China: An Interview Survey." *International Journal of Nursing Studies* 43 (2006): 193–202.

Chin, Hsien-Yu. "Colonial Medical Police and Postcolonial Medical Surveillance Systems in Taiwan, 1895–1950s." *Osiris* 13 (1999): 326–38.

China Medical Commission of the Rockefeller Foundation. *Medicine in China.* New York: Rockefeller Foundation, 1914.

"China Vows Health Care for 900 Million." *China Daily Online*, June 11, 2002. http://china.org.cn/english/China/34280.htm.

Chinese National Association for the Advancement of Education. "Statistical Summaries of Chinese Education." *Bulletins on Chinese Education* 2 (1923).

Choa, G.H. *"Heal the Sick" Was Their Motto: The Protestant Medical Missionaries in China.* Hong Kong: The Chinese University Press, 1990.

Chou Chun Yen. "The Female Body and Nationality: Vigorous Nation and Women's Hygiene in Modern China (1895–1949) (*Nüti yu guozu: Qiangguo qiangzhong yu jindai zhongguo de funü weisheng*)." PhD dissertation, Taibei, Taiwan: National Chengchi University, 2008.

Cochran, Sherman, ed. *Inventing Nanjing Road: Commercial Culture in Shanghai, 1900–1945.* Ithaca, NY: Cornell University Press, 2000.

Cody, Lisa Forman. *Birthing the Nation: Sex, Science, and the Conception of Eighteenth-Century Britons.* Oxford: Oxford University Press, 2005.

Cohen, Paul A. *History in Three Keys: The Boxers as Event, Experience, and Myth.* New York: Columbia University Press, 1997.

———. "Reflections on a Watershed Date: The 1949 Divide in Chinese History." In *Twentieth-Century China: New Approaches*, edited by Jeffrey Wasserstrom, 27–36. London and New York: Routledge, 2003.

Complaint re: Hu Hsi Obstetrical Hospital, 112 Markham Road, Shanghai International Settlement. Police Report, March 20, 1936, Shanghai Municipal Archives, Public Health Department, 1–16–1–769.

Culp, Robert. *Articulating Citizenship: Civic Education and Student Politics in Southeastern China, 1912–1940.* Cambridge, MA and London: Harvard University Asia Center, 2007.

Cunningham, Andrew, and Bridie Andrews, eds. *Western Medicine as Contested Knowledge.* Manchester and New York: Manchester University Press, 1997.

Cunningham, F., Kenneth Leveno, Steven Bloom, John Hauth, Dwight Rouse, and Catherine Spong. *Williams Obstetrics.* 23rd ed. Chicago: McGraw-Hill Professional, 2009.

Curtin, Philip D. *Disease and Empire: The Health of European Troops in the Conquest of Africa.* New York: Cambridge University Press, 1998.

Davin, Delia. "The Single-Child Family Policy in the Countryside." In *China's One-Child Family Policy*, edited by Elisabeth Croll, Delia Davin, and Penny Kane, 37–82. New York: St. Martin's Press, 1985.

DeGruche, Kingston. *Dr. D. Duncan Main of Hangchow (who is known in China as Dr. Apricot of Heaven Below).* London: Marshall, Morgan & Scott, Ltd., 1930.

Dikötter, Frank, ed. *The Age of Openness: China before Mao.* Berkeley and Los Angeles: University of California Press, 2008.

———. *Imperfect Conceptions: Medical Knowledge, Birth Defects, and Eugenics in China.* London: Hurst & Co., 1998.

———. "Race Culture: Recent Perspectives on the History of Eugenics." *American Historical Review* 103, no. 2 (1998): 467–78.

———. "Reading the Body: Genetic Knowledge and Social Marginalization in the People's Republic of China." *China Information* 13, no. 2 (1998): 1–99.

———. *Sex, Culture and Modernity in China: Medical Science and the Construction of Sexual Identities in the Early Republican Period*. Hong Kong: Hong Kong University Press, 1995.

Dingwall, Robert, Anne Marie Rafferty, and Charles Webster. *An Introduction to the Social History of Nursing*. London: Routledge, 1988.

Dirlik, Arif. "The Ideological Foundations of the New Life Movement: A Study in Counterrevolution." *Journal of Asian Studies* 34, no. 4 (1975): 945–80.

Dong, Madeline Yue. *Republican Beijing: The City and its Histories*. Berkeley: Univeristy of California Press, 2003.

"Dowager Empress Died of Apoplexy." *New York Times*, November 20, 1908.

Duden, Barbara. *Disembodying Women: Perspectives on Pregnancy and the Unborn*. Translated by Lee Hoinacki. Cambridge, MA: Harvard University Press, 1993.

———. *The Woman Beneath the Skin*. Translated by Thomas Dunlap. Cambridge, MA: Harvard University Press, 1991.

Eastman, Lloyd, Jerome Ch'en, Suzanne Pepper, and Lyman P. Van Slyke. *The Nationalist Era in China 1927–1949*. Cambridge: Cambridge University Press, 1991.

Edwards, Louise. "Policing the Modern Woman in Republican China." *Modern China* 26, no. 2 (April 2000): 115–47.

Ehrenreich, Barbara, and Deirdre English. *For Her Own Good: 150 Years of the Experts' Advice to Women*. New York: Doubleday, 1978.

Eno, Eula. "Chinese Female Pelvis: A Study in the Pelvic Measurements of 2,260 Chinese Women, with Suggestions as to the Probable Normals." *Chinese Medical Journal* 47 (1933): 179–86.

Esherick, Joseph W. "Modernity and Nation in the Chinese City." In *Remaking the Chinese City: Modernity and National Identity, 1900–1950*, edited by Joseph W. Esherick, 1–16. Honolulu: University of Hawai'i Press, 1999.

———. *The Origins of the Boxer Uprising*. Berkeley: University of California Press, 1987.

———, and Mary B. Rankin, eds. *Chinese Local Elites and Patterns of Dominance*. Berkeley: University of California Press, 1990.

Esper, Robert, and David Bovaird. *The Problem of Medical Education in Canton*, July 1915.

Fan, Zi Tian, Xue Lian Gao, and Hui Xia Yang. "Popularizing Labor Analgesia in China." *International Journal of Gynecology and Obstetrics* 98, no. 3 (September 2007): 205–7.

Farquhar, Judith. "For Your Reading Pleasure: Self-Health (*Ziwo baojian*) Information in 1990s Beijing." *Positions* 9, no. 1 (2001): 105–30.

Fee, Elisabeth. "Nineteenth-Century Craniology: The Study of the Female Skull." *Bulletin of the History of Medicine* 53, no. 3 (1979): 415–33.

First National Midwifery School, Peiping, July 1, 1932. Folder 373, box 45, series 601, RG1, RAC.

First National Midwifery School, *First Annual Report, First National Midwifery School, 1929–1931*. Annual Report, February 3, 1932.

————. *Second Annual Report, First National Midwifery School, Peiping, July 1, 1930–June 30, 1931.* Annual Report, February 17, 1932.

————. *Third Annual Report, First National Midwifery School, Peiping, July 1, 1931–June 30, 1932.* Annual Report, August 1, 1932.

————. *Fourth Annual Report, First National Midwifery School, Peiping, July 1, 1932–June 30, 1933.* Annual Report, July 15, 1933.

————. *Fifth Annual Report, First National Midwifery School, Peiping, July 1, 1933–June 30, 1934.* Annual Report, September 15, 1934.

————. *Sixth Annual Report, First National Midwifery School, Peiping, July 1, 1934–June 30, 1935.* Annual Report, 1935.

Foucault, Michel. *The Birth of the Clinic: An Archaeology of Medical Perception.* New York: Vintage, 1973.

Franklin, Sarah. "Postmodern Procreation: A Cultural Account of Assisted Reproduction." In *Conceiving the New World Order: The Global Politics of Reproduction,* edited by Faye D. Ginsburg and Rayna Rapp, 323–45. Berkeley: University of California Press, 1995.

French, Francesca. *Thomas Cochrane: Pioneer and Missionary Statesman.* London: Hoder and Stoughton, 1956.

Friedson, Eliot. *Profession of Medicine: A Study of the Sociology of Applied Medicine.* New York: Dodd, Mead & Company, 1972.

Fulton, Mary. "Hackett Medical College for Women, Canton." *Chinese Medical Journal* 23, no. 5 (1909): 324–29.

Furth, Charlotte. "Concepts of Pregnancy, Childbirth, and Infancy in Ch'ing Dynasty China." *Journal of Asian Studies* 46, no. 1 (February 1987): 7–35.

————. *A Flourishing Yin: Gender in China's Medical History, 960–1665.* Berkeley: University of California Press, 1999.

Gerth, Karl. *China Made: Consumer Culture and the Creation of the Nation.* Cambridge, MA: Harvard University Asia Center, 2004.

Glosser, Susan. "The Business of Family: You Huaigao and the Commercialization of a May Fourth Ideal." *Republican China* 20, no. 2 (1995): 80–116.

————. *Chinese Visions of Family and State, 1915–1953.* Berkeley: University of California Press, 2003.

Goldberg, Michelle. *The Means of Reproduction: Sex, Power, and the Future of the World.* New York: Penguin, 2009.

Goldman, Merle. "Restarting Chinese History." *The American Historical Review* 105, no. 1 (February 6, 2000): 153–64.

Goldstein, Joshua. "Scissors, Surveys, and Psycho-Prophylactics: Prenatal Health Care Campaigns and State Building in China, 1949–1954." *Journal of Historical Sociology* 11, no. 2 (1998): 153–83.

Gottschang, Suzanne. "The 'Becoming' Mother: Transitions to Motherhood in Urban China." PhD dissertation, University of Pittsburgh, 1998.

Gough, E. "Difficulties and Discouragements of Obstetric Work in China." *China Medical Missionary Journal* 15, no. 4 (1901): 249–54.

Grant, John B. Letter. "Letter to Dr. Victor Heiser," September 20, 1926.

————. "Letter to Victor Heiser," 1928.

——. *Midwifery Training*. Report. Peking: Peking Union Medical College, December 22, 1927. Folder 371, box 45, series 601, RG 1, RAC.

Greenhalgh, Susan. "Controlling Births and Bodies in Village China." *American Ethnologist* 21, no. 1 (1994): 3–30.

——. *Just One Child: Science and Policy in Deng's China*. Berkeley: University of California Press, 2008.

Grieg, James. "A Case of Decapitation." *China Medical Missionary Journal* 7, no. 1 (March 1893): 230–32.

Gronewold, Sue Ellen. "Encountering Hope: The Door of Hope Mission in Shanghai and Taipei, 1900–1976." PhD dissertation, Columbia University, 1996.

Guangdong Provincial Government Police Department. *Police Department announcement of draft regulations for registered western doctors, obstetrists, pharmacists, prescriptions, western hospitals and the Red Cross (Jingchating gongbu shixing suo ni xiyisheng chankesheng yaojishi tiaoji yaofang xiyiyuan chihongzihui ge li'an zhangcheng wen)*. Vol. 23. Guangdong Provincial Government, 1913.

Guo Jianyao. *Lin Qiaozhi: China's outstanding female obstetrician/gynecologist (Lin Qiaozhi: Zhongguo jiechu fuchanke nu yisheng)*. Hong Kong: Xin ya wenhua shiye youxian gongsi, 1990.

ter Haar, Barend J. *Telling Stories: Witchcraft and Scapegoating in Chinese History*. Leiden: Brill, 2006.

Handwerker, Lisa. "The Hen That Can't Lay an Egg (Bu Xia Dan de Mu Ji): Conceptions of Infertility in Modern China." In *Deviant Bodies: Critical Perspectives on Difference in Science and Popular Culture*, edited by Jennifer Terry and Jacqueline Urla, 358–86. Bloomington: Indiana University Press, 1995.

——. "The Politics of Making Modern Babies in China: Reproductive Technologies and the 'New' Eugenics." In *Infertility around the Globe: New Thinking on Childlessness, Gender, and Reproductive Technologies*, edited by Marcia C. Inhorn and Frank Van Balen, 298–311. Berkeley: University of California Press, 2002.

Harvey, Travis Anna. "The Jie Sheng Po of China." *Midwifery Today* 66 (2003): 53–54.

Hayford, Charles W. *To the People: James Yen and Village China*. New York: Columbia University Press, 1990.

Hershatter, Gail. "Birthing Stories: Rural Midwives in 1950s China." In *Dilemmas of Victory: The Early Years of the People's Republic of China*, edited by Jeremy Brown and Paul Pickowicz. Cambridge, MA: Harvard University Press, 2008.

——. *Dangerous Pleasures: Prostitution and Modernity in Twentieth-Century Shanghai*. Berkeley: University of California Press, 1997.

——. *Women in China's Long Twentieth Century*. Berkeley and Los Angeles: University of California Press, 2007.

Ho, Y.T., Marian Manly, and Gladys Cunningham. "Measurements of Chinese Female Pelvis and Fetal Heads in Relation to Labor." *Chinese Medical Journal* 48 (1934): 47–55.

Holden, Reuben. *Yale in China: The Mainland 1901–1951*. New Haven: The Yale in China Association, Inc., 1964.

Hollander, D. "Maternal Mortality Exceeds U.S. Goal; Age and Racial Differences Are Marked." *Perspectives on Sexual and Reproductive Health* 35, no. 4 (2003): 189–90.

Hong Shilu, and Wu Mai. *Childbirth and Nursing (Shengchan yu yuying)*. 1st ed. Medical Science Series. Shanghai: Shangwu yinshuguan, 1930.

Hong Youxi, and Chen Lixin. *Birth Grannies, Midwives, Obstetrician/gynecologists (Xianshengma, chanpo yu fuchanke yishi)*. Taibei shi: Qianwei, 2002.

Honig, Emily. *Sisters and Strangers: Women in the Shanghai Cotton Mills, 1919–1949*. Stanford: Stanford University Press, 1986.

Houghton, Henry S. Letter. "Letter to E.C. Lobenstein," October 11, 1937. Folder 669, box 94, RG IV2B9, RAC.

Hsieh, Winston. "The Ideas and Ideals of a Warlord: Ch'en Chiung-Ming (1978–1933)." *Papers on China: Harvard University Committee on Regional Studies* 16 (1962): 198–252.

Hsu, Shou Shang, Hsiao Lan Ou Yang, and Yoehngoo Tsohsan Wu Lew. "Education of Women in China." In *Education in China: Papers Contributed by the Members of Committees of the Society for the Study of International Education*, edited by T.Y. Teng and T.T. Lew, 1–35. Peking: Society for the Study of International Education, 1923.

Hu Caojuan. "Why I Want to Study Nursing (Wo wei shenme yao xue hushi)." In *Bethel Annual (Boteli niankan)*, 4–5. Shanghai: Shanghai Boteli yiyuan hushi chanke xuexiao bian zuan, 1936.

Hu, Dr. Hou-ki. Letter. "Letter from Dr. Hou-ki Hu to County Hospital, Shanghai," n.d. 1–16–1–772. Shanghai Municipal Archives.

Huang Qinghua. *Lin Qiaozhi: Biography of China's Famous Physician (Lin Qiaozhi: Zhongguo zhuming kexuejia zhuanji)*. Beijing: Tuanjie chubanshe, 1997.

Huang Shi. "What Is Fetal Education? (Shenme shi taijiao?)." *Ladies' Journal (Funü Zazhi)*, 1931.

Huang, Gordon. "The Development of Health Centres." *Chinese Medical Journal* 55 (June 1939): 546–60.

Huang, K. "The Medical, Cultural, and Social Life of Shanghai: A Study Based on Advertisements for Medicines in Shenbao, 1912–1926 (Cong Shenbao yiyao guanggao kan min chu Shanghai de yiliao wenhua yu shehui shenghuo)." *Bulletin of the Institute of Modern History, Academia Sinica (Zhongyan yanjiuyuan jindaishi yanjiusuo jikan)* 17, no. 2 (1988): 141–94.

Huang, Philip C.C. "Women's Choices under the Law: Marriage, Divorce, and Illicit Sex in the Qing and the Republic." *Modern China* 27, no. 1 (January 2001): 3–58.

Hui Fu. "First National Midwifery School and Director Yang Chongrui (Guoli di yi zhuchan xuexiao yu Yang Chongrui xiaozhang)." In *Wenshi ziliao xuan bian*. 30. Beijing: Beijing shi haidian qu weiyuanhui, 1986.

Hunter, Jane. *The Gospel of Gentility: American Women Missionaries in Turn-of-the-Century China*. New Haven: Yale University Press, 1984.

Huxley, Aldous. *Brave New World*. New York: Harper Perennial Modern Classics, 2006.

"Hygiene and Public Health: The First National Midwifery School, Peiping." *Chinese Medical Journal* 46 (1932): 32–33.

"Important declaration of Guangzhou Midwifery Association board member chief Pang Fu'ai (*Guangzhoushi zhuchanshi gonghui lishizhang Pang Fu'ai zhongyao shengming*)." *Daguangbao* (*Guangzhoubao*), September 13, 1947.

Information Office of the State Council of the People's Republic of China. "Children's Health and Care." *White Papers of the Government*, April 1996. www.china.org.cn/e-white/children/c-3.htm.

Jiang, Xiaoyang. "Cross-Cultural Philanthropy as a Gift Relationship: The Rockefeller Foundation Donors and Chinese Recipients, 1913–1921." PhD dissertation, Bowling Green State University, 1994.

Jie Ping. "A Discussion of Improving Marriage (*Hunli gailiang de shangque*)." *Nantao Christian Institute Bulletin* (*Puyi zhoukan*), December 4, 1924.

Jin Wuzhou. "How to be a Good Republican Citizen" (*Zen yang zuo yi ge zhonghua minguo de lianghao gongmin?*)." *Nantao Christian Institute Bulletin* (*Puyi zhoukan*), March 20, 1925.

Johnson, Kay Ann. *Women, the Family, and Peasant Revolution in China*. Chicago: University of Chicago Press, 1983.

Johnson, Tina Phillips. "Yang Chongrui and the First National Midwifery School: Childbirth Reform in Early Twentieth-Century China." *Asian Medicine: Tradition and Modernity* 4, no. 2 (2009): 280–302.

Jordan, Brigitte. *Birth in Four Cultures: A Crosscultural Investigation of Childbirth in Yucatan, Holland, Sweden, and the United States*, edited by Robbie Davis-Floyd. 4th ed. Prospect Heights, IL: Waveland Press, 1993.

Judge, Joan. "Citizens or Mothers of Citizens? Gender and the Meaning of Modern Chinese Citizenship." In *Changing Meanings of Citizenship in Modern China*, edited by Merle Goldman and Elizabeth J. Perry, 23–43. Cambridge, MA: Harvard University Press, 2002.

Jun, Jing, ed. *Feeding China's Little Emperors: Food, Children, and Social Change*. Stanford: Stanford University Press, 2000.

Jun, Sheng. *Index of Living Cost in Shanghai*. Shanghai: The National Tariff Commission, 1930.

Kanazu, Hidemi. "The Criminalization of Abortion in Meiji Japan." Translated by Marjan Boogert. *U.S.-Japan Women's Journal* 24 (2003): 35–57.

Kansas State Historical Society. "Dr. Williams' Pink Pills for Pale People." *Cool Things*, n.d. http://www.kshs.org/cool3/pinkpills.htm.

Kartchner, Robin, and Lynn Clark Callister. "Giving Birth: Voices of Chinese Women." *Journal of Holistic Nursing* 21 (June 2003): 100–16.

Kazuko, Ono. *Chinese Women in a Century of Revolution, 1850–1950*. Stanford: Stanford University Press, 1989.

Kerber, Linda. "Foreword." In *Chinese Visions of Family and State, 1915–1953*, by Susan Glosser, ix–xiv. Berkeley: University of California Press, 2003.

King, Gordon, and Yu Teh T'ang. "Obstetrical Criteria in North China: The Weights and Measurements of the Mature New-Born Child." *Chinese Medical Journal* 52 (October 1937): 501–6.

Kingston, Maxine Hong. *Woman Warrior: Memoirs of a Girlhood among Ghosts.* New York: Vintage, 1976.

Kirby, William C. "Engineering China: Birth of the Developmental State, 1928–1937." In *Becoming Chinese: Passages to Modernity and Beyond,* edited by Wen-hsin Yeh, 137–60. Berkeley, Los Angeles, London: University of California Press, 2000.

Kwok, D.W.Y. *Scientism in Chinese Thought, 1900–1950.* New Haven and London: Yale University Press, 1965.

Lamson, Herbert D. "Educated Women and Birth Control in China." *China Medical Journal* 44, no. 11 (1930): 1100–109.

———. "Family Limitation among Educated Chinese Married Women: A Study of the Practice and Attitudes of 120 Women." *Chinese Medical Journal* 47 (1933): 493–503.

Lao She. *Camel Xiangzi.* Translated by Shi Xiangzi. Bilingual edition. The Chinese University Press, 2005.

Larson, Magali Sarfatti. *The Rise of Professionalism: A Sociological Analysis.* Berkeley and Los Angeles: University of California Press, 1977.

League of Nations Health Organization. *Collaboration with the Government of China: First Report of the Central Field Health Station,* May 10, 1934.

———. *Health.* Geneva, Switzerland: League of Nations Health Organization Information Section, 1931.

Leavitt, Judith Walzer. *Brought to Bed: Childbearing in America, 1750 to 1950.* New York: Oxford University Press, 1986.

Lee, Edward Bing-Shuey. *Modern Canton.* Shanghai: The Mercury Press, 1936.

Lee, Leo Ou-fan. "The Cultural Construction of Modernity in Urban Shanghai: Some Preliminary Explorations." In *Becoming Chinese: Passages to Modernity and Beyond,* edited by Wen-hsin Yeh, 31–61. Berkeley, Los Angeles, London: University of California Press, 2000.

Lei, Sean Hsiang-Lin. "Habituate Individuality: Framing of Tuberculosis and Its Material Solutions in Republican China" presented at the Annual Meeting of The Association for Asian Studies, Chicago, IL, April 2, 2005.

Leung, Angela Ki-che. "Organized Medicine in Ming-Qing China: State and Private Medical Institutions in the Lower Yangzi Region." *Late Imperial China* 8, no. 1 (1987): 134–66.

———. "Women Practicing Medicine in Premodern China." In *Chinese Women in the Imperial Past: New Perspectives,* edited by Harriet T. Zurndorfer, 101–34. Leiden: Brill, 1999.

Li Ting'an. *The Problem of Rural Health in China (Zhongguo xiangcun weisheng wenti).* Shanghai: Shangwu yinshuguan, 1935.

Li Xiaojiang, ed. *Birth: Tradition and Modernization (Shengyu: Chuangtong yu xiandaihua).* Henan: Henan renmin chubanshe, 1997.

———. "Preface: Why Do We Use Cultural Anthropology As a Starting Point in Our Research? (Xu: Women wei shenme yi wenhua renleixue wei yanjiu *qidian?*)." In *Birth: Tradition and Modernization (Shengyu: Chuangtong yu xiandaihua)*, edited by Li Xiaojiang, 3–15. Henan: Henan renmin chubanshe, 1997.

———. *Women Speak for Themselves (Rang nuren ziji shuohua)*. Beijing: Shenghuo, dushu, xinzhi san lian shudian, 2003.

Lieberman, Sally Taylor. *The Mother and Narrative Politics in Modern China*. Charlottesville: University of Virginia Press, 1998.

Lien, Ling-ling. "Leisure, Patriotism, and Identity: The Chinese Career Women's Club in Wartime Shanghai." In *Creating Chinese Modernity: Knowledge and Everyday Life, 1900–1940*, edited by Peter Zarrow, 213–40. Studies in Modern Chinese History 4. New York, Berne, Frankfurt am Main: Peter Lang, 2006.

———. "Searching for the "New Womanhood": Career Women in Shanghai, 1912–1945." University of California at Irvine, 2001.

Lim, Khati (Lin Qiaozhi). "Obstetrics and Gynecology in the Past Ten Years." *Chinese Medical Journal* 79, no. 5 (November 1959): 375–83.

Lin Yutang. *A History of the Press and Public Opinion in China*. Chicago: University of Chicago Press, 1936.

Lipkin, Zwia. *Useless to the State: "Social Problems" and Social Engineering in Nationalist Nanjing, 1927–1937*. Cambridge, MA: Harvard University Asia Center, 2006.

"Liu Hanzhen, Female Physician (Liu Hanzhen, nu yishi)." *Guo huabao*, July 27, 1936.

Liu Xiang. "Scroll 1, Mothers of Zhou (Juan yi, Zhou shi san mu)." In *Biographies of Exemplary Women (Lienu zhuan)*, 18 BCE. http://etext.lib.virginia .edu/chinese/lienu/browse/scroll1.html.

Liu, Chung-tung. "From san gu liu po to 'caring scholar': the Chinese nurse in perspective." *International Journal of Nursing Studies* 28, no. 4 (1991): 315–24.

Liu, J. Heng (Liu Ruiheng). "The Chinese Ministry of Health." *National Medical Journal of China* 15 (1929): 135–48.

———. "National Health Organization." In *The China Christian Yearbook, 1936–37*, edited by Frank Rawlinson, 336–55. Glendale, CA: The Arthur H. Clark Co., 1937.

———. *Report Given at the 1937 League of Nations-Health Organization Intergovernmental Conference of Far Eastern Countries on Rural Hygiene*. Geneva, Switzerland: League of Nations Health Organization, 1937.

Loudon, Irvine. *The Tragedy of Childbed Fever*. Oxford: Oxford University Press, 2000.

"Low-Cost Midwifery Offered to Qinghai Women." *China Daily Online*, November 2, 2004. http://china.org.cn/english/2004/Nov/110984.htm.

Lu Xun. "What is Required to be a Father Today (Women xianzai zenyang zuo fuqin)." *Xin Qingnian* 6, no. 6 (1919): 558–59.

Lu Yu. "The Fangbian Hospital of Canton (Guangzhou de fangbian yiyuan)." *Guangdong wenshi ziliao* 8 (1963): 139–50.

Lucas, AnElissa. *Chinese Medical Modernization: Comparative Policy Continuities, 1930s–1980s*. New York: Praeger Publishers, 1982.

MacGillivray, Donald. *A Century of Protestant Missions in China*. Shanghai: American Presbyterian Mission Press, 1907.

MacKinnon, Stephen R. "Toward a History of the Chinese Press in the Republican Period." *Modern China* 23, no. 1 (January 1997): 3–32.

Macklin, W.E. "Notes on Cases." *The China Medical Missionary Journal* 7, no. 1 (1893): 101–3.

MacPherson, Kerrie L. *A Wilderness of Marshes: The Origins of Public Health in Shanghai, 1843–1943*. Hong Kong and New York: Oxford University Press, 1987.

Manly, Marian. "Outpatient Obstetrics in China: A Review of 1000 Cases." *Chinese Medical Journal* 51 (1937): 237–44.

Mann, Susan. "The Cult of Domesticity in Republican Shanghai's Middle Class." *Historical Research on Modern Chinese Women (Jindai zhongguo funü shi yanjiu)* 2 (1994): 179–201.

———. *Precious Records: Women in China's Long Eighteenth Century*. Stanford: Stanford University Press, 1997.

Manning, Kimberley Ens. "The Gendered Politics of Woman-work: Rethinking Radicalism in the Great Leap Forward." *Modern China* 32, no. 3 (2006): 349–84.

Mao Zedong. "On the United Front in Cultural Work." In *Selected Readings*, 185–86. Peking: Foreign Language Press, 1967.

Martin, Emily. *The Woman in the Body: A Cultural Analysis of Reproduction*. Boston: Beacon Press, 1992.

Maxwell, Dr. J. Preston. "On Criminal Abortion in China." *Chinese Medical Journal* 16 (January 12, 1928): 1–8.

———. *Scheme for a Six Months' Course in Midwifery for Midwives in Training*, 1926. Folder 601, box 45, Series 371, RG 1, RAC.

———, and J.L. Liu. "Ta Sheng P'ian: A Chinese Household Manual of Obstetrics." *Annals of Medical History* 5, no. 2 (1923): 95–99.

———, and Dr. Lee M. Miles. "Osteomalacia in China." *The Journal of Obstetrics and Gynaecology of the British Empire* 32, no. 3 (1925): 433–41.

———, and Amos K. Wong. "On Puerperal Mortality and Morbidity." *National Medical Journal of China* 16 (1930): 684–703.

Mayer, Tamar. "Gender Ironies of Nationalism: Setting the Stage." In *Gender Ironies of Nationalism: Sexing the Nation*, edited by Tamar Mayer, 1–22. London and New York: Routledge, 2000.

MCH-PH Visiting Report. Health Station Annual Report, 1931. Folder 472, box 67, RG IV2B9, RAC.

Menzies, James. "Some Interesting Obstetric Cases." *China Medical Missionary Journal* 20, no. 1 (1906): 1–5.

"Midwifery Association Dispute: Pang Fu'ai Issues Another Statement (*Zhuchanshi gonghui jiufen an: Pang Fu'ai zai fa shengming*)." *Qianduo ribao*, September 16, 1947.

"Midwifery Phased out in China's Rural Areas." *People's Daily Online*, September 30, 2002. http://english.people.com.cn/200209/30/eng20020930_104171 .shtml#.

Minden, Karen. "The Development of Early Chinese Communist Health Policy: Health Care in the Border Region, 1936–1949." *American Journal of Chinese Medicine* VII, no. 4 (1979): 299–315.

Minutes of the Peiping Union Medical College Committee on the Hospital. Plan of Cooperation Between the Department of Obstetrics and the Health Station, November 22, 1932. Folder 669, box 94, RG IV2B9, RAC.

Mittler, Barbara. *A Newspaper for China? Power, Identity, and Change in Shanghai's News Media, 1872–1912.* Cambridge, MA: Harvard University Asia Center, 2004.

More, Ellen S. *Restoring the Balance: Women Physicians and the Profession of Medicine, 1850–1995.* Cambridge, MA: Harvard University Press, 1999.

"Mother's Association in Nanking." *Chinese Medical Journal* 47 (1933): 418.

Na, Jiang. "The 'New Virtuous Wife and Good Mother': Women Intellectuals' Group Identity and the Funü Zhoukan (Women's Weekly), 1935–1937." *Women's History Review* 16, no. 3 (July 2007): 447–61.

Nakajima, Cheiko. "Health and Hygiene in Mass Mobilization: Hygiene Campaigns in Shanghai, 1920–1945." *Twentieth-Century China* 34, no. 1 (November 2008): 42–72.

Nathan, Carl F. "The Acceptance of Western Medicine in Early 20th Century China: The Story of the North Manchurian Plague Prevention Service." In *Medicine and Society in China*, edited by John Z. Bowers and Elizabeth F. Purcell, 55–75. New York: Josiah Macy, Jr. Foundation, 1974.

Neal, Dr. James Boyd. "Training of Native Women in Midwifery." *China Medical Missionary Journal* 15, no. 3 (1901): 221–22.

Neizhengbu nianjian bianzuan weiyuanhui. *Yearbook of Internal Affairs (Neizheng nianjian)*. Vol. 4. Shanghai: Shangwu yinshuguan, 1936.

Neubauer, W. "Social Gynaecology in China." *Chinese Medical Journal* 51 (June 1937): 825–32.

Niles, Mary W. "Native Midwifery in Canton." *China Medical Missionary Journal* 4 (1890): 51–55.

Perry, Elizabeth J. *Shanghai on Strike: The Politics of Chinese Labor.* Stanford: Stanford University Press, 1993.

Pfeiffer, Stefani. "Epistemology and Etiquette: Bargaining, Self-Disclosure, and the Struggle to Define the Patient Role at PUMC Hospital, 1921–1941" Presented at the Association for Asian Studies Annual Meeting, Chicago, IL, April 2, 2005.

Poulter, Mabel. "Obstetrical Experiences in a Chinese City." *China Medical Journal* 30, no. 2 (1916): 75–89.

"Profile of Ob-Gyn Practice." American Congress of Obstetricians and Gynecologists, 2003. http://www.acog.org/from_home/departments/practice/ProfileofOb-gynPractice1991–2003.pdf.

Public Health Department. "Kai Mai Commoners' Obstetrical Hospital (*Ning Shao pingmin chanke yiyuan*)." Shanghai Municipal Archives, 1933. 1–16–1–770. Shanghai Municipal Archives.

———. "San Ming Obstetrical Hospital (*Sanmin chanke yiyuan*)." Shanghai Municipal Archives, 1935. 1–16–1–771. Shanghai Municipal Archives.

————. "Shanghai Hospital for Women and Children (*Shanghai furu chanke yiyuan*)." Shanghai Municipal Archives, 1935. 1–16–1–856. Shanghai Municipal Archives.

————. "Shanghai West Gate Hospital for Women and Children (*Shanghai ximen furu yiyuan*)." Shanghai Municipal Archives, 1937. 1–16–1–866. Shanghai Municipal Archives.

————. "Women's Hospital (*Chanfu yiyuan*)." Shanghai Municipal Archives, 1935. 1–16–1–773. Shanghai Municipal Archives.

————. "Zung Wei Obstetrical Hospital (*Renhui chanke yiyuan*)." Shanghai Municipal Archives, 1935. 1–16–1–772. Shanghai Municipal Archives.

Pyenson, Lewis. *Cultural Imperialism and Exact Sciences: German Expansion Overseas 1900–1930.* New York, Berne, Frankfurt am Main: Peter Lang, 1985.

Qian, Xu, Helen Smith, Li Zhou, Ji Liang, and Paul Garner. "Evidence-Based Obstetrics in Four Hospitals in China: An Observational Study to Explore Clinical Practice, Women's Preferences and Provider's Views." *BioMed Central Pregnancy and Childbirth* 1, no. 1 (2001).

Que Lianyu. "The Creation and Historical Significance of the Sanitary Police in the Late Qing Dynasty (*Qingmo weisheng jingcha de chuangli ji lishi zuoyong*)." *Zhonghua yishi zazhi* (*Chinese Journal of Medical History*) 18 (1988): 97–98.

Rawski, Evelyn S. *Education and Popular Literacy in Ch'ing China.* Ann Arbor: University of Michigan Press, 1979.

Rayburn, W.F., B.L. Anderson, J.V. Johnson, M.A. McReynolds, and J. Schulkin. "Trends in the Academic Workforce of Obstetrics and Gynecology." *Obstetrics and Gynecology* 115 (2010): 141–46.

Reeves, Caroline Beth. "The Power of Mercy: The Chinese Red Cross Society, 1900–1937." PhD dissertation, Harvard University, 1998.

Regulations of the First National Midwifery School. Beiping: First National Midwifery School, 1930. Folder 372, box 45, series 601. RAC.

Renshaw, Michelle. *Accommodating the Chinese: The American Hospital in China, 1880–1920.* New York Routledge, 2005.

Rich, Adrienne. *Of Woman Born: Motherhood as Experience and Institution.* New York: Bantam Books, 1977.

Rogaski, Ruth. "Hygienic Modernity in Tianjin." In *Remaking the Chinese City: Modernity and National Identity, 1900–1950*, edited by Joseph W. Esherick, 30–46. Honolulu: University of Hawai'i Press, 1999.

————. *Hygienic Modernity: Meanings of Health and Disease in Treaty-Port China.* 1st ed. Berkeley: University of California Press, 2004.

Rong Wangxi. "The Life of a Nurse in the Old Days (*Jiu shehui hushi de shenghuo*)." In *Hua County Gazetteer* (*Huaxian wenshi ziliao*), 5:100–103. Henan sheng, Huaxian: Zhengxie huaxian weiyuanhui wenshi ziliao yanjiu weiyuanhui bian, 1989.

Rosebury, Theodor. *Microbes and Morals; the Strange Story of Venereal Disease.* New York: Viking Press, 1971.

Schneider, Laurence. *Biology and Revolution in Twentieth-Century China.* Asia/Pacific/Perspectives. Lanham, MD: Rowman & Littlefield Publishers, Inc., 2003.

Schwarcz, Vera. *The Chinese Enlightenment: Intellectuals and the Legacy of the May Fourth Movement of 1919*. Berkeley, Los Angeles, London: University of California Press, 1986.

Scott, Dr. Annie V. "Well Baby Clinic: Its Organization and Aim." *Chinese Medical Journal* 50 (1936): 620–22.

Shao, Qin. *Culturing Modernity: The Nantong Model, 1890–1930*. Stanford: Stanford University Press, 2004.

Shemo, Connie. "'An Army of Women': The Medical Ministries of Kang Cheng and Shi Meiyu, 1873–1937." PhD dissertation, SUNY Binghamton, 2002.

———. "'How Better Could She Serve Her Country?' Cultural Translators, U.S. Women's History, and Kang Cheng's 'An Amazon in Cathay.'" *Journal of Women's History* 21, no. 4 (2009): 111–33.

Shen, Jiaying. "Report on the School and Lying-in Hospital (*Ben xiao chanyuan liang zhou shixi zhi jingkuang*)." *Shanxi shengli zhuchan xuexiao niankan* (1935): 91–92.

Shi Gu. *Man May Live Two Hundred Years (Rensheng erbainian)*. 1st ed. Shanghai: Shangwu yinshuguan, 1929.

Shields, Stephanie A. "The Variability Hypothesis: The History of a Biological Model of Sex Differences in Intelligence." *Signs: Journal of Women and Culture in Society* 7 (1982).

Sommer, Matthew Harvey. *Sex, Law, and Society in Late Imperial China*. Stanford: Stanford University Press, 2000.

Spence, Jonathan D. *The Search for Modern China*. New York and London: W.W. Norton, 1990.

Stapleton, Kristin. *Civilizing Chengdu: Chinese Urban Reform, 1895–1937*. Cambridge, MA: Harvard University Press, 2000.

Steger, Brigitte. "From Impurity to Hygiene: The Role of Midwives in the Modernisation of Japan." *Japan Forum* 6, no. 2 (1994): 175–87.

Stevens, Sarah E. "Making Female Sexuality in Republican China: Women's Bodies in the Discourses of Hygiene, Education, and Literature." PhD dissertation, Indiana University, 2001.

Stewart, Agnes. "Gynaecological Practice in China." *China Medical Journal* 22, no. 3 (May 1908): 145–50.

Stinson, Mary H., MD. *Work of Women Physicians in Asia*. Norristown, NJ: J.H. Brandt, 1884.

Stockard, Janice. *Daughters of the Canton Delta: Marriage Patterns and Economic Strategies in South China, 1860–1930*. Hong Kong: Hong Kong University Press, 1989.

Stone, Mary (Shi Meiyu). "Obstetrical Outfit in China." *China Medical Journal* 26, no. 6 (November 1912): 347–50.

Strand, David. *Rickshaw Beijing: City People and Politics in the 1920s*. Berkeley: University of California Press, 1989.

Su, Tsu-fei, and Chueh-ju Liang. "Growth and Development of Chinese Infants of Hunan Province." *Chinese Medical Journal* 58 (July 1940): 104–12.

Sze, Szeming. *China's Health Problems*. Washington, DC: Chinese Medical Association, 1944.

Tang, Chindon Yiu. "Woman's Education in China." *Bulletins on Chinese Education* 9, no. 2 (1923): 1–36.

T'ao, Lee. "Some Statistics on Medical Schools in China for 1932–1933." *Chinese Medical Journal* 47 (1933): 1029–39.

Tao, S.M. "Medical Education of Chinese Women." *Medical and Professional Woman's Journal* (1934): 73–76.

Tatchell, W. Arthur. "The Training of Male Nurses." *China Medical Journal* 26, no. 5 (1912): 269–73.

Taylor, Edward Stewart. *History of the American Gynecological Society 1876–1981 and American Association of Obstetricians and Gynecologists 1888–1981*. St. Louis: C.V. Mosby Company, 1985.

Taylor, Kim. *Chinese Medicine in Early Communist China, 1945–63: A Medicine of Revolution*. London: RoutledgeCurzon, 2005.

Terazawa, Yuki. "Gender, Knowledge, and Power: Reproductive Medicine in Japan, 1690–1930." PhD dissertation, UCLA, 2001.

———. "The State, Midwives, and Reproductive Surveillance in Late Nineteenth- and Early Twentieth-Century Japan." *U.S.-Japan Women's Journal* 24 (2003): 59–81.

Thomson, Jos. C. "Native Practice and Practitioners." *China Medical Missionary Journal* 4, no. 3 (1890): 185–91.

Tien, Hung-Mao. *Government and Politics in Kuomintang China 1927–1937*. Stanford: Stanford University Press, 1972.

Tomes, Nancy. *The Gospel of Germs: Men, Women, and the Microbe in American Life*. Cambridge, MA: Harvard University Press, 1999.

———. "The Private Side of Public Health: Sanitary Science, Domestic Hygiene, and the Germ Theory, 1870–1900." In *Sickness & Health in America: Readings in the History of Medicine and Public Health*, edited by Judith Walzer Leavitt and Ronald L. Numbers, 506–28. Madison: University of Wisconsin Press, 1997.

Topley, Marjorie. "Marriage Resistance in Rural Kwangtung." In *Women in Chinese Society*, edited by Margery Wolf and Roxane Witke, 67–88. Stanford: Stanford University Press, 1975.

Tsin, Michael. *Nation, Governance, and Modernity in China: Canton 1900–1927*. Stanford: Stanford University Press, 1999.

Tucker, Sara Waitstill. "The Canton Hospital and Medicine in Nineteenth Century China 1835–1900." PhD dissertation, Indiana University, 1983.

Tuqiang Advanced Midwifery School. *Record of the 50th Graduating Class of Tuqiang Advanced Midwifery School (Tuqiang gaodeng zhuchan xuexiao #50 jie biye tongxue lu)*. Guangzhou: Dongya zhongxi yinwuju, 1936.

Uttley, K.H. "The Birth Weight of Full Term Cantonese Babies." *Chinese Medical Journal* 58 (November 1940): 582–91.

Van Hollen, Cecilia. *Birth on the Threshold: Childbirth and Modernity in South India*. Berkeley: University of California Press, 2003.

Verdery, Katherine. "From Parent-State to Family Patriarchs: Gender and Nation in Contemporary Eastern Europe." *East European Politics and Societies* 8, no. 2 (1994): 225–55.

Wakeman, Frederic. *Policing Shanghai 1927–1937*. Berkeley, Los Angeles, London: University of California Press, 1995.

Wang Yugang, and Qu Shaoheng. "Script for The Moment of Life and Death (*Sheng si guantou juben*)." In *Shengsheng Midwifery School Yearbook*, 49–64. Shanghai: Shengsheng Midwifery School, 1935.

Wang, Bin, Qi Shi, Yan Wang, Nan Li, and Ling Shi. "National Survey on Midwifery Practices in Health Facilities in China (*887 suo yiliao baojian jigou zhuchan jishu shishi xiankuang de fenxi*)." *Chinese Journal of Obstetrics and Gynecology (zhonghua fuchanke zazhi)* 42, no. 5 (May 2007): 305–8.

Wang, K.Y. *A Report of Hsiang-Ya Medical College & Hospital*. Archival material, January 1930. Series 601A, RG 1, RAC.

Wang, Shumin. "My Reflections on Entering Bethel Obstetrics School (*Wo ru Boteli chanke xuexiao de ganxiang*)." In *Bethel Annual (Boteli niankan)*, 16–17. Shanghai: Shanghai Boteli yiyuan hushi chanke xuexiao bian zuan, 1936.

Watt, John. "Breaking into Public Service: The Development of Nursing in Modern China, 1870–1949." *Nursing History Review* 12 (2004): 67–96.

White, Tyrene. "The Origins of China's Birth Planning Policy." In *Engendering China: Women, Culture, and the State*, edited by Christina Gilmartin, Gail Hershatter, Lisa Rofel, and Tyrene White, 250–78. Cambridge, MA: Harvard University Press, 1994.

Witz, Anne. *Professions and Patriarchy*. London and New York: Routledge, 1992.

Wong, Amos. "Committee on Contraception." *Chinese Medical Journal* 51 (1937): 770–71.

Wong, K. Chimin, and Lien-Teh Wu. *History of Chinese Medicine: Being a Chronicle of Medical Happenings in China from Ancient Times to the Present Period*. Tientsin, China: The Tientsin Press, Ltd., 1932.

Wong, Ling-ling. "Tso yüeh-tzu: The Post-Natal Ritual of Han Chinese Women in Taiwan." University of Oxford, 1998.

Woo, Margaret Y.K. "Chinese Women Workers: The Delicate Balance between Protection and Equality." In *Engendering China: Women, Culture, and the State*, edited by Christina Gilmartin, Gail Hershatter, Lisa Rofel, and Tyrene White, 279–95. Cambridge, MA: Harvard University Press, 1994.

Woodhead, H.G.W, ed. *The China Yearbook 1935*. Shanghai: The North China Daily News and Herald, Ltd., 1935.

World Health Organization. *World Health Statistics 2009*. Geneva, Switzerland: World Health Organization, 2009.

Wright, David. *Translating Science: The Transmission of Western Chemistry into Late Imperial China, 1840–1900*. Leiden: Brill, 2000.

Wu, Liande. *Plague Fighter: the Autobiography of a Modern Chinese Physician*. Cambridge, England: W. Heffner, 1959.

Wu, Yi-Li. "The Bamboo Grove Monastery and Popular Gynecology in Qing China." *Late Imperial China* 21, no. 1 (June 2000): 41–76.

———. "Ghost Fetuses, False Pregnancies, and the Parameters of Medical Uncertainty in Classical Chinese Gynecology." *Nan NÜ* 4, no. 2 (2002): 170–206.

———. "Introducing the Uterus to China: Benjamin Hobson's New Treatises on Women's and Children's Diseases (Fuxing xinshuo), 1858" presented at the Association for Asian Studies Annual Conference, Chicago, IL, March 22, 2001.

———. *Reproducing Women: Medicine, Metaphor and Childbirth in Late Imperial China*. Berkeley and Los Angeles: University of California Press, 2010.

———. "Transmitted Secrets: The Doctors of the Lower Yangzi Region and Popular Gynecology in Late Imperial China." PhD dissertation, Yale University, 1998.

Wu, Zhuochun, Kirsi Viisainen, Xiaohong Li, and Elina Hemminki. "Maternal Care in Rural China: A Case Study from Anhui Province." *BMC Health Services Research* 8, no. 55 (March 10, 2008). http://www.biomedcentral.com/1472–6963/8/55.

Xiao Wenwen. "The History of Modern Obstetrics in Western Medicine in China (*Zhongguo jindai xiyi chanke xueshi*)." *Zhonghua yishi zazhi* (*Chinese Journal of Medical History*) 25, no. 4 (1995): 204–10.

Xie Ruiyi. "First Anniversary Report (*Yi zhounian huiwu baogao*)." *Guangzhou shi zhuchanshi gonghui tekan* (1947): 21–22.

Xie Siyan. "The Question of Women's Physical Culture (*Nüzi tiyu wenti*)." *Ladies' Journal* (*Funü zazhi*) 9, no. 7 (1923): 2–5.

Xu, Xiaoqun. *Chinese Professionals and the Republican State: The Rise of Professional Associations in Shanghai, 1912–1937*. Cambridge: Cambridge University Press, 2001.

———. "'National Essence' vs. 'Science': Chinese Native Physicians' Fight for Legitimacy, 1912–1937." *Modern Asian Studies* 31, no. 4 (1997): 847–77.

Xu, Yamin. "Wicked Citizens and the Social Origins of China's Modern Authoritarian States: Civil Strife and Political Control in Republican Beijing, 1928–1937." PhD dissertation, University of California, 2002.

Yan Renying, ed. *Dr. Yang Chongrui: 100 Year Commemoration* (*Yang Chongrui boshi: Danchen bai nian ji nian*). Beijing: Beijing yike daxue, zhongguo xiehe yike daxue lianhe chubanshe, 1990.

Yang Chongrui. "My Autobiography (*Wo de zizhuan*)." In *Dr. Yang Chongrui: 100 Year Commemoration* (*Yang Chongrui boshi: Danchen bai nian ji nian*), edited by Yan Renying, 143–53. Beijing: Beijing yike daxue, zhongguo xiehe yike daxue lianhe chubanshe, 1990.

Yang Nianqun. "The Establishment of Modern Health Demonstration Zones and the Regulation of Life and Death in Early Republican Beijing." Translated by Larissa Heinrich. *East Asian Science, Technology, and Medicine*, no. 22 (2004): 69–95.

———. "The Transformation of Space and Control of Birth and Death in Early Republican Beijing (*Minguo chunian beijing de shengsi kongzhi yu kongjian zhuanhuan*)." In *Space, Memory, Society: A Collection of New Historical Cultural Research* (*Kongjian, jiyi, shehui zhuanxing: 'xin shehui shi' yanjiu lunwen jingxuan*), edited by Yang Nianqun. Shanghai: Shanghai renmin chubanshe, 2001.

Yang, Cui, and Brian G. Southwell. "Dangerous Disease, Dangerous Women: Health, Anxiety and Advertising in Shanghai from 1928 to 1937." *Critical Public Health* 14, no. 2 (June 2004): 149–56.

Yang, Marion (Yang Chongrui). "Birth Control in Peiping: First Report of the Peiping Committee on Maternal Health." *Chinese Medical Journal* 48 (1934): 786–91.

———. "Control of Practising Midwives in China." *Chinese Medical Journal* 44, no. 5 (1930): 428–31.

———. Letter. "Letter [to John B. Grant?]," 1928.

———. Letter. "Letter to the Editor." *China Medical Journal* 42 (1928): 554.

———. Letter. "Letter to Dr. Frank E. Whitacre," June 8, 1948.

———. Letter. "Letter to Dr. W.A. Sawyer," January 21, 1937. Folder 374, box 45, series 601, RG 1, RAC.

———. Letter. "Letter to Miss Mary Beard," November 7, 1930.

———. "Midwifery Training in China." *China Medical Journal* 42 (1928): 768–75.

———. *Report of the Training and Supervision for Midwives*, February 1929. Folder 371, box 45, series 601, RAC.

———. "The Training of Midwives." *China Medical Journal* 42 (1928): 554.

———, and I-Chin Yuan. "Report of an Investigation on Infant Mortality and its Causes in Peiping." *Chinese Medical Journal*, 47 (1933): 597–604.

Yao Changxu. *Essentials of Obstetrics (Taichan xuzhi)*. 6th ed. Medical Series. Shanghai: Shangwu yinshuguan, 1929.

Ye, Weili. ""Nu Liuxuesheng": The Story of American-Educated Chinese Women, 1880s-1920s." *Modern China* 20, no. 3 (1994): 315–46.

Ye, Xiaoqing. *The Dianshizhai Pictorial: Shanghai Urban Life, 1884–1898*. Ann Arbor: University of Michigan Press, 2003.

Yeh, Wen-hsin. "The Paradox of Autonomy: Nation, Revolution, and Women through the Chinese Looking Glass." In *Women in China: The Republican Period in Historical Perspective*, 40–56. Germany: LIT Verlag Munster, 2005.

———. "Shanghai Modernity: Commerce and Culture in a Republican City." *China Quarterly* 150 (June 1997): 375–94.

Yen, Hsiao-pei. "Body Politics, Modernity and National Salvation: The Modern Girl and the New Life Movement." *Asian Studies Review* 29 (2005): 165–86.

Yip, Ka-che. *Health and National Reconstruction in Nationalist China: The Development of Modern Health Services, 1928–1937*. Monograph and Occasional Paper Series. Ann Arbor: Association for Asian Studies, Inc., 1995.

Yong Ze. "English Doctor Ma Gen-Jia and Ma Doctor Hospital (*Yingyi Ma Genjia yu Tianjin Ma Daifu Yiyuan*)." *Jinwanbao: jinri tianjin huakan*, December 16, 2003.

Yu, Chien-Ming. "Midwives During the Japanese Occupation." In *Research on Women in Modern Chinese History*, 1: 49–89. Taipei: Academia Sinica, Institute of Modern History Publications, 1993.

Yuan, I.C. Letter. "Letter to Dr. John B. Grant," March 21, 1939.

Yun Long, ed. *Administrative Records of Kunming (Kunming xingzheng jishi)*. Vol. 22. Kunming: Yunnan zezhengting yinshua, 1943.

Yun Qin. "Hygiene and Fetal Education during Pregnancy (*Renshen de weisheng yu taijiao*)." *Far Eastern Miscellany (Dongfang Zazhi)* 34, no. 7 (1937): 257–60.

Yuval-Davis, Nira. "Women and the Biological Reproduction of 'the Nation.'" *Women's Studies International Forum* 19, no. 1 (1996): 17–24.

Zhang Xiaohuai. "Translator's Preface (*Yi zhe xu*)." In *Fumu zhi dao*, 1–2. Shenzhou guo guang she chuban, 1930.

Zhang Zaitong, and Cheng Rijin, eds. *Selected Republican-Era Medical and Public Health Legislation (Minguo yiyao weisheng fagui xuanbian, 1912–1948)*. Shandong: Shandong Daxue Chubanshe, 1990.

Zhongde Professional Midwifery School Association (*Zhongde gaoji zhuchan zhuanye xuexiao weiyuanhui*), ed. *Zhongde Professional Midwifery School 15th Anniversary Commemorative Publication (Zhongde gaoji zhuchan zhuanye xuexiao 15 zhounian jinian kan)*. Shanghai, 1940.

Zhu Dan. "How to Manage Midwife Training (*Zenyang ban jiesheng xunlianban*)." *New Woman of China (Xin zhongguo funü)* (November 1949): 9.

Zhu Wenyin. "Fetal Education and Eugenics (*Taijiao yu youshengxue*)." *Ladies' Journal (Funü zazhi)* 17, no. 8 (1931): 11–19.

Zi Yun (pseud.). "Childbirth Customs in My Hometown: Beijing (*Wu xiang de shengchan fengsu: Beijing*)." *Ladies' Journal (Funü zazhi)* 11, no. 7 (1925): 1173–1200.

Glossary of Chinese Terms

angzang 肮脏
ban shen bu sui 半身不遂
Beijing xiehe yixueyuan 北京协和医学院
Beijingshi sili gongyi gaoji zhuchan zhuanye xuexiao 北京市私立公益高级助产专业学校
Beiping shili gonganju baoying shiwusuo 北平市立公安局保婴事务所
Beipingshi gong'anju di yi weisheng shiwusuo 北平市公安局第一卫生事务所
Boji yiyuan 博济医院
chanfu huli 产妇 护理
chanfu yiyuan 产妇医院
chankesheng 产科生
chanpo 产婆
chanpo xunlianban 产婆训练班
Chen Duxiu 陈独秀
Chen Zhiqian 陈志潜
cun 村
daixia 帶下
danwei 单位
Dasheng bian 達生遍
Datong shu 大同书
Dianshizhai huabao 点石斋华报
Dingxian 定县
Dongfang zazhi 东方杂志
dongya binfu 东亚病夫
Fangbian yiyuan 方便医院
fangbiansuo 方便所

fuchanke 婦產科
fuke 妇科
Fumu zhi dao 父母之道
funü jibing 妇女疾病
Funü zazhi 妇女杂志
Furen renzi, qin bu ze, zuo bu bian, li bu bi, bu shi xie wei, bu zheng bu shi, bu zheng bu zuo 妇人任子，寝不侧，做不边，立不跸，不食邪味，不正不食，不正不坐
fuying menzhen 妇婴门诊
fuying weisheng 妇婴卫生
Gaoqiao xiangcun weisheng mofan qu 高桥乡村卫生模范区
gei ying'er kai lu 给婴儿开路
gonganju 公安局
gongde 公德
gonggong weisheng hushi 公共卫生护士
gonggong weisheng renyuan xunlianban 公共卫生人员训练班
gonggong weisheng yishi 公共卫生医师
Gongyiyuan 公医院
Guangdong gaoji hushi zhuchan zhuanye xuexiao 广东高几护士助产专业学校
Guangdong wenshi ziliao 广东文史资料
Guangzhou de fangbian yiyuan 广州的方便医院
Guangzhou shi shili yiyuan baogao shu 广州市市立医院报告书
Guangzhou shi zhuchanshi gonghui 广州市助产士工会
Guangzhoushi zhuchanshi gonghui tekan 广州市助产士公会特刊
Guohuabao 国华报
guomin zhi mu 国民之母
Hangzhou guangji yiyuan fushe zhuchan xuexiao 杭州广济医院附设助产学校
Hu Shi 胡适
Hunan chanyuan 湖南产院
hushi 护士
Huxi pingmin chanke yiyuan 沪西平民产科医院
Jiangning zizhi shiyan xian 江宁自治实验县
Jiangsu sheng hui weisheng shiwusuo 江苏省会卫生事务所
jiating fangshi 家庭访视
Jiating xingqi 家庭星期
jiesheng 接生
jieshengpo 接生婆
Jingchating gongbu shixing suo ni xiyisheng chankesheng yaojishi tiaoji yaofang xiyiyuan chihongzihui ge li'an zhangcheng wen 警察厅公布施行所拟西医生产科生药剂师调剂药方西医院赤红字会各立案章程文

jinshi 进士

jiqi you shen, mu bu jian shi e se, er bu ting yin sheng, kou bu chu ao yan, neng yi taijiao 及其有娠, 目不见视恶色, 耳不听淫声, 口不出敖言, 能以胎教

Jiu yu xin 旧与新

jixiang laolao 吉祥姥姥

kang 炕

Kang Cheng 康成

Kang Youwei 康有为

keyi liwen liang jiao 可以立稳两脚

kuai ma qing che, mou shi shou xi 快马轻车，某氏收洗

laolao 姥姥

Lao Huaigu 劳怀古

Lao Taitai 老太太

Lao Ye 老爷

Li Hongzhang 李鸿章

Li Shufen 李树芬

Li Tingan 李廷安

liangqi xianmu 良妻贤母

Liangyou huabao 良友华报

Liang Qichao 梁启超

Lienü zhuan 烈女传

Liji 礼记

Lin Qiaozhi 林巧稚

Liu Hanzhen 刘汉真

Liu Ruiheng 刘瑞恒

Lu Xun 鲁迅

minban 民办

minzhengting 民政厅

minzhong 民众

modeng nüzi 摩登女子

mu 亩

muqin hui 母親會

neike 内科

Neize 内则

Neizheng nianjian 内政年鉴

Ningshao pingmin chanke yiyuan 宁绍平民产科医院

pingmin chanyuan 平民产院

poshangfeng 破伤风

Pou fu chu er 剖腹出儿

Puyi zhoukan 普益周刊

qi 气

qing xing jibing 轻性疾病
Qinghe shiyanqu 清河试验区
quanguo jingji weiyuanhui 全国经济委员会
Renhui (Zung wei) chanke yiyuan 仁惠产科医院
Renshen de weisheng yu taijiao 妊娠的卫生与胎教
Sanmin chanke yiyuan 三民产科医院
Shanghai Boteli yiyuan hushi chanke xuexiao 上海伯特利医院护士产科学校
Shanghai furu chanke yiyuan 上海妇孺产科医院
Shanghai shengsheng zhuchan xuexiao 上海生生助产学校
Shanghai sili gongde zhuchan xuexiao 上海私立同德助产学校
Shanghai ximen furu yiyuan 上海西门妇孺医院
Shanghai zazhi gongsi 上海杂志公司
Shanghai zhongde gaoji zhuchan zhuanye xuexiao 商海中得高几株产专业学校
shanren 善人
Shangwu yinshuguan 商务印书馆
Shenbao 申报
Shengchan yu yuying 生产与育婴
Shenghuo shudian 生活书店
Shenjue weisheng gongzuo zai xiangcun zhi zhongyao 深觉卫生工在鄉村之重要
Shengsi guantou juben 生死关头剧本
sheng weisheng chu 省卫生处
sheng weisheng shiyanchu 省卫生实验处
shi 士
Shi Meiyu 石美玉
shousheng laolao 收生姥姥
shouyao dianji zhenzhifa 手摇电机诊治法
Shunde 顺德
side 私德
Sili minguo gaoji zhuchan zhuanye xuexiao 私立民国高级助产专业学校
sui (age) 岁
sui (break) 碎
Sun Fo (Sun Ke) 孫科
Sun Zhongshan boshi yixueyuan 孙中山博士医学院
Taichan xuzhi 胎产须知
taijiao 胎教
Taixian xianli yiyuan 台县县立医院
Tan Sitong 谭嗣同
tuijin ju guanli quan sheng zhuchan gongzuo zhi zhongxin jiguan 推进及管理全省助产工作之中心机关

Tuqiang gaodeng zhuchan xuexiao 图强高等助产学校
wa (frog) 蛙
wa (cry) 哇
waike 外科
weisheng 卫生
weisheng fensuo 卫生分所
weisheng mofan qu 卫生模范区
weisheng shiyan chu 卫生试验处
weishengsuo 卫生所
weisheng weiyuanhui 卫生委员会
weisheng xuanchuan 卫生宣传
weishengyuan 卫生院
wenming 文明
Wenpingxian 宛平县
wenpo 稳婆
wenyan 文言
Wu xiang de shengchan fengsu: Beijing 吾乡的生产风俗: 北京
xian 县
xiao jiating 小家庭
xiezhu yishi 协助医师
xin nuxing 新女性
Xin zhongguo funü 新中国妇女
xisan 洗三
xiyao 西药
xueduzheng 血毒症
xuetang 學堂
xuexiao 學校
xunlianban 训练班
Yan Yangchu 晏阳初
Yang Chongrui 杨崇瑞
ying'er huli 婴儿护理
Yingyi Ma Genjia yu tianjin ma daifu yiyuan 英医马根济与天津马大夫医院
yixue zhuanmen xuexiao 医学专门学校
yiyao 医药
yuesao 月嫂
yufang zhushe 预防注射
Yunnan xingzheng jishi 云南行政纪实
Zeng Guofan 曾国藩
Zhabei qu 闸北区
Zhang Renjun 張人駿
Zhang Xiaogang 张晓刚

Zhejiang shengli zhuchan xuexiao 浙江省立助产学校
zhengchangchan 正常产
zhiliaosuo 治疗所
zhiye zhuyi 职业注意
zhongfeng 中风
Zhonghua di er zhuchan xuexiao 中华第二助产学校
Zhonghua fuchanke zazhi 中华妇产科杂志
Zhongyang gaoji hushi zhuanye xuexiao 中央高级护士专业学校
Zhongyang hushi xuexiao 中央护士学校
zhongyao 中药
Zhuchan jiaoyu weiyuanhui 助产教育委员会
zhuchan xuexiao 助产学校
zhuchanshi 助产士
zhuliyuan 助理员
Zung wei (Renhui) chanke yiyuan 仁惠产科医院
zuo yuezi 坐月子

Index

abortion, 16, 148, 173
Academia Sinica, xxiii
acupuncture, xvi, 148, 177
Afshar, Haleh, 125
age, calculating, 164n140
All-China Women's Federation, 170,
172
analgesia, xvi, xxxixn4
Andrews, Bridie, xxv
apoplexy, 1

Barefoot Doctors, 170, 176
Beiping Child Health Institute, 92–
93; *jieshengpo* courses, 93, 95–97;
traditional midwives overseen by,
92, 95, 96
Beiping Health Demonstration
Stations, 144–45
Beiping Municipal Private Welfare
High Ranking Midwifery School,
147
biological determinism, 38–42
biomedicine, xxii–xxv; applications,
xxxiii; pathogenic theory of, xxiii
birth attendants: importance of, 102;
lay, 175; sex of, xxxiv
birth control, 149. *See also*
contraception services
birth dates, 177
birth defects, xx

birth models: biomedical, xxxiv, xix,
xxxii; intellectual, 49; traditional,
xxxiii–xxxiv; Western, 49
birth registration, 100, 151
Borçic, Berislav, 138
Boxer Indemnity money, 80
Boxer Rebellion, 12, 15, 77
Bray, Francesca, 48
breast binding, 155
breech birth, xvi
Bureau of Health, 18

caesarean section, xxviii, 177;
illustration of, 50; planned, xvi,
xxxixn3; rates, xix
Canton Hospital, 11, 127
CCP. *See* Chinese Communist Party
Central Field Health Station, 133,
140–41, 146
Central School of Nursing, 135
Chen, C.C. *See* Chen Zhiqian
Chen, P.C. Frank, 22
Chen Duxiu, xxv
Chen Heyun, 7
Chen Huipu, 7
Chen Jianshan, 41
Chen Zhiqian (C.C. Chen), xxvii,
132, 143, 158
Chiang Kai-shek, xxiii, 107, 132;
Madame Chiang Kai-shek, 133

childbirth: aseptic, xxvii, 94–100, 156; biological processes, xxxii; breech, xvi; complications, xx, 14; consumerism and, 175; cosmologically resonant, xxxvi, 48, 172–73; culture and, xix–xxi; environment, modern, xxxiv; gender and approaches to, 49; germ theory and, xxviii; as illness, xxvii, xxxii–xxxiii; images, 50; interventions, 12; in Japan, 16; medicalization of, xxxii–xxxv, 174–77; new birth method, 171; options, 52–54; organizational control, 105; pathogenic theory of medicine and, xxiii; practices, xliin40; process, xviii, xx; psychoprophylactic painless childbirth method, 172–73; in Republican China, xx–xxi; routine procedures, 177; spacing of births, 148–49; standardizing, 149–56, 153; state-controlled, 157; surgical interventions, 12; traditional, 59; vaginal, xvi; written accounts, xxxv
Childbirth and Nursing (Hong Shilu and Wu Mai), 52
childbirth reform, xxv; areas of, xxxvi–xxxvii; CCP and, 169; Guomindang, 126–27, 149–50, 157–58; Nationalist era, 149–50, 158
child care, xxxvi, 43, 54; importance of, 35; modern methods, 60–63; national, 88; PRC and, 170; reform, xxii; strength of country and, 8; Western medicine, xxvii
Child Health Bureau, 111
China: childbirth process in, xviii; educational policy, xxix; foreign philanthropists in, 12; health care, xix; Japanese invasion, 168; Japan's occupation, 16; medical profession in, 74; medicine in, 74; public health in, criticisms of, 9; racial makeup, 39; Sino-Japanese War, 77, 168; Taiwan's occupation, 16; twentieth-century, reproduction in, 167–82; wartime, 168–70; Western ideas in, xxiii, 8; Western medicine in, entry of, 2–3; women in, xxi
China Medical Board, xxxviii, 131
China Medical Journal (China Medical Missionary Journal), 11, 13, 50–51, 63, 105, 148
Chinese Career Women's Club, 104
Chinese Communist Party (CCP), 126, 180n41; childbirth reforms, 169; civil war, 168; Guomindang and, xxxviii–xxxxix; midwifery training, 169; population policies, 173–74; public health policies, 169; reproductive health and, 167; traditional Chinese medicine and, 169–70; traditional midwives and, 171; women in, 171–73
Chinese Medical Association, 48, 83–84
Chinese medicine. *See* "Traditional Chinese Medicine"
Chinese Midwifery Association, 104
Chinese People's Political Consultative Conference, 170
Choa, G.H., 2
Christianity, xx, 4, 10. *See also* missionaries; Nantao Christian Institute; Shanghai Bethel Nursing and Obstetrics School
Chujoto, 44, 46
cities, modern, 14–19
Cixi, Empress Dowager, 4
Cochran, Thomas, 4
co-education, 79. *See also* education
Cohen, Paul, xxxviii
Committee on Contraception, 149. *See also* contraception services
Confucianism, 39
consumerism: childbirth and, 175; nationalism and, 19; reproduction and, 19–24, 172

consumption, culture of, 43
contraception services, 148–49
cosmologically resonant childbirth, 172–73
Culp, Robert, 155
culture: biology and, 64; modernity and, 24–25

Datong shu (Kang Youwei), 39
delivery methods, 13–14. *See also* childbirth
Demerol, xvi
Deng Xiaoping, 19, 173
diazepam (Valium), xvi
Dikötter, Frank, 38
Dingxian Mass Education Movement, 139–40. *See also* education
Dingxian Rural Health Station, 132, 143
disease prevention, 18
dissection, 68n64
doulas (lay birth attendants), xvi, 175
Dr. Wei's Red Pills, 44, 47
Dr. Williams' Pink Pills for Pale People, 43–44, *45*
Duchess De, 4
Duden, Barbara, 52

education: gender and, 79; policy, xxix, 77; rural, 137–43; sex, 148; women's, xxix, 7–8, 52, 77, 80. *See also* fetal education; medical training
electrotherapy treatment, 1
En Shou, 5
episiotomy, xvi, xxxixn7
Esherick, Joseph, xxiii
Essentials of Obstetrics (Yao Changxu), 52
eugenics, xxvi, 38–42
evolution, 38–39
eye infections, 62

family structure, 19–20; nuclear, 20, 41; patriarchal, 24

Fangbian Hospital (*Fangbian yiyuan*), 6–7
Feng Yuxiang, 133, 160n40
fertility, 64. *See also* infertility
fetal development: anatomy and, 48–49; images, *51*, 51–52, *53*
fetal education (*taijiao*), xvii, xxxiv, 38–42, 156; modern, 40–41; theory of, 39–40; women's responsibility for, 39
fetal health care, xix. *See also* child care
First National Midwifery School (FNMS), xxvii, xxxvi, 73–74, 113; admittance to, 151; clerkships, 91–92; curriculum, 57, 86–87; fellowships, 90; founding of, 84; Graduate Courses for Nurses and Midwives, 88–90; growth of, 85; higher-level courses, 87; infant/maternal mortality, 156; National Midwifery Board and, 134; practical experience, 90–91; PUMC and, 51, 74; purpose of, 84; Six-Month Graduate Course, 91; tuition, 87, 118n74; Two-Month Refresher Course, 91, 92; Two-Year Midwifery Course, 87–89; during wartime, 168–69; Yenching University Department of Sociology and, 141–42
FNMS. *See* First National Midwifery School
foot binding, 155
forceps, xxviii
fuke, 48
Fulton, Mary, 7, 11, 24
Furth, Charlotte, xxxiii, 48
Fu Wei, 174

Gaoqiao Village Public Health Model District, 145–46
Gates, Frederick T., xxvi, xliin43
gender: of birth attendants, xxxiv; childbirth approaches and, 49; of children, 40; fertility and, 64;

identity, xxix, 80; infertility and, 43–44; medical profession and, 74; medicine and, 7–8; modern medicine and, 64; nursing and, 74; orphans and, 173; physician's, xxxvi, 1, 7; relations, 49; reproduction and, 64; roles, 25–26
germ theory, xxviii
Glosser, Susan, 20, 43
Goldstein, Joshua, 172, 173
Gongyiyuan, 6
Grant, John B., 81–82, 132, 134; Beiping First Health Demonstration Station, 144
Greater Shanghai Bureau of Public Health, 145
Greig, James A., 14
Guangdong Medical College for Women, 11. *See also* Hackett Medical College for Women
Guangdong Provincial High Grade Nursing and Midwifery Professional School, 147
Guangzhou: Bureau of Health, 18; Midwifery Association, 105; Municipal Hospital Maternity Department, 54, *55*; Three-Year Plan, 146; Tuqiang Midwifery School, 147
Guomindang: capitol, 132; CCP and, xxxviii; central government, 126; childbirth reform, 126–27, 149–50, 156–57; city administrations, 15; control of private matters by, 157; legislation, 126–27; midwifery legislation, 126–30, 151; New Life Movement, 153–55; public health goals, xxxi, 128–29; PUMC and, 132–33
Gu Shi, 42

Hackett Medical College for Women, 7, 81, 112
Handwerker, Lisa, 177
Han dynasty, 40

Hangzhou Guangji Hospital Midwifery School, 147
Heiser, Victor, 81
Hershatter, Gail, xxxvi, 110, 171
Hobson, Benjamin, 12, 63
Hodgman, Gertrude, 107
home births, xvi, xxxiii. *See also* childbirth
Hong Shilu, 52, 133
Honig, Emily, 75, 104
Hormotone, 44
hospitals: births, xxvii, 57–59, 174; charity, 9–10; cost of, 23–24; maternity, 149–50; native place ties of, 22–23; regulation, 149–50; sliding scale payment, 23; socioeconomic class and, 20, 22; support of, 17–18; unlicensed, 21–22; Western-style, 3; workplace ties of, 22–23. *See also specific hospitals*
Howard, Leonora, 1, 7, 10, 26
Huang Gongkun, 54
Huang Shi, 41
Hu Caojuan, 109
Hu Hsi Commoners' Obstetrical Hospital, 21–22
Hunan Yu Chun Educational Association (HYCEA), 6
Hu Shi, xxv
Huxley, Aldous, 19
HYCEA, 6
hygienic modernity, xxxi, 9

infant care, 61–63
infant mortality rates, xx, xxv–xxvi; causes, 130–31; declined, 176; FNMS, 156; modern childbirth and, 176; tracking, 100; U.S., xxxii, 181n55
infections: eye, 62; umbilical cord, xxv–xxvi
infectious diseases, 9
infertility, 20, 43–44
inoculation, 18, 139, 144, 147. *See also* vaccinations

International Children's Day, 172
International Health Division, 82, 130, 140
interventions, medical, 12, 49
Irwin, A., 1
Isabella Fisher Hospital, 10

Japan: childbirth in, 16; infant/ maternal mortality rates, 181n55; invasion of China, 168; medical education, 77; midwifery in, 16; occupation, 16; public health reform in, 16; Sino-Japanese War, 77, 168
jieshengpo, xvii; Beiping Child Health Institute classes for, 93, 95–97; birth outcomes, 110–11; criticism of, 117n60; current, 174–75; demise of, 101; equipment, 98; fees, 97–98; image of, 108; regulation of, 101, 150–51; responsibilities, xvii–xviii; retraining, 93–102, *96*, *97*; ritual functions, 102; supervision of retrained, 99–100; uniform, 98, *99*; *zhuchanshi* v., 85–86, 101, 113, 151–52
Johns Hopkins School of Medicine, 74, 83, 130
Joint Conference of Education and Industry, 79
Jordan, Brigitte, xxxii, xlivn70

Kahn, Ida. *See* Kang Cheng
Kang Cheng (Ida Kahn), 5, 76
Kang Youwei, xxv, 66n31; *Datong shu*, 39
Kawashima, 15–16
Kirby, William, 103
Koch, Robert, xxiii
Kung Yee Society (*Gongyiyuan*), 6

labor: arrested, xvi; complications, xx; positions, massage and, xviii; prolonged, 57; protracted, 13–14
labor-inducing drugs, xvi

Lao She, xxv
Law on Maternal and Infant Health care, 174–75
League of Nations Health Organization (LON-HO), xxvi, 130–31, 137
Lee, Leo Ou-fan, 36
Liang Qichao, 17, 107, 175
Lien Ling-ling, 104
Lienü Zhuan, 40
Li Hongzhang, 1–2, 4, 15, 77; Lady Li Hongzhang, 1–2, 26
Liji, 40
Lim, S.K., 50
Lin Qiaozhi, 76, 170, 180n41
Li Shufen, 6
literacy, 37–38, 43–44
Li Ting'an, 100, 158
Liu, J. Heng. *See* Liu Ruiheng
Liu Chung-tung, 107
Liu Ruiheng (J. Heng Liu), xxvii, 130, 132, 158; Central Field Health Station, 140; LON-HO report, 137; National Health Administration report, 136; National Midwifery Board, 133
Li Xiaojiang, xx, 59, 171
LON-HO. *See* League of Nations Health Organization
Lu Sandong, 5
Lu Xun, xxv, 25

Mackenzie, John Kenneth, 1–2
MacPherson, Kerrie L., 143
Main, Duncan, 4–5
Major, Ernest, 50
male heirs, 25, 48
Mao Zedong, 169, 172
Martin, Emily, 64
massage, xvi, xviii
maternal health care, xix, xxxvi; importance of, 35; national, 88; PRC and, 170; reform, xxii; socioeconomic status and, 177–78; strength of country and, 8; Western medicine, xxvii

maternal mortality rates, xx, xxv–
xxvi; causes, 130–31, 181n55;
FNMS, 156; modern childbirth
and, 176; tracking, 100; U.S.,
xxxii, 181n55
Maternity Hospital, Hangzhou, 4–5
Maxwell, J. Preston, 148
May Fourth era, 106
medical documentation, 92
medical images, 50–51, 51
medical missionaries, xxvi, 2–3,
9–10; traditional Chinese
practices and, 13
medical profession(s), 74, 76–77,
102–13; development of, 75;
gender and, 74. See also specific
professions
medical schools, xxvii, 78–80. See
also specific schools
Medical Special Colleges, 78
medical specialization, xxvii, 10–11
medical training, xxviii–xxix;
Chinese, xxiv; in Japan,
77; modernization and, 10;
specialization, 10–11; Western,
xxiv, 3; for women, 76–81; Yang
Chongrui's, 82–83, 132
men: medical schools for, 79–80;
physicians, xxxvi, 49, 114,
123n176; roles of modern, 25–26.
See also gender
Menzies, James, 13–14
middle class, 19
midwife/midwives: birth registration
by, 151; forensic examinations
done by, 101; government
regulation of, 18; image of, 84;
local, xvii; modern childbirth
ideas and, 54; physicians and,
xxxvi, 74, 152; professional,
74; registered, 126, 128, 157;
socioeconomic status of, 111–12.
See also specific midwives
midwifery: equipment, 54–56, 56;
infant mortality and, xxv–xxvi;
in Japan, 16; legislation, xxxv,

126–30, 151; license, 151–52;
maternal mortality and, xxv–
xxvi; Nationalist era and, 114;
organizations, 103–5; professional,
xxix–xxx, 73–123, 75–76, 84;
regulation, xxxi, 73, 114, 127;
reputation of, 113, 128; social
support of, 112–13; writings
about, xxxvi. See also modern
midwifery/midwives; traditional
midwifery/midwives
midwifery reform, xxi, 83;
Guomindang, 126–27, 151;
National Midwifery Board and,
134; Yang Chongrui and, 83,
134–35
midwifery training, xxxv, 20–21,
57; CCP and, 169; cost, 21;
mandatory, 88; modern, 85–93;
municipal, 143–47; National
Midwifery Board's regulation of,
152–53, 154; old-style, 94–97,
96, 97, 142–43; private, 143–47;
provincial, 135–37; rural, 137–43;
schools, 107–8; unregistered, 20–
22; Yang Chonguri and, 11, 82–84,
96–97, 137–38. See also medical
training; specific schools
Milbank Memorial Fund, 139–40
Minden, Karen, 170
Ministry of Education, 78
Ministry of Health, 130
miscarriage, 142
missionaries, 4, 12. See also medical
missionaries
Mittler, Barbara, 37, 43–44
modern childbirth, xxv, 35–71, 176;
midwives and, 54; techniques of,
12; utilization of, 19. See also
childbirth
modernity/modernization: of cities,
14–19; concept of, 8; cultural
ideals and, 24–25; fetish of, 15,
126; health, xxvi; health care
reform and, xxii; hygienic, xxxi,
9; localized, 15; medical training

and, 10; medicine and, 8–14;
nationalism v., xxiii; print media,
36–37; public health and, 8–9; in
Republican China, xxi–xxii, xxx–
xxxi; Westernizing v., xxii–xxiv, 8;
women, 43
modern medicine, xxii, 8–14;
access to, xxxv; gender and, 64;
terminology, xxiii–xxiv. See also
biomedicine
modern midwifery/midwives,
xviii, xxxiv–xxxv; candidates,
151; cleanliness and, xxxiv;
development of, xxx–xxxi;
employment possibilities for, 111;
equipment, 56, 56–60; image of,
108, 155; professionalism, 75;
profession of, 112; tools, xxxiii;
training, 85–93; use of, 156–57.
See also zhuchanshi
mothercraft classes, 156
motherhood, modern, 60–63
mothers as citizens, xxii
Mother's Association, 61
Mothers' Clubs, 60–61, 62, 142, 156
mothers-in-law meetings, 61

Nanchang Women's and Children's
Hospital, 5
Nanjing Central Midwifery School,
111, 135, 146
Nantao Christian Institute, 38
National Board of Health (National
Health Administration), 18,
130; FNMS fellowships, 91; Lui
Ruiheng's report on, 136
National Child Welfare Association,
146
National Department of Internal
Affairs and Public Health, 146
National Economic Board, 146
National Health Administration. See
National Board of Health
nationalism, xxiii, 19
Nationalist era, xxix–xxx, 73–74,
133; childbirth reform, 149–50,

158; midwifery regulation in, 114;
professionalism in, 103–4
The National Medical Journal of
China, 50–51
National Midwifery Board,
xxxi, 88, 113–14, 133–35, 146;
FNMS and, 134; midwifery
reform and, 134; midwifery
schools/training programs
regulated by, 152–54
Neal, James Boyd, 11
Neo-Confucianism, 48
Neubauer, W., 148
neural tube defects, xx
new birth method, 171
New Culture Movement, xxii
New Life Movement, xxiii, 107,
153–55; hygienic modernity and,
xxxi; public health care reforms
and, 130; public health goals,
155–56; women and, 155
New Policies, 15, 77
New Woman, 19, 25, 106
New Women of China (magazine),
172
Ning Shao Commoners' Obstetrical
Hospital, 22
North Manchurian plague epidemic,
xxix
nurse-midwives, xvi, 88–90
Nurses' Association of China, 104–6
nursing: associations, 103–4; gender
and, 74; profession, 77; training,
112, 135, 146–47

obstetrics, 7
opium poisoning, 5
osteomalacia, xx
overpopulation, 149

parasitic diseases, 9
Pasteur, Louis, xxiii
Peiping Committee on Maternal
Health, 149
Peking First Health Demonstration
Station, 132

Peking Union Medical College (PUMC), xxvi; Beiping First Health Demonstration Station, 144–45; FNMS and, 51, 74; graduates, 132; Guomindang government and, 132–33; Hygiene department, 135; improving public health and, 131–32; OB/GYN at, 92–93, 103, 135; Public Health department, 135; Rockefeller Foundation and, 74; Yang Chongrui and, 83

People's Republic of China (PRC), xxxviii; child health in, 170; early, 170–73; maternal health in, 170

pethidine (Demerol), xvi

Pfeiffer, Stefani, 92

philanthropy/philanthropists: foreign, 12; gentry, 3–8; secularization, 12; western, public health and, 130–33

Phillips, Mildred, 5

physicians, xvi; Chinese-trained, xxiv; female, 1, 7, 10–11, 114, 123n176, 152; home visits by, 10–11; male, xxxvi, 49, 114, 123n176; midwives and, xxxvi, 74, 152; protracted labor and, 13–14; "Traditional Chinese Medicine," xxiv; training, 146–47; Western-trained, xxiv, 3

placenta, xviii

population policies, 173–74

postnatal care, xx

postpartum period, xvi, 102, 175

PRC. See People's Republic of China

pregnancy, 40–41, 48; diet during, xvii; emotions and, 41; fetal education theory and, 39–40; as illness, xxvii, xxxii–xxxiii; modern views on, 86; Qing dynasty and, 40; regulation, xxv; secret, 173; tests, xln10; women's responsibilities during, 40–41

prenatal care, xv, xvii, xx, 157

print media, 36–37; advertisements, 44–48

private maternity hospitals, 20, 22–24. See also hospitals

professionalism, 103–4

protracted labor, 13–14

Provincial Education Associations, 79

psychoprophylactic painless childbirth method, 172–73

public health, xxvi; administration, 16–17; CCP, policies, 169; clinics, 138; criticisms of China's, 9; global competitiveness and, 8–9; Guomindang's goals for, xxxi, 128–29; modernization and, 8–9; New Life Movement and, 130, 155–56; programs, xxx–xxxi, 18; provincial, 136; PUMC and, 131–32, 135; reforms, xxix, 16, 130; Western philanthropy and, 130–33

Public Health Experimental Station, 148

puerperal sepsis, xxv, 12, 83, 143

PUMC. See Peking Union Medical College

qi, 48

Qing dynasty: education in, 77; fall of, 24; New Policies, 77; philanthropists, 3; pregnancy during, 40; Western medicine in, 4–7

Qinghe public health program, 141–42

Qinghua University, 80

Qin Shao, 43

Qu Shaoheng, 110

race, 39, 181n55

religion, xxvi–xxvii; Christianity, xx, 4, 10; Confucianism, 39

reproduction, xxxi; commodities of, 42–48; consumerism and, 19–24, 172; gender and, 64; government policies regarding, 125; laws related to, xviii; modern, 175; national, in Republican China,

125–66; print media related to, 36–37; reforms, xxxiii–xxxiv, 126–27; science, 54; sources of, xxxiv–xxxvii; state control over, xxxi–xxxii; technology, 172; theory, xxxii–xxxiv, 35–71; in twentieth-century China, 167–82; visualizing, 48–56; women and, 25, 42, 176–77
reproductive health, 43; CCP and, 167; Chinese notions, 48; legacy of, 173–75; policies, 18; reforms, twentieth-century, 167–68
Republican China, xix, 73–74; childbirth in, xx–xxi; local leadership, 15; modernity in, xxi–xxii, xxx–xxxi; national reproduction in, 125–66; provincial governments in, 135; reproduction reforms in, xxxiii–xxxiv; women's work in, 76
Republic of China Private High Ranking Midwifery School, 147
Richardson, Frank Howard, 60
rituals, xviii, 102
Rockefeller Foundation: China Medical Board, xxxviii, 131; International Health Division, xxvi, 82, 130, 140; PUMC and, 74
Rogaski, Ruth, xxxi, 9, 143

Sanger, Margaret, 148
sanitation, 9, 17–18
San Ming Obstetrical Hospital, 23, 24
Schneider, Laurence, xxii
Semmelweis, Ignaz, xxiii, xlin28
sex education, 148
sex of fetus, xv, xvii
sexually transmitted diseases (STDs), 20, 148
Shanghai Bethel Nursing and Obstetrics School, 109
Shanghai Maternity Hospital, 23–24
Shanghai Private Tongde Midwifery School, 147

Shanghai public health centers, 145–46
Shanghai Shengsheng Midwifery School, 110
Shanghai West Gate Women and Children's Hospital, 24
Shanghai Zhongde Professional Midwifery School, 109, 147
Shi Meiyu (Mary Stone), 5, 13, 76
silk industry, 106
silver nitrate, 54, 59, 62, 153, 171
Sino-Japanese War, 77, 168
Snow, John, 9
socioeconomic status, 19; hospitals and, 20, 22; maternal health care and, 177–78; of midwives, 111–12
Sommer, Matthew, 101
Song dynasty, 48
Spencer, Herbert, xxi–xxii, 39
St. John's University College of Medicine, 112
Stapleton, Kristin, 15
STDs. See sexually transmitted diseases
sterilization, 156, 173
Stewart, Agnes, 14
stillbirths, xx, 142
Stockard, Janice, 106
Stone, Mary. See Shi Meiyu
Strand, David, 15
Sun Fo, 6
Sun Keh-chi, 133
Sun Yat-sen, 6, 129
Suzhou Women's Hospital, 5
Sze Szeming, 48

Tai County Hospital, 141
taijiao. See fetal education
Taiwan, 16
Tang dynasty, 3
Tan Sitong, 17
Taylor, Kim, xxiv, 170
telegony, 39, 41–42
tetanus, xxv, 83; neonatorum, 143; umbilical cord care and, 61, 142–43

Tianjin Massacre, 4
Tien, Hung-mao, 132, 135
Todd, Paul, 6
Topley, Marjorie, 106
"Traditional Chinese Medicine,"
xxii–xxv; CCP and, 169–70;
medical missionaries and, 13;
physicians, xxiv; practitioners,
170; terminology, xxiv; Western
anatomy adopted into, xxv
traditional midwifery/midwives,
xviii, 75; Beiping Child Health
Institute overseeing, 92, 94, 95;
CCP and, 171; discrimination
against, 174; malpractice, 174;
modern v., xxxv; retraining,
93–102, 96, 97; social functions of,
101; tools, xxxiii; training, 94–97,
96, 97, 142–43; use of, 156. See
also jieshengpo
Training Home for Midwifery,
Hangzhou, 4–5
Tsin, Michael, 6–7, 17
Tuqiang Advanced Midwifery
School, Guangzhou, 108, 147

ultrasound, xv
umbilical cord: cutting of, 13;
infection and, xxv–xxvi; tetanus
and, 61, 142–43
Union Medical College, 79
United States, infant/maternal
mortality rates, xxxii, 181n55
University Act (1912), 78
uterine prolapse, 14

vaccinations, 5, 18
Valium xvi,
venereal illness, xxvii, 139
Verdery, Katherine, 125
vitamin deficiency, maternal, xx

Wang Shumin, 109
Wang Yongwei, 109
Wang Yugang, 110
Well-Baby Clinics, 60–61

Westernizing, xxiii; modernizing v.,
xxii–xxiv, 8
Western medicine, xxiv–xxv; child
care, xxvii; in China, entry of,
2–3; Li Hongzhang's support of, 2,
4, 15; maternal health care, xxvii;
Qing dynasty and, 4–7; support
of, 15
Williams, J. Whitridge, 74
women: biology and, 42; as birth
attendants, xxxiv; CCP and,
171–73; education, xxix, 7–8, 52,
77, 80; employment, 76, 107;
femininity and, 155–56; fetal
education responsibilities of, 39;
illnesses, 44–48; literacy, 37–38;
male heirs and worth of, 25;
married, 106–7; in medical field,
xxx, 80–81; medical missionaries
and, 10; medical training for, 76–
81; medicine and, 48; modern, 25,
43; New Life Movement and, 155;
occupations, 19; as physicians,
1, 7, 10–11, 114, 123n176, 152;
pregnancy and responsibilities
of, 40–41; reproduction and, 25,
42, 176–77; Republican China
and work of, 76; roles of modern,
25; submissiveness, 39. See also
gender
Women's Hospital, Shanghai, 23
Wu, Yi-Li, xix, 48, 172; midwifery
writings, xxxvi; study of
reproduction, 40
Wu Lai Chua, 133
Wu Mai, 52

Xiangya Medical College and
Hospital, 5–6, 147
xian health stations, 138–39, 141
Xiaozhuang Rural Health
Demonstration Program, 143
Xia Zenan, 5
Xie Siyan, 40–41
xisan, xviii
xuetang, 78. See also education

xuexiao, 78. *See also* education
Xu Xiaoqun, 75, 103
Yale-China Association, 5–6, 147
Yandell, A.E., 5
Yang Chongrui (Marion Yang), xxvii, xxxviii, 76, 113, 158; CCP and, 180n41; FNMS, 81; Gaoqiao Village Public Health Model District and, 146; Johns Hopkins School of Medicine and, 83; medical training, 82–83, 132; midwifery reform and, 83, 134–35; midwifery training and, 11, 82–84, 96–97, 137–38; National Midwifery Board, 133–34; Peiping Committee on Maternal Health, 149; professionalism of midwifery and, 105; PUMC and, 83
Yang Nianqun, 101–2
Yan Yangchu. *See* Yen, James
Yao Changxu, 52
Yeh, Wen-hsin, 104
Yen, F.C., 133
Yen, James (Yan Yangchu), 139–40
Yen, L.C., 133
Yenching University Department of Sociology, 141–42

yin/yang, 49
Yip, Ka-che, 100, 107
yiyao, xxiii
Yong Hong, 77
You Huaigao, 20, 43, 60
Yuan Shikai, 15–17
yuesao, 175
Yun Qin, 41

Zeng Guofan, 2, 77
Zhang Cha, 17
Zhang Jian, 17
Zhang Renjuin, 7, 15
Zhang Xiaogang, 19, 60
zhiye zhuyi. *See* professionalism
zhongyao. *See* "Traditional Chinese Medicine"
Zhu Baosan, 5
zhuchanshi, 74–75; employment opportunities, 111; *jieshengpo v.*, 85–86, 101, 113, 151–52; support of, 150–51; term, 85–86. *See also* modern midwifery/midwives
Zhu Xiaxian, 109
Zung Wei Obstetrical Hospital, 21–22, 23
zuo yuezi, xvi, xxxiv, 175

About the Author

Tina Phillips Johnson is assistant professor in the Department of History and director of Chinese Studies at Saint Vincent College in Latrobe, Pennsylvania. Her research interests include historical examinations of reproductive health, the intersections of state and gender, and changes in cultural medical practices.